Bitten

Also by *Pamela Nagami*

The Woman with a Worm in Her Head

Pamela Nagami, M.D.

Bitten

**True
Medical
Stories
of
Bites
and
Stings**

ST. MARTIN'S GRIFFIN   NEW YORK

Design by Judith Stagnitto Abbate / Abbate Design

www.stmartins.com

Library of Congress Cataloging-in-Publication Data

Nagami, Pamela.
Bitten : true medical stories of bites and stings / by Pamela Nagami.
p. cm.
Includes bibliographical references (p. 297) and index (p. 339).
ISBN 0-312-31822-7 (hc)
ISBN 0-312-31823-5 (pbk)
EAN 978-0-312-31823-9
1. Bites and stings. 2. Bites and stings—Treatment. I. Title.
RD96.2 .N34 2004
617.1—dc22   2003027210

10   9   8   7   6   5   4   3

Note to
Readers

To Glenn

Contents

Preface xi
Acknowledgments xiii

1 Invincible Invaders 1
2 Fangs in the Dark 18
3 Stingers from the Sea 40
4 Beautiful, Deadly Cones 56
5 The Limbless Ones 66
6 Silent Stowaways 87
7 Nightmare 101
8 Sponge Face and Black Fever 126
9 New York, Summer 1999 153
10 "The Jaws That Bite" 169
11 Rage 191
12 Bitten 207
13 Menagerie 221
14 Monkey Business 244
15 Human Bites 268

Conclusion 287
Glossary 289
References 297
Index 339

Preface

We live in an age of ecotourism, in which it is not only possible but fast and easy to book an African safari, a trek through Brazil, or a retreat in far north Queensland online. But within a few weeks, the virtual reality of a Web page may become the real experience of sleeping sickness, leishmaniasis, or the Irukandji syndrome.

Whether we journey far from home or just sit on our back porch and swat mosquitoes, we need to look up and see what's out there. This book is an introduction to the biters and stingers with which we share our world, and a work of grateful homage to the people—past and present—who try to understand the animals, save the injured, and ultimately protect us from *being BITTEN*.

Acknowledgments

It is a pleasure to acknowledge the following colleagues, patients, friends, and family: Sylvan Cohen, who shared both his knowledge of dangerous animals and his considerable library, my subjects "Helene and Albert Eliah," my son Paul Nagami for skillful editing and topic suggestions, my daughter Ellen Nagami for the book's title, librarians Elliott M. Gordon, Marsha L. Edenburn, and Annette Wolfson, dermatologist Paul Wolfish and pathologist Jeffrey Shiffer, Susan Novak and Michael Collier for laboratory support, my clinic assistant Zoraida Medina, and the staff of the Infusion Center at the Kaiser Foundation Hospital in Woodland Hills.

Special thanks to Frank Steurer and James Mcguire at the Centers for Disease Control and Prevention, to my agent B. J. Robbins, and to my editor Marie Estrada.

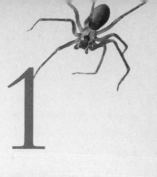

1

Invincible
Invaders

In a chronic-care facility in Houston, Texas, on a routine morning check, nursing home attendants discovered one of their patients—a ninety-year-old woman who suffered from a weak heart and "moderately severe" dementia—fully conscious but covered with thousands of rice-sized insects. The tiny creatures had been crawling in and out of her mouth and swarming over her body, conceivably for hours. However, due to the woman's general debility, she had been unable to summon help. After the attendants washed away the creatures, they discovered multiple welts all over her body. Over the next six hours, the reaction spread to her lungs, and, despite attentive hospital care, she died.

The red fire ant, *Solenopsis invicta,* the species responsible for the woman's death, is one of over eight thousand species of ants worldwide. All ants are social insects, living together in colonies.

They are heat-loving creatures—only a few species live in Alpine or arctic regions. The first fossil ants appear in European and North American rock strata dating back about sixty million years, around the same time that the dinosaurs were dying out.

Ants have large heads and oval abdomens joined to the thorax by a narrow waist. The antennae have an elbowlike bend, and the mouth is equipped with two sets of jaws, the outer pair for carrying and digging and the inner set for chewing. Like their close relatives, the bees, many species have a powerful stinger at the tip of the abdomen, which in ants can be used repeatedly without damaging the owner.

Solenopsis invicta is not native to North America. It arrived on ships from South America in the 1930s through the port of Mobile, Alabama. Since then, fire ants have invaded the southern and southeastern United States and Puerto Rico. Every year, between 30 and 60 percent of people living in these areas experience their painful stings. The ant grasps the skin with its tiny, powerful jaws, arches its body, and then injects venom through the stinger. If allowed to do so, the ant will rotate itself about its anchored head and create a whole circle of stings. There's an immediate burning sensation, followed by hours to days of intense itching. Virtually everyone who is stung by a fire ant reacts with a red welt that, over several days, turns into a pus-filled pimple. Up to half of the victims will experience larger local reactions, and occasionally surgical drainage and amputation are necessary because of complicating infections.

Fire ant venom may be toxic to the nervous system, as illustrated by two cases reported by Dr. Roger Fox and his colleagues at the University of South Florida in 1982. The first patient was a thirty-nine-year-old tree trimmer who was cutting palm trees when roughly one hundred fire ants bit his arms and shoulders. Ten months later, about two hundred fire ants attacked his arms and shoulders, and the next workday about the same number of ants bit him again. Following this final attack, his right hand and forearm gradually became numb, and over the next thirty-six hours his wrist became weak. The hand returned to normal in a month, but no further information on the patient was available; after the last attack, he moved and left no forwarding address.

The other patient in Dr. Fox's report was a four-year-old boy who was with his father, a neurosurgeon, when he was stung by twenty red fire ants on his right foot. A half hour later the child had two convulsions, from which he recovered without ill effects.

The most dangerous physical response to a fire ant sting is called an anaphylactic reaction, which is the same kind of reaction some people have to bee stings. This is not surprising, since ants belong to the same insect order as bees, the Hymenoptera.

An anaphylactic reaction begins with faintness, itching, chest tightness, and wheezing, and ends with a precipitous fall in blood pressure and sometimes death. In parts of the southern United States where fire ants are prevalent, fatal allergic reactions to their venom are more common than deaths from bee stings. In sensitive people, only a sting or two is necessary to provoke the reaction.

A typical case was that of the thirty-one-year-old man who arrived in an emergency department in Augusta, Georgia, thirty minutes after a fire ant stung him on the thumb. He told the doctors that within two or three minutes of the sting he had a strange metallic taste in his mouth. Then there was a sudden pain in his temples—he called it "the worst headache of [his] life." He felt shaky and had a sensation of pins and needles all over his body. His heart pounded, and his face turned red. This man, however, had the presence of mind to swallow two tablespoons of Dimetapp before he came to the emergency room. The liquid antihistamine got into his bloodstream quickly enough to save his life.

Others have not been as fortunate. In 1989, Dr. Robert Rhoades and his colleagues reported the case of a thirty-two-year-old junior high school teacher who succumbed to anaphylaxis following fire ant stings. The patient had suffered a severe reaction to a sting in the past and had consulted an allergist, who recommended a course of desensitizing injections to prevent another reaction. She had declined treatment and, some time later, she sustained ten stings to her feet and ankles. Immediately she began gasping for breath as the air passages in her lungs squeezed shut. Although she was still alive on arrival to the emergency room, an electrocardiogram showed signs of severe heart strain and lack of oxygen. Shortly thereafter, her heartbeat stopped. The doctors were unable to resuscitate her.

This young teacher had such a severe allergy to fire ant venom that even one sting would likely have proved fatal. If such a highly allergic victim were to succumb immediately as the result of one or two stings, it is conceivable that, in the absence of history, the cause of death could remain unknown. Physicians in areas where fire ants are plentiful speculate that a certain percentage of unexplained cases of cardiac arrest may be caused by unseen fatal allergic reactions to stings.

Although lethal reactions to fire ant venom are uncommon, they are only the smallest part of a larger problem. A 1971 survey of physicians in Alabama, Georgia, and Mississippi revealed that over a three-year period doctors treated ten thousand patients for fire ant stings. Probably at least ten times that number were stung but did not seek medical attention. An estimated one half to one percent of fire ant stings result in severe allergic reactions, and a 1989 survey of 29,300 physicians practicing in fire ant–infested areas identified thirty-two confirmed deaths due to sting-induced anaphylaxis. It is probably safe to say that this figure is an underestimation. In some patients, as in the elderly woman in the nursing home, whose case opened this chapter, it is difficult to determine whether their deaths occurred as a result of allergic reactions or simply from a lethal dose of venom due to multiple stings. In small children suffering a large number of stings, this distinction may be impossible to make, as in this tragic case, also reported by Dr. Rhoades.

A healthy, sixteen-month-old girl was "bumped by the family dog" and fell into a fire ant mound. The child suffered innumerable stings over her entire body. Her mother, a registered nurse, brushed off as many ants as she could and then bathed the child to remove those remaining, but it was already too late. The girl began gasping, and the mother started mouth-to-mouth breathing and dialed 911. By the time she arrived in the emergency room, the toddler was in full cardiac arrest. After she spent six days on a ventilator machine without signs of brain recovery, life support was stopped, and the child died.

But fire ants are more than a medical menace. They threaten agriculture, animal husbandry, native plants and animals, and even roadways and electrical installations. To understand this invading insect enemy, it is necessary to return to its homeland, the Pantanal. The Pantanal is the vast flood plain of the headwaters of the Paraguay River, which includes areas in southwest Brazil, eastern Bolivia, Paraguay, and northern Argentina.

In the Pantanal, fire ants build four- to six-inch mounds along roadsides. One egg-laying queen controls each mound, and is supported by one to two hundred thousand sterile female workers. Unlike bees, which use their venom only for defense, foraging fire ants are stinging predators. They subdue other invertebrates, consume their body fluids, and return with these nutrients to the nest. Fire ants are omnivorous and adaptable. They are efficient scavengers, feeding on dead animals, plant tissues, seeds, and sap flows. Where aphids are plentiful, they may turn from hunters to herders, tending and milking these tiny insects for their sweet secretions.

However, in their homeland, fire ant populations are limited by competition from other species of ants and by disease-producing parasites. When baits were set up in the fire ant's habitat in Brazil, only thirteen percent of the traps with ants contained *Solenopsis invicta*. Other species of ants were equally common.

Over twenty species of viruses, fungi, protozoa, roundworms, and flies attack fire ants in South America. *Thelohania,* a one-celled animal, or protozoan, multiplies inside the abdomen of worker fire ants, filling them with debilitating cysts. A tiny roundworm may also infect the stomach of the ant. However, the most bizarre of the South American fire ant parasites are the gnat-sized phorid flies. The females dive-bomb fire ants and inject their eggs into the animal's body. When the larva hatches, it burrows into the ant's head, where it releases enzymes that cause the host's head to fall off. Inside the detached head, the larva continues to grow until it emerges as a mature fly.

But between 1930 and 1940, some lucky colonies of red fire ants left all of this behind. Their nests were loaded, most likely as ballast, onto cargo ships carrying lightweight agricultural goods from South America to Mobile, Alabama. In Mobile, the accidental stowaways were unloaded so that heavy machinery could be stowed in the ship's hold for the return trip.

Upon its arrival in the Mobile, Alabama, area, *Solenopsis invicta* found the soil already colonized with native ants as well as an earlier arrival from South America, *Solenopsis ricteri,* the black fire ant. By 1950, the native species had all but disappeared; black ants had been pushed out of many of their habitats or had formed hybrid tribes with the invaders.

Fire ant mounds are bigger in the United States than in South America, and often stand a foot and a half high, with tunnels that may radiate out over a hundred feet. Colonies are larger, numbering up to four hundred thousand individuals, and there are about nine times as many mounds in infested areas of Alabama as there are in similar habitats in Brazil.

The red fire ant is known as a "tramp" or "weed" species. It thrives in recently opened or disturbed areas. Following World War II, there was rapid population growth in the "Sunbelt," and fire ants quickly invaded land cleared for homes, recreational areas, and industry. A survey of the infestation in 1950 showed that ants had spread from the port area halfway up the border between Mississippi and Alabama. In 1957, the United States Department of Agriculture attempted to quarantine the species, but overlooked the spread of the ants hiding in nursery stock. By 1989, *Solenopsis invicta* had invaded all the southern states.

The red fire ant can survive in areas where the average minimum temperature is 10 degrees Fahrenheit (about negative 12 degrees Celsius). They have recently been reported in California and, based on annual average temperatures, they could spread from Arizona, through Southern California, and along the West Coast as far north as the Canadian border.

But it was not only the welcoming climate and lack of competition and of diseases that allowed the wildfire spread of *Solenopsis invicta* across the south. The red fire ant itself was changing in ominous ways, probably as a result of genetic mutations.

Every fire ant colony begins with a queen, a winged, half-inch-long female who has mated with a winged male while in flight. Upon landing, the mated female sheds her wings and burrows three to ten inches into the earth, sealing the entrance with soil. Within one day she lays ten to twenty eggs, which give rise to the first workers, her attendants. If many newly mated females land in the same area, they may aggregate and found a colony together. However, as the colony becomes established, the workers will eventually execute all the queens but one. The workers then fiercely defend the area around their mound from the incursions of workers from neighboring mounds. The number of mounds in a given area is thus strictly limited by the territorial instincts of red fire ant workers.

However, in the early 1970s scientists in several locations began to report colonies with multiple queens. These colonies contain workers who, despite being genetically unrelated, cooperate over extended areas without territorial hostility. Mound densities increased three to ten times, and some mound systems contain millions of individuals.

Once the red fire ants in a given area evolve these multiple-queen—or polygyne—colonies, other species of invertebrates cannot compete, and the ecological diversity of that environment is severely damaged. Sanford Porter and Dolores Savignano at the University of Texas in Austin studied a 32-hectare tract at the Brackenridge Field Laboratory near that city, using pitfall and bait traps to measure invertebrate abundance and diversity. At infested sites, the investigators found a ten- to thirtyfold increase in the total number of ants, of which over 99 percent were *Solenopsis invicta*. The abundance of isopods, mites, and scarab beetles declined severely, leaving the field to a few types of roaches, ground crickets, and beetles adapted to life with ants. Overall, there were a third fewer different species of invertebrates, and individual populations dropped to one quarter of their original size, pointing to severe ecological disruption by this foreign invader.

Although red fire ants sometimes feed on agricultural pests, the damage they do to crops, particularly seeds and germinating seedlings, outweighs their beneficial role as insect predators. In addition, the presence of fire ant colonies in a field can lower crop yields, because the cutting bars of harvesting machinery have to be raised to avoid damage from the hard, heaped-up mounds.

Fire ants will attack and kill a newborn calf, bird hatchling, disabled animal, or any confined animal that cannot avoid their stings. Furthermore, livestock may starve in the field when swarms of fire ants render their food inaccessible. Animals have been blinded by their attacks or suffered bites in mouth, rectum, or pre-existing wounds. Even fish are not immune to the ant invasion; thousands of trout have died of venom poisoning after eating swarms of winged males and queens that have flown into lakes.

Fire ants attack not only plants and animals. Attracted to the heated asphalt, they build mounds under rural roads, which then collapse as the undermined soil subsides. In 1977, a survey of forty miles of roadway in North Carolina revealed an average of twenty fire ant colonies per mile, with some undermining of the road at each location.

Solenopsis invicta, the most pragmatic of creatures, has one peculiar trait. It is attracted to anything electrical. Fire ants, like bees, have tiny deposits of iron in their bodies and are, in fact, slightly ferromagnetic. But scientists are puzzled as to why fire ants enjoy being shocked by electric currents so much. Researchers at the University of Texas in El Paso set up special electric boxes, each with sixteen sets of copper points. They then put about four hundred worker fire ants in each box and turned on the current. Whether AC or DC, once the voltage reached fifty, the ants started swarming over the points. Even three hundred and fifty volts of direct current was not too hot for them. But it had to be electricity—electromagnetic fields, ozone, or wire insulation left the ants indifferent.

In areas where they are plentiful, red fire ants will accumulate in the proximity of any exposed electric field. According to entomologist S. Bradley Vinson, "their numbers build up slowly on powered bare wires, contact points, and around fuses and switches." The ants not only swarm over wiring, they fill the devices with dirt. Fire ants have caused short circuits in telephone junction and switching equipment, traffic control cabinets, power company transformers, airport landing lights, computers, flood control equipment, home wall plugs, and even car electrical systems. They foul contact surfaces, inhibit mechanical functions, and can cause electrical fires.

Even homes are not safe. In South America, fire ants invade human habitations mainly during times of flooding or drought. But in the United States, perhaps because of the presence of wiring in walls, *Solenopsis invicta* nests are increasingly turning up in homes and apartments. In 1995, Drs. Richard de Shazo and David Williams reported the case of a thirty-nine-year-old woman and her nine-year-old daughter in Tampa, Florida, who, along with their dog and cat, were suffering repeated fire ant stings indoors. The family lived on the second floor of a wooden, three-story apartment complex. Despite repeated visits by the exterminator, fire ants persisted. When Dr. Williams, an entomologist, visited the building, he found colonies of red fire ants in the soil beneath the concrete slab foundation of the structure and also above the slab, in a first-floor corridor. Inside the apartment, the ants swarmed everywhere. Then Dr. Williams discovered along the wall of the living room a lump that had previously gone unnoticed. When he pulled back the carpet, he found a large mound of dirt—a colony of about fifty thousand ants.

When fire ants build nests in homes or invade them on their foraging expeditions, a true ant horror can result. Fire ants make no distinction between a newborn calf and a newborn baby. They will attack any prey that cannot escape their stings, as in the following 1992 case from Birmingham, Alabama.

A five-day-old boy was placed in a playpen six inches from the floor. The following morning, his parents found him pale, limp, and covered with ants. After quickly rinsing the ants off, they rushed him to a local emergency room. On arrival he was in cardiac arrest. When the emergency room doctors inserted a plastic tube into his airway, they found ants in the back of his throat.

After five minutes of resuscitation, the baby's heart began to beat. His doctors gave him epinephrine and antihistamines for anaphylactic shock and admitted him to the intensive care unit. He had approximately two thousand fire ant stings, and on one area of his forehead there was so much damage that a patch of his skin came off. The child was kept on a ventilator, but for the first sixteen hours he didn't move or try to breathe on his own. The infant's treatment was long and difficult. After five weeks in the hospital he was able to take formula from a bottle but was slightly spastic and did not follow objects well with his eyes. Six months after the attack, though the boy seemed to have recovered, he had some "mild delay in achieving motor milestones."

In the seven decades since its arrival in the United States the red fire ant has defied all methods of eradication. This species, which has had various scientific names, was officially designated *invicta*, meaning "invincible," by the late W. F. Buren in 1965, because he felt that the species would prove almost impossible to manage.

Dr. Buren's prediction has been abundantly borne out. Frantic farmers have poured gasoline onto fire ant mounds and set them on fire, but to no avail. Environmentally friendly but ineffectual home remedies have included wood ashes, citrus peels, watermelon rinds, vinegar, and grits poured or stuffed into mounds. In a review of the problem, Dr. Williams, the entomologist, records such "high-tech" solutions as microwave radiation, electrical probes, and explosives. Another remedy, he notes, is to dig up a mound and place it on top of another mound with the expectation that the ants will fight, eliminating both colonies. Without a bulldozer, this last scheme would be hard to implement without incurring hundreds of stings.

Chemical control has been and continues to be the main weapon in the ant wars and, in fact, the fire ant crisis helped to create the environmental movement in this country. In August 1957, the U.S. Congress appropriated $2.4 million for imported fire ant control and, in October of that year, the Department of Agriculture began to show farmers how to drench ant mounds with the chlorinated hydrocarbon heptachlor. During the cold, wet winter of 1957–58, thousands of gallons of heptachlor were poured into the environment. Shortly afterward, wildlife and cattle began to die.

In a 1961 effort to reduce the amount of pesticide needed to kill the ants, scientists at the Department of Agriculture Methods Development Laboratory in Gulfport, Mississippi, developed toxic baits. The researchers dissolved the powerful chlorinated hydrocarbon mirex in soybean oil, which they then used to soak corncob grits. Field studies showed that repeated applications of this pesticide resulted in excellent control of fire ant infestations.

Then, in 1962, Rachel Carson published *Silent Spring*. Her warning of the adverse environmental impact of all chlorinated hydrocarbon pesticides, including mirex, led to studies in the late 1960s that showed that this pesticide biodegraded only very slowly. In 1970, environmental groups requested a court injunction to halt the use of mirex. Although their request was denied, that year the U.S. Department of the Interior banned its use on public lands they managed. Persistent pressure by environmental groups on the issue of pesticides led, in 1973, to the formation of the Environmental Protection Agency. In 1976, Allied Chemical Corporation voluntarily discontinued manufacture of mirex baits. A government nonprofit agency took over the factory and produced mirex until 1977, when the EPA was able to stop its use completely.

But even before mirex was banned, it was clear that the red

fire ant would never be contained, much less eradicated, from North American soil by chemical means. Control efforts still rely on baits laced with insecticide, but scientists have always hoped that biological methods of control might be brought to bear. Unfortunately, attempts to harness the known protozoan and fungal parasites of the fire ant have failed so far, because it has proved impossible to spread these diseases in ant colonies under experimental conditions. All ants are meticulous housekeepers and personal groomers. They recognize anything foreign in the colony and remove it immediately. In addition, some of the protozoan parasites are probably spread to the ants by some, as yet unidentified, intermediate host.

Recently researchers in Florida have begun studying the phorid flies that lay eggs inside fire ants and make their heads fall off. If effective, they could be released into the wild. However, releasing one new species to attack another may backfire. The phorid flies could attack native insects or, separated from their own natural enemies, they, too, could multiply out of control.

It seems, then, that the invincible fire ants will never be vanquished and will continue to extend their range in the United States. Patients and the doctors who treat them will have to be prepared for the consequences of their stings.

Fire ant venom is a watery solution of organic compounds loosely termed alkaloids. They have a direct toxic effect on the membranes of mast cells. Paul Ehrlich, who later became famous for developing drug treatments for syphilis, discovered these curious cells in the 1870s. He found one form circulating in the blood stream and another living in the tissues. Stuffed with dense, blue-staining granules filled with histamine, both types act like tiny land mines. When a mast cell in the nose, for example, encounters a pollen grain, it explodes. The histamine provokes all the familiar allergic symptoms: runny, itchy nose and eyes, and sneezing. If the allergen—from strawberries, for example, or shellfish—arrives via the blood stream, histamine release from mast cells in the skin causes hives. In the lungs, histamine provokes more serious reactions: spasmodic constriction of the bronchial passages with wheezing, coughing, and, in severe cases, an asphyxiating blockage of all airflow.

Fire ant alkaloids are allergic mimics. They trigger histamine release from mast cells by direct membrane damage. No preexisting allergy is required. When stung by a fire ant, everyone develops the same kind of welts. In many people this local reaction, however massive, is all that occurs, as in the following patient.

In 1971, two doctors from Houston, Texas, described the case of a forty-nine-year-old alcoholic who was brought to the hospital at two a.m. one Sunday morning. The man had been drinking all day and all night on Saturday and was on his way to a friend's house when he was overcome with drowsiness. Arriving in the dark at the ditch in front of the house he "selected a fire ant mound as his pillow." When his friend discovered him a few hours later, he had thousands of small black fire ants crawling on him. After the ants were washed off, the emergency room physicians found approximately five thousand fire ant welts on his face, torso, and extremities. Other than a strong odor of alcohol on his breath, the welts were the only abnormal finding on examination, and he survived without any other ill effects. The authors concluded, "After a night on the town, one should make an all-out effort to return home, for the fire ant is quite reluctant to share his bed with strangers."

Life-threatening anaphylactic reactions are almost always triggered by substances that have a protein component. Bee sting venom, for example, is a complex mixture of various proteins, to which individuals become highly allergic after repeated exposures. For many years, ant-sting anaphylaxis was a medical mystery, because fire ant venom seemed to lack proteins. But it only takes an infinitesimal amount of allergen to trigger a fatal anaphylactic reaction and, in fact, there are proteins in fire ant venom, though they make up only one tenth of one percent of its weight.

In 1979, Dr. Harold Baer and colleagues reported a meticulous chemical analysis of the contents of the venom sacs of *Solenopsis invicta*. It is possible to obtain minute amounts of venom by milking fire ants and collecting the fluid in tiny tubes. The investigators used Sephadex column chromatography, a method of analyzing solutions in which venom extracts are poured over beads to separate the different components. They found tiny amounts of the same set of enzyme proteins that bees have in their venom, and serum samples from patients with fire ant allergy showed strong binding of allergy-specific antibodies to several of the venom proteins. However, the specific proteins that trigger fire ant allergy are different from the proteins that trigger dangerous reactions to bee stings, which explains why patients who react to bee venom may or may not react to fire ant stings, and vice versa.

The best treatment for anaphylaxis is by aborting the reaction by early treatment with epinephrine. Patients who have had severe reactions to fire ant stings should be prescribed epinephrine for self administration. Products such as Epi-pen contain a dose of epinephrine preloaded into a pen-shaped syringe that can be administered subcutaneously with the push of a button. If the victim or the parent of a child with fire ant allergy can act quickly enough, a fatal allergic reaction can be diminished or delayed until paramedics arrive.

It is better to prevent the reaction from occurring at all, and the most effective preventive measure for hypersensitive people who coexist with fire ants is immunotherapy. Already proven effective for bee sting allergy, immunotherapy for fire ant allergy was pioneered by Dr. R. Faser Triplett and reported in the *Southern*

Medical Journal in 1973. Dr. Triplett enrolled eighteen patients from the Mississippi Allergy Clinic in Jackson, each with a previous severe reaction to fire ant stings. Eight patients were under the age of four years. Of the eighteen patients, four had a past history of skin allergy or asthma before their first serious fire ant reaction, or had an anaphylactic reaction to a bee sting, and one had almost died following a wasp sting. The remaining twelve patients had nothing in their past histories to suggest a dangerous allergic tendency, but had received a warning with the first sting—hives, swelling of the lips or tongue, tightness in the chest, wheezing, or a fall in blood pressure.

Because fire ant venom is so difficult to harvest in quantity, Dr. Triplett used an extract made from whole ants. In a series of injections lasting up to two years, patients received gradually increasing doses either once or twice weekly. Their bodies reacted by producing blocking antibodies that prevented the allergic chain reaction. Fire ants stung eight of the eighteen patients again, and all survived their repeat encounter without any dangerous symptoms.

Immunotherapy with whole body extracts (WBE) of *Solenopsis* is now an accepted practice. But as immunotherapy is cumbersome, expensive, and time-consuming, doctors will usually perform a skin test to confirm allergy. Selected patients can be given an accelerated course of shots to provide protection faster, but the injections must still be given every year to maintain protection. For children and adults who must coexist with *Solenopsis invicta* despite serious allergy, these shots can mean the difference between life and death.

No government agency or private concern will ever eradicate the red fire ant from the United States. And it is invading other countries, as well. In February 2001, fire ants attacked a workman at a container facility at the mouth of the Brisbane River in

Australia. According to genetic tests, the ants were a North American strain of *Solenopsis invicta*. Simultaneously, authorities discovered infestations several miles away in Brisbane's western suburbs. This strain of red fire ants came from South America, suggesting two separate incursions.

For millions of years the red fire ant lived in the heart of the South American continent, cut off from contact with the outside world. Its life was supported and its population balanced within the ecosystem in which it evolved. But this isolation ended when North Americans, eager to exploit the region, breached the natural barriers, bringing their machines with them. There they encountered an invincible little adversary, as ruthless and resourceful as they were. And then, by accident, they brought it home.

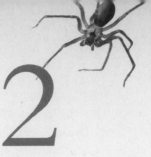

2

Fangs in
the Dark

November 9, 1966. A sixty-three-year-old retired farm worker living in Arkansas visited his physician's office complaining of fever, pain in the left side of his chest, and dark urine. His doctor found nothing abnormal except for a "peculiar dusky color" to his skin. The doctor gave the farm worker some antibiotic tablets and sent him home. Two days later, the farm worker returned to the doctor's office in early shock. His blood pressure was low, his lips were blue, and there was a large bruise on the left side of his chest.

The doctor arranged for the farm worker's admission to the University Hospital in Little Rock. There, the examining physicians found a "slender, irrational man with a peculiar dark slate gray color to his skin." In addition, the victim had two small necrotic areas on his chest, surrounded by a large bruise.

The doctors inserted a catheter into the farm worker's bladder, and the urine that flowed out was dark red. However, when the urine was examined under the microscope, there were no intact red cells; he was not bleeding into his urine, which would be a signal that he had kidney stones.

The hospital laboratory spun a sample of the patient's blood in a centrifuge. In a healthy person, the red blood cells would be thrown to the bottom of the tube. At the bottom third to one half of the tube, it would form a red layer surmounted by a layer of straw-colored plasma. In this man, there was only a tiny pellet of intact red blood cells and the plasma was almost black.

Red blood cells are basically bags of hemoglobin, the oxygen-carrying protein, surrounded by a fatty membrane. In this man, eighty percent of his red blood cells had exploded, turning the plasma dark and the urine red. Unable to transport oxygen from his lungs to his tissues, he had turned blue-gray from asphyxia and had gone into shock. The hemoglobin pigment, which is so helpful *inside* the red blood cells, was extremely toxic to the kidneys. Urine flow slowed to a trickle, and his kidneys had shut down. Despite dialysis and blood transfusions, the farm worker died after nine days in the hospital. At autopsy, the skin ulcer showed the telltale signs of necrotic arachnidism.

Throughout the world, there are approximately 34,000 known species of spiders. The Araneida, the order of spiders, is ancient. Fossil spiders first appear in red sandstone deposits dating nearly 395 million years ago.

Today, spiders are found on every continent except Antarctica, and range in size from the dwarf spider, no bigger than the period at the end of this sentence, to the enormous South American tarantula. Unlike insects, which have six legs and three body segments, all spiders have eight legs and two body segments, are predatory flesh-eaters, and nearly all are venomous. And because they are also cannibals, humans have yet to succeed in raising spiders for their extremely strong silk.

However, despite their ferocity, spiders cannot ingest solid food. The spider pumps digestive enzymes from its intestine into its prey and then sucks up the liquefied tissue and body juices. Some spider venom, like some snake venom, act by destroying tissue and, therefore, may have evolved to aid in digestion. A rattlesnake, which swallows its prey whole, and a spider, which ingests only liquids, both produce venom that kills and digests the living tissue of its victim.

Spider venoms that produce severe local damage are responsible for the syndrome of necrotic arachnidism. Necrosis means tissue death, and arachnidism refers to the arachnids, the class of invertebrates that includes spiders and scorpions.

Until the 1940s the only venomous spider recognized in the United States was the black widow. But as far back as the nineteenth century, farmers in the Midwest had known about a type of painful, deep-skin ulcer that took anywhere from weeks to months to heal and left a white scar. People didn't seem to get the ulcer more than once—after one attack, they were immune. Despite what was written in the medical textbooks, physicians practicing in these rural areas suspected that these ulcers were really spider bites. In Missouri in the 1940s, there were reports of isolated clinical cases of ulcers following the bites of an unidentified species of "brown spider." In July 1957, three researchers from the University of Missouri published a short article in the journal *Science,* pointing out the striking similarity between the spider-inflicted wounds in Missouri and the "gangrenous spot" of Chile, Uruguay, and other South American countries. They cited the work of a Dr. Macchiavello, who in 1937 had shown that the bite of the Chilean brown spider, *Loxosceles laeta,* caused the South

American ulcer. The authors of the article in *Science* deduced that a spider common in the Midwest, *Loxosceles reclusa,* probably caused necrotic arachnidism in the United States.

Loxosceles reclusa, or brown recluse spider, is a half-dollar-sized brown spider that lives in houses—on the floor or behind furniture. The spider is easily overlooked, as its body is small and its legs, though long, are hairless and very thin. Also known as the fiddleback, it is best identified by the dark, violin-shaped band on its back, extending from behind its six eyes to the end of its first segment, the cephalothorax. *Loxosceles reclusa* lives in the fifteen central states from the eastern half of Texas to the western corner of Georgia and as far north as Ohio. It's not aggressive and usually only bites defensively—when crushed between folds of clothing or bedding and the body of a person, often a sleeper.

A typical uncomplicated case of brown recluse spider bite, or *loxoscelism,* was published as a series of six color photographs in the *New England Journal of Medicine* in 1998. Dr. Edwin Masters of Cape Girardeau, Missouri, reported that a brown recluse, later recovered and identified, bit a forty-six-year-old woman on the underside of her left arm. Twenty-four hours later the patient had a moderately painful area of redness about four inches across. She applied cold packs and took codeine and aspirin for pain. Three days later the wound had turned into a saucer-sized open ulcer, which showed the classic "red, white, and blue sign" of necrotic arachnidism. Viewed from the outer edge to the center, there was first a wide circle of redness from inflammation, then a narrower ring of pallor from blocked blood flow to the skin, and, in the center, a blue circle of dying tissue. Two days later, Dr. Masters admitted this patient to the hospital with fever, severe pain, and a red rash over her entire body. Her upper arm was swollen from fluid seeping into the tissues around the bite. He treated the woman with dapsone pills, an antileprosy drug with anti-inflammatory effects, as well as with antibiotics, to prevent infection of the open wound. Eight days after the bite the patient's pain had lessened, but there was a thick, black scab of dead tissue in the wound, which was surgically removed on the tenth day. On day twenty-four, the patient still had a saucer-sized ulcer, which did not completely heal until sixty-seven days after the spider bite.

The exact mechanism by which the bite of a small spider can produce such extensive tissue damage is not completely understood. One component of recluse venom is the enzyme *sphingomyelinase D,* which attacks and dissolves cell membranes. This enzyme and probably other components of the venom set off a chain of chemical reactions in the blood vessels of the skin that turns the patient's inflammatory defenses against his or her own tissues. The patient's infection-fighting white blood cells are activated by a venom false alarm. These white blood cells normally act like kamikazes to destroy bacterial invaders. After a recluse bite, they surge through the blood vessel walls, move into the tissues, and blow themselves up releasing other enzymes that destroy the patient's own flesh. Clots form inside the tiny blood vessels nourishing the skin, which dies for lack of oxygen and nutrients, and a deep ulcer is left. The reaction, once set off, takes weeks or even months to subside.

Brown recluse spider bites are painful and debilitating, but when the reaction is limited to the skin, they are usually not life-threatening, unless the bite is in a particularly bad location, as in the following case.

A seven-year-old boy was awakened from sleep by a sharp pain in the front of his neck. The next day the patient's family brought him to his pediatrician, along with a spider they had found in his bed. The doctor identified the spider as *Loxosceles reclusa.* He found two small round spots under the left side of the boy's jaw, surrounded by a three-inch area of tender swelling. He gave the boy a return appointment for the next day and sent him home. A few hours later, the patient began to have fever and increased swelling in his neck.

The boy's family rushed him to the emergency room of a local hospital. On examination, the patient was alert but had a racing pulse and a temperature of almost 104°F. Swelling now extended from jaw to collarbone on the left. He was admitted to the hospital. The next day the swelling had spread to the upper chest, and the patient was having trouble breathing and swallowing. His doctors decided to transfer him by helicopter to the University of Texas Southwestern Medical Center in Dallas.

On arrival in the pediatric emergency room, the boy was alert but frightened, and his breathing was labored and rapid. The swelling now involved the entire front of the neck and extended to the level of the nipples. X-rays showed extensive swelling of the tissue around his windpipe. He was admitted to the intensive care unit.

Over the next two days, the boy's neck and chest swelling gradually subsided, and his breathing eased. However, by the third day, a deep blistering ulcer had appeared at the site of the original bite. He was given dapsone and soothing dressings and was able to go home on the fifth day, but did not return for his subsequent appointments.

On rare occasions, recluse spider venom may escape the bite site, get into the blood stream, and punch holes in the victim's red blood cells, causing them to explode. Between 1939 and 1958, thirty-nine cases were reported of spider-bite hemolysis, as the process is called; six proved fatal. Two physicians at the University of Arkansas in Little Rock reported the fatal case that opened this chapter.

. . .

Although species of *Loxosceles* are found around the world, they are not found outside the Midwest and southeast states in this country. However, physicians practicing in the Pacific Northwest had been reporting an increasing number of cases of apparent necrotic arachnidism. The offending spider was a mystery until the late 1980s, when Dr. Darwin K. Vest of Washington State University implicated the hobo spider, *Tegenaria agrestis*. Investigating thirty cases of necrotic arachnidism in Washington, Oregon, and Idaho, Dr. Vest was able to show that the syndrome only occurred in regions where this spider was common.

Tegenaria agrestis, a brown spider with a one- to two-inch leg span, is native to Europe. It was accidentally introduced into the Seattle area in the 1920s and early 1930s and has subsequently spread as far as central Utah and the Alaskan panhandle.

Hobo spiders build funnel-shaped webs in moist, dark areas such as woodpiles, crawl spaces, and basements. They wait in the narrow end of the web until they feel the vibration of an insect crossing the strands. Then the spider dashes out, at the intimidating speed of a meter per second, seizes the prey, bites it, and drags it back into the web. During midsummer through fall, the more venomous male hobo spiders leave their webs and wander in search of females. These fast-moving spiders are not unusually aggressive but will bite if provoked or threatened.

Besides a chronic, painful skin ulcer the bite causes, a classic symptom of *Tegenaria agretis* envenomation is severe, persistent headache. The following case in an adult illustrates the debilitating effects of the hobo spider's venom.

On September 26, 1983, a thirty-four-year-old man was installing insulation in the wooden floor joints beneath a mobile home north of Idaho Falls, Idaho. At about twelve-thirty p.m. he felt a momentary pinch on his right forearm. He "shook the arm of his coverall, and the crushed body of a brown, long-legged spider fell to the floor." The man continued working, but within ten minutes his right hand and his tongue began to tingle, he became dizzy, and felt short of breath. His coworkers pulled him out from beneath the mobile home and took him to a hospital.

On arrival, he was confused, disoriented, and complained of a severe headache. The examining doctors noted a four-inch zone of redness around the bite site. After an hour and a half, the patient was breathing easily, but the headache persisted. Two hours after the bite, he was tired, weak, and having some visual blurring, but as his blood tests were normal, and the redness around his wound was subsiding, his doctors sent him home.

At first the victim felt better, but by nine-thirty that evening he said he "felt weird"; he had pains in his joints and complained of a pounding headache. By the next day, the bite had raised a white blister, and in addition to the joint and head pain, he was incoherent. He made his way back to the emergency room that afternoon and received a Demerol injection. He felt better and again went home. However, by eight p.m. that evening his headache had returned and was accompanied by nausea, profuse sweating, and inability to eat.

The next morning, the blister at the spider bite burst, leaving an ulcer, but the patient felt so much better that around five p.m. he drank a can of beer. Almost immediately, he felt a tingling of his scalp and tongue, and a moderate headache returned. Later that evening, he had distorted vision with "light flashes" and heard a high-pitched squeal. After a final sick headache on October 1 he gradually recovered, and his ulcer healed after a month.

When the authors of this paper inspected the crawl space under the mobile home, they found hobo spiders in "literally every crack or indentation of the foundation." Although none of the thirty patients in this series actually brought the biting spider with them to the hospital, one victim picked *Tegenaria agrestis* out of a lineup of ten live spiders, insisting that the *Tegenaria* specimen was the same kind of spider he discovered in his bedsheets.

Unique among spiders, *Tegenaria* may on rare occasions kill the patient by attacking the bone marrow factory. In late January 1986, a "bug" bit a fifty-six-year-old resident of Spokane, Washington, on her right thigh. Within twenty-four hours she developed severe headache, nausea, and confusion. She did not see a doctor until February 16, when she began to bleed from "her ears and other orifices." On admission to the hospital, she had the typical scabbed ulcer of necrotic arachnidism, but, in addition, the counts of all three blood elements—red blood cells, white blood cells, and platelets—were drastically reduced. Her physicians determined that her bone marrow had stopped functioning. Despite transfusion therapy, the patient bled internally and died in early March. Inspectors found abundant hobo spiders adjacent to her home.

In the seventy years since *Tegenaria agrestis* invaded Seattle, it has spread to six states and to southwestern Canada. Like other ecological opportunists, the spider proliferates namely because it left its natural enemies behind. In cities like Moscow, Idaho, and Pullman, Washington, *Tegenaria* is easily the most common large spider found and is present in most houses.

Necrotic arachnidism is a worldwide problem with no consensus on the best treatment. Dapsone therapy remains popular, although this drug can itself cause red cell destruction. One patient with a recluse bite to the penis seemed to respond favorably to high-pressure (hyperbaric) oxygen, but animal studies of this modality have been inconclusive. Most physicians now agree that the old remedy of surgically cutting out the ulcer is not helpful. No antivenins have been developed for the effects of these bites.

In Australia, necrotic arachnidism is an area of active research interest. The white-tailed spider, *Lampona,* and the black *window* spiders, genus *Badumna,* are thought to cause the syndrome. In addition, two species of *Loxosceles* have been accidentally introduced into the country in recent years. To better delineate the clinical syndromes produced by each of these species, Australians anywhere in the country are encouraged to capture the offending spider and "Call NASTY!"—the acronym for a study of necrotic arachnidism at the Australian Venom Research Unit and the Monash Medical Center. For the duration of the study, an investigator is on call twenty-four hours a day to enroll patients and to identify the offending spiders.

The other venomous spiders of medical importance inject toxins that target the victim's nervous system. The most notorious, though not the most deadly, spiders of this type are the widows, genus *Latrodectus.* This name derives from the Greek and means roughly "robber-biter." There are some forty species of *Latrodectus* spiders, all dangerously venomous. They live from southern Canada through South America, and from France south, including most of Africa and Australia. Male widows are very small, variably colored, and do not bite. Females are small to medium-sized, with globular bodies, and, in many species, beautiful red markings on the underside of the abdomen. Despite their name, they don't always eat their husbands after mating. The most common widow in the United States, *Latrodectus mactans,* has a jet-black abdomen and sports a red hourglass on the underside of her belly. Widow spiders in other countries have distinctive local names, sometimes descriptive of their markings.

In Mexico, *Latrodectus mactans* is known as *araña capulina,* the "cherry spider." In the West Indies, it is called *cul rouge,* "red-tail," or *veinte cuatro horas* "twenty-four hours." A very toxic widow spider in Corsica is called the *malmignatta* or "bad leech." In southern Africa, one name for their widow is the *knoppiespinnekop,* or "shoe-button spider." The Australians have *L. hasseltii,* the redback spider.

The symptoms of latrodectism, or widow-spider bite, have been known for centuries and people have learned to identify the local *Latrodectus* species unerringly.

Although *Latrodectus* may be found in wild areas, like abandoned rodent burrows, it prefers to live a commensal existence with humans. These spiders are attracted to the structures people build and the clutter that surrounds human habitation, favoring outbuildings like garages, barns, storage sheds, and privies. During cold weather, widows may migrate indoors and take up residence in closets, cupboards, and bed frames. *Latrodectus mactans* is especially plentiful in southern California. After I wrote the last paragraph, I conducted a ten-minute nighttime search under my travel trailer, which is parked in my driveway, and found one large and two small black widow spiders perched motionless, upside down in the center of their messy webs. At the first flash of light, two of them clambered away and disappeared into the shadows.

The black widow waits in its web until it detects the telltale vibration of enmeshed prey. It throws sticky silk over the victim and then cautiously descends and gives it a paralyzing bite. When the prey becomes quiet, the spider again descends and bites the victim several more times, pumping it with digestive enzymes, liquefying its body contents.

Female widow spiders are shy, nocturnal creatures that never leave their webs and do not bite people unless provoked or confused. In the days of the outhouse, most black widow bites involved a confused spider. A privy is a magnet for insects, and widows will take advantage of the draft coming through the seat hole to build a web either across it or just underneath. The spider then waits out of sight. When a person, most often a male, sits on the privy seat, the spider feels an exciting vibration and dashes out to bite the "prey" with excruciating results for the accidental victim. In his book *The Red Hourglass,* Gordon Grice writes that his grandmother, who grew up in rural Oklahoma, told him that some people would take a stick to the privy and scrape under the seat. The widow's web is supposed to make a sound when it is broken, like paper crackling in fire.

In areas where the privy has disappeared, most widow-spider bites occur among people working outdoors with their bare hands. Farmers are at risk during harvesting and when they work along fences or outbuildings. In urban environments, widows bite people clearing rubbish, or working in gardens, hot metal sheds, or along metal fence lines. Sometimes a large number of widows will infest a small area, when the successive progeny of one spider take up residence in a favorable location. Although they are inveterate cannibals, individual widows can live close to one another because, once established, they do not leave their webs. Spider-bite epidemics have occurred when a group of people, usually a military troop, camps in such an area.

The first sign of widow bite is a trivial pinprick sensation as the spider's twin fangs pierce the skin, followed by a little pause— from a few minutes to a half-hour—until the venom reaches the nerves and begins to take effect. *Latrodectus* venom is complex, with many components active only against invertebrate prey. The business end of the venom for people is a large protein, alpha latrotoxin. This toxin stimulates various nerves to release chemical substances, like acetyl choline, that trigger other nerves to fire. The result is a chaotic neural storm in which muscles are stimulated to contract painfully and cells become depleted of transmitter compounds. Sometimes voluntary muscles can't function, which leads to profound weakness. Sensory nerves are painfully stimulated. The autonomic nerves, which handle automatic functions, discharge. Blood pressure climbs; the victim sweats profusely and vomits. The heart first races and then may slow to a dull thud, leaving the patient in a state of ashen collapse.

In some victims the toxin affects the brain. They may feel extremely anxious, "speeded up," even manic, or become forgetful, suffer amnesia, or even become psychotic. But the cardinal symptom of latrodectism is agonizing pain, as in this patient, whose case was reported in 1996.

An eight-year-old boy living in North Carolina experienced a bite on his left elbow while putting on his shirt. Almost immediately he felt pain at the bite site, which quickly spread to his abdomen. When the boy's mother removed his shirt, she saw a spider fall to the floor. She killed it and saved it. She then called 911, and paramedics transported both the boy and the spider to the emergency room.

On arrival, the boy told the doctors through a teeth-chattering chill that his stomach hurt. The examining physicians found that the boy's abdominal muscles were locked in a rigid, boardlike spasm. No bite site was apparent, but the spider was definitely a black widow. The doctors started an intravenous drip of saline and glucose, and then gave the child two doses of calcium gluconate. Calcium solutions are a time-honored method of reducing pain in envenomations. As a precaution, he received a tetanus shot. After five hours of observation, the boy felt well and was sent home.

The next day, the child's family brought him to their physician's office, because his abdomen was hurting again. The doctor gave him acetaminophen and Benadryl. However, throughout the rest of the day, the boy's condition declined. His abdomen and legs were racked with cramps. He became feverish and nauseated and began vomiting. He complained of blurry vision.

Twenty-four hours after the spider bite, the victim's mother brought him back to the emergency room. He was panting, and his blood pressure was elevated. At the bite site there was now a one-inch firm and tender area. Over the next two days, he received intravenous fluid, calcium, and Demerol. The skin lesion disappeared, his condition improved, and, after two days, he was able to go home.

Latrodectism, while agonizing, is rarely fatal in the United States, with estimated death rates ranging from one to five percent. However, these figures are probably an overestimate, as most nonfatal attacks are almost never reported. Infants and toddlers, the elderly, and people with other serious conditions, such as heart disease, are at highest risk for death. One famous example was the actor Harry Carey, who was working on the movie *Red River* when it was reported that he had died of a heart attack following a black widow spider bite.

In Australia, the death rate from redback spider bites is higher, and patients frequently require treatment with antivenin. The Australian Commonwealth Serum Laboratory makes antivenin by injecting horses with increasing doses of redback venom and then harvesting the antibody-rich horse serum. A similar product is available in the United States, which works against *Latrodectus mactans* and other American species.

To make antivenin, one must first obtain venom by milking spiders. Unanesthetized widows can be milked by being carefully picked up and teased to discharge their venom into a small glass tube. Sometimes mild electric currents are applied about the head and fangs to provoke venom discharge.

Doctors rarely resort to black widow spider antivenin in the United States, because of the risk of severe, immediate, allergic reactions to it. In addition, within a week or two of its use, patients may come down with serum sickness, a prolonged reaction consisting of fever and joint pains. However, antivenin can be useful in severe or protracted cases, such as that of the thirteen-year-old boy, recently described in the *New England Journal of Medicine*.

After being bitten on the neck by a black widow, this patient was brought to a local hospital with severe pain at the bite site and muscle cramps in his chest, abdomen, and legs. Doctors gave him calcium gluconate and Demerol. After twenty-four hours he was still too weak to walk, but, despite this, he was sent home with a prescription for Vicodin.

Three days later, the patient sought care at a second hospital. His heart beat slowly when he was lying down, but raced when he tried to stand up. His blood pressure was elevated. Because of weakness and muscle cramping, he was unable to walk. Doctors in the second emergency room obtained and administered one vial of *Latrodectus mactans* antivenin. Ten minutes after the infusion was complete, the patient was able to dress himself. His pulse became steady, and he was able to walk with assistance.

In the United States, the only neurotoxic spider is the black widow. In Brazil, there are three species of *Latrodectus,* and, in that warm climate, they are plentiful. One investigator, working along a three-kilometer beach, was able to capture 1,400 widows in one week. But, despite this rich supply, Brazilians do not consider the widow to be their most important venomous spider. That honor goes to *Phoneutria,* the wandering spider. These are big, hairy, aggressive spiders that grow up to thirteen inches across. When threatened, wandering spiders do not run away. Instead they rise on their two pairs of hind legs, lift the long forelegs, and bristle their red underhairs. Accompanying an aggressor's movements, they will maneuver to stay in front. If they are not killed by the first swat of a broom, they may climb rapidly up the stick and are not reluctant to bite. At the Instituto Butantan in São Paulo, Brazil, these spiders are always milked by two people working together and only after the spider has been lightly anesthetized with ether.

Phoneutria nigriventer, the species accounting for the most bites in Brazil, lives along the eastern coast of the country. Wandering spiders do not construct webs, but instead hunt at night for insects and other spiders. They live beneath fallen trees, in banana plants, palms, and bromeliads. They invade construction refuse, and, especially during the mating season, enter homes and garages. In the cool months of March and April, shoes and trunks are daytime hiding places. Occasionally, they are inadvertently transported thousands of miles from home in shipments of bananas.

Wandering-spider bites are extremely common in the São Paulo area. At the Hospital Vital Brazil, for example, in the ten-year period between 1970 and 1980, there were 7,087 *Phoneutria* bites, accounting for over twenty percent of all admissions to that hospital. But, while frequent, they are never routine. As in latrodectism, pain is the most common symptom in phoneutrism. The composition of the spider's venom is complex, but it causes the same kind of uncontrolled neural discharge as the widow venom and with similar symptoms. Priapism, or spontaneous erection due to massive release of the nerve transmitter acetyl choline, is very common in children bitten by this spider and may be a harbinger of fatal neurological collapse. Irregular heart rhythms and pulmonary edema, in which the lungs fill with fluid, account for most of the other fatalities.

Doctors treating *Phoneutria* bites in Brazil frequently use anesthetic nerve blocks to relieve pain. Less than five percent of cases at the Hospital Vital Brazil are severe enough to require antivenin. Death is rare with proper care and occurs mainly in children under the age of seven and in the elderly.

Most people unfortunate enough to experience the bite of the recluse, the widow, or the wandering spider of Brazil will suffer, often profoundly, but they will live to tell the tale. This is not the case with the Australian funnel web spider, which delivers a bite so lethal that the doctor-scientist who developed the first antivenin, Dr. Struan K. Sutherland, became something of a hero in Australia. Funnel web spiders, much like their cousins the harmless tarantulas, are hairy and heavy, measuring up to two inches across. When stepped on, their bodies are said to crunch like a chicken bone. The most important species is *Atrax robustus,* or the Sydney funnel web, whose home range is limited to within a 150-mile radius of Sydney. These spiders build silk-lined burrow retreats with an open entrance and irregular silk triplines radiating out over the ground. The spider forages near the entrance and seizes prey that blunders over a tripline. Most bites occur when the male funnel web spiders leave their webs permanently to search for mates. In their travels they often enter houses and may find their way into clothing and footwear. They can be aggressive when encountered.

The lethal component of funnel web venom is called atrotoxin or robustoxin. Human beings, other primates, and newborn mice are sensitive to its affects, but other laboratory animals, such as rabbits, are resistant. The funnel web's large fangs inject the venom, which travels through the lymphatic system—a network of tiny vessels—and then binds to nerve endings throughout the body. Atrotoxin triggers explosive nerve cell discharges, especially in the autonomic nervous system, resulting in wide swings in pulse and blood pressure, fever, irregular heart rhythm, muscle damage, and shifts of fluid into the lungs. Death may occur from fifteen minutes to as long as six days after a bite. The average survivor spends fourteen days in the hospital if he or she does not receive antivenin. A survivor from the days before antivenin, one C. A. Monticone, a forty-two-year-old doctor of laws, wrote an objective, yet vivid account of his experience.

"Monday, 20th June, 1927, 6:10 a.m. While doing physical culture exercises in pyjamas [sic] and bare feet . . . I felt something under my left foot. It was dark at the time and I rubbed my foot on the carpet, thinking it was a button or other small object. Suddenly I felt a severe prick as from a pin. I looked and saw something dark and wrenched it off with some effort."

Monticone killed the spider and then noticed two small punctures.

"6:45 a.m. A peculiar numbness of tongue and loss of taste is noticed, and a twingeing [sic] pain in the tongue and lips similar to that of a strong electric current running through the throat.

"7:30 a.m. About this time the pain extended to both hands and feet, with a strange sensation as though something cold was touching the skin.

"8:00 a.m. (approximately). I felt pains in both arms and legs and had annoying and excessive salivation, necessitating continuous spitting. I had also a discharge of mucous matter from my nose . . . The most troublesome symptoms were the twitching of all facial muscles, especially the lips . . . My face felt as though the whole surface were a boil ready to burst . . .

"10:00 a.m. About this time I felt considerable depression, my eyes lachrymating [tearing] and I was able to control my eyelids with difficulty . . . strong feeling of nausea, a choking sensation in the throat and obstruction of nasal passages. About 10:30 a.m. my vision became very blurred so that several images appeared . . . I had a certain amount of difficulty in controlling my limbs, hands, and feet, all being very numb and extremely sensitive to cold.

"11:30 a.m. . . . Symptoms . . . more and more severe . . . impossible to write a word on the typewriter . . .

"1:30 p.m. . . . Had a small lunch, and went to bed . . . All symptoms continued until late in the night.

"Tuesday, June 21, 1927. The sneezing, spitting and belching subsided, but the tingling remained . . . tired, depressed, numb.

"Thursday, 23rd June. No further symptoms except a drowsy and tired feeling."

C. A. Monticone survived his encounter with the funnel web spider, but many people are not as fortunate. Tragically, some patients, after an initially severe course, seem to be recovering when they suddenly succumb. Dr. Sutherland reported the following patient in the *Medical Journal of Australia*.

At 8:20 a.m. on December 28, 1970, a seventeen-year-old girl who was twenty-eight weeks pregnant was walking with friends at Caves beach in the Sydney area when something dropped from a tree into her blouse. She screamed, clutched her right breast, and a spider fell to the ground. It was later identified as a male funnel web. She was admitted to the hospital at 10:30 that morning, delirious and frothing from the mouth. Fluid flooded her lungs, and her lips had turned blue from lack of oxygen.

The girl was thrashing so wildly in her delirium that her doctors had trouble giving her intravenous drugs and had to sedate her with Valium. However, seven hours after her bite, the victim's condition was "clearly improving." By midnight she was breathing freely and "fully cooperative."

Then, at 2:30 a.m., just after talking to the nursing sister and without any warning signs, she had a sudden cardiac arrest. For about fifteen minutes, it seemed her doctors might be able to revive her. But then her heart stopped beating a second and final time, and soon thereafter the fetal heart tones ceased as well.

Dr. Struan K. Sutherland was the head of immunology research at the Commonwealth Serum Laboratories in Melbourne at the time he wrote this report. He has spent almost his entire career as a twenty-four-hour-a-day consultant, helping medical professionals manage dangerous bites and stings in Australia. As a laboratory and clinical scientist, he headed a team that developed life-saving methods of diagnosis and treatment for these envenomations. However, it was his conquest in 1981 of the terrible funnel web syndrome that made him a household name in Australia.

In 1980, Dr. Sutherland and his colleagues showed that a simple first-aid measure could delay the onset, and even attenuate the severity, of funnel web poisoning in macaque monkeys. The investigators injected the animal's limb with venom, wrapped it with a stretchy crepe bandage, using the same pressure as for a sprain, and then immobilized the limb with a splint. The wraps stop the venom from spreading through the lymphatic system to the rest of the body and allow some of it to be inactivated locally. This technique was then applied to human victims with excellent results. Ordinary Australians now learn the Sutherland pressure/immobilization technique and apply it for snake, as well as for spider, bites. If a crepe bandage is not available, panty hose has been found to be a sufficient substitute. In the bush, the technique allows rescuers the precious time needed to transport victims to clinics and hospitals for antivenin treatment.

But the pressure/immobilization technique could not save everyone. Dr. Sutherland writes in his autobiography, *A Venomous Life,* that it was the death of two-year-old James Culley in January 1980 that fueled his determination to develop an effective antivenin for funnel web bites. James had put his little hand into his tracksuit when he suddenly cried out, "Needle, needle!" He slipped into a coma, and three days later he died. Dr. Sutherland, who himself had young children, was deeply affected.

However, developing a funnel web antivenin would not be easy; all past efforts had failed. Obtaining the venom is fairly straightforward but dangerous. The spider is placed in a small glass jar. When the lid is taken off the jar, the spider, its fangs dripping with venom, rears up to bite. The intrepid investigator sucks venom off each fang with a Pasteur pipette attached to a suction line. The problem with this technique, according to Dr. Sutherland, is that sometimes the spider had made a fine web "around the side of the jar which it could run up quickly and escape." Occasionally a spider would "blatantly march straight up the pipette." The funnel webs had bitten two of Dr. Sutherland's assistants while being milked, but luckily, in both cases, the biter was the much less dangerous female. Eventually, the team devised a safety lid to work through when milking the male spiders.

Since rabbits are resistant to atrotoxin, they made good subjects in which to raise antibodies to the venom. However, repeated attempts to produce an effective antivenin failed. After much painstaking work, Dr. Sutherland's team at last discovered the reason for the previous failures. Most of the atrotoxin was sticking to the laboratory glassware and being lost before it could be injected into the rabbits. After the team solved this problem, an effective antivenin was ready for testing in primates and then in bite victims. In November 1981, Dr. Sutherland's team reported their first successes in two patients, one a small boy who would have certainly died without the new treatment.

On May 3, 1981, at 11:40 a.m. a male *Atrax robustus* bit a three-year-old boy named Liam Trehy on the left big toe. His mother, who was with him in the backyard, "prised the spider from his foot and killed it." She then applied an arterial tourniquet to her son's foot from a commercial 'spider bite kit' and took him to Gosford District Hospital.

Except for a bit of pain in his toe, the child looked well on arrival. Doctors placed a pressure/immobilization wrap and released the arterial tourniquet. Within minutes, saliva began to pour out of the child's mouth, and tears ran from his eyes. He dripped sweat, and his hairs stood on end. The boy's heart began racing, his blood pressure climbed, and straw-colored fluid filled his lungs and frothed from his mouth. He turned blue and became delirious. Despite intravenous atropine and hydrocortisone, his breathing failed, and he had to be attached to a ventilator machine.

At 12:45 p.m., one hour after being bitten, he received one teaspoon of antivenin intravenously. By two p.m. he was off the ventilator and breathing on his own. By four p.m., his delirium had resolved. Two days later and fully recovered, he went home to his family.

Of the approximately 34,000 venomous spiders in the world

only a few make venom powerful enough to injure human beings. After all, their prey is usually not much larger than they are. In fact, for years, scientists have puzzled over the evolutionary advantage, if any, conferred by the terrible toxins, since their painful bites often result in the death of the spider at the hands of the human victim. Perhaps it is that surviving spiders benefit from the fear that the few dangerous ones inspire in people.

On a warm winter afternoon in southern California I arm myself with a short metal rod and a pair of gloves and make a second visit to my parked trailer. The black widow webs are easy to recognize because of the leaves and other debris sticking to their strong strands. The spiders I had seen earlier are now out of sight, hiding close by in the shadows. I wait for an airplane to fly overhead and for a car to pass. Then, putting my ear as close to the web as I dare, I slowly drag the rod across, breaking the strands. I hear the unmistakable crackling sound—the sound of paper in fire.

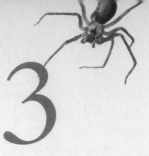

3

Stingers from the Sea

On December 19, 1987, a healthy forty-five-year-old scuba instructor on a night dive at the Pacific Reef off Miami, Florida, surfaced from a depth of nine meters without a handheld lamp. He was handing a lobster from each hand to the boat captain when he felt a mild pricking pain on his left cheek. Suddenly, he felt a "vicious burning sensation" on his torso. The diver had surfaced directly under a large Portuguese man-o'-war. He rolled in the water attempting to get away, but instead managed to wrap the animal around his neck and head. The diver then sprang onto the diving platform and doused himself with a solution of vinegar and alcohol.

Intense and increasing pain lashed his chest, lower back, and right upper arm. Within five minutes, all of his muscles went into jerking spasms so severe that he had trouble breathing. A rescue boat ferried him to a helicopter and during the flight to the hospital he lost consciousness.

On his arrival, physicians administered adrenaline, Valium,

and Benadryl injections as well as four liters of fluid by vein. By the next day he was well enough to go home, although he had purplish-blue welts on his hands, face, and neck.

By ascending with a lobster instead of a light in each hand, this victim had broken the standard diving axiom "look up, reach up, come up." Had he ascended with a light while looking toward the surface with one arm extended, he might have seen and deflected the man-o'-war so that the tentacles made contact only with the wet-suited arm.

That same year, a sixty-seven-year-old local was swimming in waist-deep water at Riviera Beach, an inlet of the Atlantic Ocean near Palm Beach, Florida. She was a large woman who weighed over two hundred pounds, but, with the exception of mild high blood pressure and borderline diabetes, was generally healthy and a frequent swimmer.

Suddenly, the woman rushed out of the water. Wrapped around her entire right and lower left arms were a blue float and tentacles. Immediately, lifeguards and two friends sprayed a solution of the enzyme papain over the tentacles and then peeled them off using paper towels.

Within minutes, she was in extreme pain, had trouble breathing, and lost consciousness. When the ambulance arrived just three minutes later, she had stopped breathing. Two minutes after, her pulse slowed almost to a standstill. Cardiopulmonary resuscitation was started and continued as she was rushed to the hospital.

On arrival, twenty-six minutes after the sting, the woman had no heartbeat. After one hour of resuscitation her heart began beating again, but she was still unconscious. After five days on a ventilator machine the woman died. At autopsy, the pathologist found over twenty red welts on her right arm, which under the microscope revealed numerous stinging cells of the Portuguese man-o'-war, *Physalia*.

The Portuguese man-o'-war is a member of a primitive animal phylum, the coelenterates. Other animals in the man-o'-war group are the sea anemones, the corals, and the true jellyfish. *Physalia* inhabits tropical and subtropical waters around the world. It is plentiful in Australia, where it is known as the bluebottle.

In spite of its appearance, the Portuguese man-o'-war is not a true jellyfish but a colony of tiny animals whose members are specialized to perform different functions. Some of the animals form the blue, gas-filled float, which can be as big as a basketball. Others are involved in reproduction, while a third group develops into the stinging tentacles.

The Portuguese man-o'-war floats on the surface of the sea, often in large groups of colonies also called navies. Each colony has at least one fishing tentacle that measures up to fifty feet long, and a large number of short, frilled tentacles. Like the true jellyfishes, *Physalia* is a predator. Its tentacles are armed with thousands of stinging cells, called nematocysts, and inside each nematocyst is a minute, coiled, spring-loaded syringe filled with venom. When a fish comes in contact with the long tentacle, the nematocysts fire, either stunning or killing the fish. The long tentacle then draws the victim to the short tentacles and into the opening at the bottom of the float, where it is digested.

Portuguese man-o'-war venom consists of a complex mixture of proteins. The principal component, physalitoxin, is a large protein molecule with a small admixture of carbohydrate. After receiving a lethal dose by injection, lab mice show signs of agitation, become tremulous, and finally are paralyzed. Within forty-eight hours, the mice die. Human victims of man-o'-war stings, however, rarely succumb. In fact, the unfortunate woman described above suffered one of the few documented fatal *Physalia* stings.

But the stings are immediately and intensely painful. Red lines with welts appear, which resemble a string of beads. Soon the pain takes on an agonizing, aching quality. Moving the stung body part increases the victim's suffering. In severe cases the welts may blister. Occasionally, victims will have headache, vomiting, and abdominal pains. Sometimes the symptoms are far worse, as in the story of the scuba diver that opened this chapter. Thousands of man-o'-war stings occur every year worldwide, producing intense pain that lasts several hours. The best procedure is for the stings and any adherent tentacles to be immediately washed with seawater and to never be rubbed with sand, because the resultant friction only causes more stinging cells to discharge. Vinegar, which inactivates nematocysts of other jellies, may have the opposite effect on *Physalia* and should not be used. Freshwater and alcohol also worsen stings, and papain is probably ineffective. The best procedure is to apply an ice pack to the stung area. For severe pain a topical anesthetic cream, like lidocaine, may be applied, and the patient may be given painkiller pills or injections for the first day or two.

The Australians, whose country can boast the greatest number of venomous species on land and sea, have the dubious honor of living side by side with the deadliest jellyfishes in the world. European immigrants, who had suffered terrible and sometimes lethal stings, did not know the identities of the most dangerous species. Until the 1950s, they blamed the ubiquitous bluebottle, the Australian species of *Physalia,* for fatal stings, even though these large jellies were often conspicuously absent from the scene of the crime. The search for the true culprits is one of the great detective stories of zoology.

Although the aboriginal peoples of Australia had undoubtedly suffered jellyfish fatalities since prehistoric times, the first recorded death from an Australian jellyfish sting occurred nearly 120 years ago.

On December 30, 1884, around seven-thirty a.m., in the estuary of Ross Creek, Queensland, an eleven-year-old boy swimming with his elder brother screamed, threw his hands up in the air, and then went under. John Kelly, a seaman whose house was nearby, dashed into the water and found the child lying on the bottom. The boy was "covered with some living matter, looking like transparent string and clinging tight to the body and arm."

Kelly carried the boy ashore. As his father came running, the boy was already pulseless and could not be revived with artificial respiration. Over his abdomen and chest were livid, purple-red marks.

By the 1930s, dozens of fatal jellyfish stings had been reported, most notably from the warm coastal waters of Northern Australia. In 1935, the British Medical Association held a conference in the city of Cairns, Queensland. As a result of the conference, the Registry of Injuries Caused by Plants and Animals was established.

The registry sent detailed questionnaires to all physicians practicing in tropical Queensland, while the Cairns Queensland Ambulance and Transport Brigade contributed reports of stings.

At the head of these efforts was Dr. Hugo Flecker, a Cairns physician who, in a letter published in the *Medical Journal of Australia* on January 27, 1945, reported the results of the registry's investigations. "It was soon very evident," he wrote, "that the great majority of the injuries were produced, certainly not by the *Physalia*, [but] by some other as yet unknown agent . . ."

By 1952, it had become clear to Dr. Flecker that there were

actually two distinct jellyfish sting syndromes occurring off the northern Australian beaches. In the first syndrome, which was sometimes fatal, the jellyfish always left a quarter-inch wide livid wheal, like a whiplash. Sometimes the marks had a very specific sign: a layer of white "frosting" shaped like a ladder.

But the second, even more common syndrome was entirely different. These patients had little or no initial skin signs of a sting, other than a small puncture. The patient complained of a local sensation, like a bee sting, or was unaware of any mishap, but would then be stricken with intense backache, retching and vomiting. Agonizing spasms racked the muscles; the abdomen hardened to boardlike rigidity.

In an article published in the *Medical Journal of Australia* in July 1952, Dr. Flecker wrote a short account of the two syndromes, giving generous credit to the case descriptions of his colleague Dr. R. V. Southcott. He proposed that the second sting syndrome, characterized by muscle pain without wheals, be designated the Irukandji syndrome, after the name of an aboriginal tribe "which formerly inhabited the coastal region between the Mowbray River to the north and the Trinity Inlet around Cairns to the south." This name was adopted, and the search for the causative agents of the two syndromes began.

Dr. Southcott knew that a relatively large jellyfish caused the lethal syndrome, because victims often had tentacle fragments stuck to their wheals. Although some fifty fatal jellyfish stings had at that time been reported in Australia, only once had a jellyfish been captured at the site and preserved. That occurred on March 13, 1938, at Darwin, in the Northern Territories.

The victim, a "half-caste boy aged 12 years . . . bathing in the local swimming baths," dove into the water, then came up in great distress. After crawling onto the beach, he collapsed and died. There were wheals on his left arm, the left side of his chest, and his neck. As the boy staggered out of the water, witnesses had been able to recover a jellyfish still sticking to his body. The specimen was preserved in the museum of the School of Public Health and Tropical Medicine in Sydney.

Dr. Southcott examined the specimen, which was mutilated and poorly preserved but obviously not a Portuguese man-o'-war. Box-shaped, with four bundles of long tentacles streaming out from the bottom corners of its bell, it clearly belonged to an entirely different group of true jellyfish. He returned to the waters off North Queensland and began to collect and study specimens of box-shaped jellyfish. They were large, pale-blue creatures, and their bells weighed up to thirteen pounds.

Southcott also studied autopsy specimens of patients' skin wheals in fatal stings. Under the microscope, he could see the spent stingers anchored to the skin. Comparing the shapes of these nematocysts with those of his collected specimens, he found a match with a species of the box jellyfish, *Chironex,* which had not been previously described or named. In 1956, Dr. Southcott christened the killer *Chironex fleckeri,* after Dr. Hugo Flecker.

To confirm the presence of venom in *Chironex,* Dr. S. Weiner at the Commonwealth Serum Laboratories in Melbourne made extracts of the frozen tentacles of the jellyfish and injected them into mice and guinea pigs. The injected animals developed paralysis of their hind limbs. Then they slipped into coma, stopped breathing, and died. Boiling the tentacle extract completely inactivated the toxic principal, suggesting that the poison was a protein, like physalitoxin.

The source of the Irukandji syndrome proved much more elusive than that of the box-jelly syndrome. Flecker and Southcott enlisted ambulance-bearers, lifesavers, and the bathing public in the search. They stationed observers in the water during the height of the jellyfish season, but while some observers became

Irukandji victims, none of them got a glimpse of the offending jellyfish.

The two investigators tested marine weeds and fish larvae. They filtered buckets of seawater and examined the deposits. On one occasion, the seawater of the Cairns City Baths was drained through a mesh because one of the patrons had a suspicious illness, but nothing was found.

Flecker never gave up his search, but at the time of his death in 1957 he still hadn't found the organism responsible for the Irukandji syndrome. "As a mark of respect" to Flecker, "that assiduous and able man," the medical practitioners of Cairns arranged for the research to continue under Dr. Jack H. Barnes.

Unfortunately, Dr. Flecker's personal notes were not available to Dr. Barnes, nor was the Registry of Injuries, established in 1935 and maintained by Flecker. Both Flecker's notes and the registry records had mysteriously disappeared about the time of his death.

However, Dr. Barnes knew that the agent must be very small and probably transparent, because no one had been able to get a glimpse of it, even as they were being stung. It was not microscopic, though, because many victims experienced some sensation of touch just before the actual stinging. Yet it was small enough to be contained in very limited volumes of shallow water, as illustrated by the following case.

A six-year-old girl was sitting on the sand at the water's edge when a wavelet washed between her legs. She complained of an immediate pain on the inside of her left thigh. Eight minutes later she had full-blown Irukandji syndrome, and small wheals appeared on her left leg.

Dr. Southcott suggested to Dr. Barnes that he start his investigation by trying to recover stinging cells from the skin of victims, a method that had been successful with *Chironex fleckeri.*

Since the Irukandji syndrome is not fatal, instead of collecting autopsy material, Dr. Barnes scraped the stung skin of patients and examined the material under the microscope. There were no nematocysts. He even went over victims' swimming apparel with a magnifier, looking for tentacle fragments, but again he found nothing.

Dr. Barnes then experimented with clear, transparent objects and found that while they could rarely be seen from above the water's surface they might be more visible if viewed from below. He found that a diver wearing a glass facemask could see transparent jellies if they were viewed with oblique lighting against a dark background. Dr. Barnes designed a black screen that could be held at arm's length and a simple device for capturing small specimens underwater. These preparations were in place when the 1961–62 summer jellyfish season began in December in the Palm Beach area of North Queensland.

The first sting occurred on Sunday, December 3, near dusk, in murky water. No search was attempted. On the afternoon of December 9, further stings were noted, but a search revealed nothing of value. On the morning of December 10, there was a south-going current of clear water inshore that "abounded in marine life of a pelagic nature." Dr. Barnes felt sure that the Irukandji agent, a small motile creature of the open ocean, was streaming toward the beach. The divers took their positions about eighteen inches under the water. At last they captured a small carybdeid medusa, which was first seen only as a set of four tentacles moving obliquely across the current. Dr. Barnes writes that the bullet-shaped body of the medusa, which was only about an inch long, remained invisible until it was brought in actual contact with the faceplate of his mask. In a glass container the jelly could be seen clearly, pulsing rapidly and traveling at a speed of about two knots.

The divers brought this first specimen ashore and showed it to the people on the beach. Soon many swimmers joined in the search and, an hour later, a second jellyfish of the same type was captured by lifesaver Don Ludbey, who caught it in his cap. The only reason he had even seen the jellyfish was that he had noticed the wobbly motions of a small fish snagged on one of its tentacles.

Now that they had captured the jellyfish, there was only one way to find out if the little jellyfish were the answer to the Irukandji puzzle: test them on human subjects. The first jellyfish was tested on Dr. Barnes and a nine-year-old boy, N.B.; the second on "a robust young lifesaver, C.R." The three volunteers wetted the inner surface of their upper arms with seawater and held jellyfish in light contact with the area until stinging became uncomfortably severe. Interestingly, the three subjects were not stung on the fingers holding the sea creature, probably because the skin on the undersurface of the fingers is thicker than that of the inner arm.

Twelve minutes after being stung "the lad reported mild abdominal pain." Two minutes later the boy's armpits began to ache. The abdominal pain worsened, and his back began to hurt. Within twenty minutes, the two adults had the same symptoms.

All of the subjects were then seized with a remarkable restlessness. They were in constant movement, swinging their arms, stamping about, twisting and writhing. They complained of trouble concentrating and became clumsy in handling objects. When their muscles were palpated, they were found to be in spasm. The author compared their postures to "that of an infant with a full nappy."

During the twenty-minute drive to Cairns, the victims' distress was heightened by the necessity of remaining seated. By forty minutes after the stinging, the abdominal muscles of the investigators were in rigid, boardlike spasm. Breathing was difficult. At about the same time, the victims began coughing and retching. Seventy-five minutes after the experiment started, the three subjects arrived at the hospital and were treated with intravenous narcotics, repeated doses of which were necessary to control their symptoms. Twenty-four hours later, they had recovered completely.

Dr. Barnes reported his findings in the *Medical Journal of Australia* in 1964 and, in 1966, Dr. Southcott named the Irukandji agent *Carukia barnesi* in his honor. *Carukia* is a member of the same class of jellyfish as *Chironex fleckeri,* but belongs to a different family, the Carybdeidae. Although its bell is only an inch long, the four tentacles may reach up to forty-five inches. The venom of *Carukia* causes overstimulation of the sympathetic nervous system with release of adrenaline (epinephrine). In rare cases, this adrenaline release leads to dangerous elevations of blood pressure or to heart failure with leakage of fluid into the lungs.

One victim, a twenty-four-year-old woman who was stung while snorkeling at Michaelmas Cay northeast of Cairns, became critically ill with heart weakness and wet lungs a day after being hospitalized, but survived with treatment in the intensive care unit.

Life-threatening illness following *Carukia* stings is thankfully rare, which is in contrast to the lethal syndrome caused by the larger jellyfish, *Chironex.* In 1970, antivenin to *Chironex* became available through the Commonwealth Serum Laboratories. To produce this antivenin, sheep are injected with increasing doses of *Chironex* tentacle extracts, and the antibody-rich serum is harvested. *Chironex* antivenin may well have saved the life of the following patient, as reported in 1980.

A husband and his twenty-year-old wife, who was thirty-four weeks into her pregnancy, entered the sea in front of a caravan park near Townsville in Queensland. It was a fine, hot morning in March, near the end of the jellyfish season, and radio warnings of large numbers of box-jellyfish being sighted had gone unnoticed by the couple. While they were sitting in two feet of cloudy water, the wife suddenly shrieked and stood up, plucking at numerous tentacles sticking to her left thigh and left lower abdomen.

Screaming with pain, she walked with her husband's help to the beach. He, too, was in pain from having been stung. The woman became irrational, pale, and unable to stand. The husband set out for help, and by the time he reached the caravan park kiosk 150 feet away, he, too, was unable to stand.

The caravan park superintendent threw ethanol over the husband's stings, then rushed to the woman. She was "lying still," he said later, "there was no visible breathing, and her face and limbs were black." He doused the stings and adherent tentacles with two liters of ethanol and, despite having no previous experience, "had a go" at mouth-to-mouth resuscitation. After a few puffs he observed that "her earlobes had gone pink, and she began to breathe." He then rushed across to the caravan park and summoned a trained nursing sister, who also happened to be thirty-seven weeks pregnant.

By the time the nurse had arrived, the woman had stopped breathing again, and her face had turned blue. The patient had also vomited, so the nurse cleared the airway and began mouth-to-nose respiration. After forty seconds, the victim began to breathe and to thrash from side to side. Both rescuers received some stings from the tentacles on the victim.

When they arrived at the hospital, aside from the large sting area with some tentacle still attached, the husband was alert. When the doctors removed the tentacle, they saw the classic, frosted-ladder pattern of *Chironex* stings. After giving the still-unconscious wife two ampoules of *Chironex* antivenin, they admitted her to intensive care on a ventilator machine. As her stung skin turned dark with gangrene, her caregivers telephoned Dr. Jack Barnes in Cairns, who recommended giving another vial of antivenin by vein, to minimize scarring.

The next morning the woman was awake but drowsy, and had slurred speech. Her doctors checked her blood-alcohol level and found that she was drunk from the fumes of the alcohol packs that had been applied to her stings. Over the next twenty-four hours she sobered up and, four days after admission into the hospital, was discharged. Nine weeks later, the woman gave birth to a healthy girl by cesarean section.

In their discussion of this extremely close call with *Chironex,* the authors considered shortcomings in the care of jellyfish stings and possible solutions. First, they emphasize the extreme importance of having people at the beach who are able to administer cardiopulmonary resuscitation. Second, in North Queensland, it is seldom possible for any victim to reach the hospital within thirty minutes of envenomation. Hoping to shorten the delay in treatment, two of the authors had begun training members of the Surf Life Saving Association on the administration of *Chironex* antivenin to seriously ill victims. Since the injection of antivenin can, on occasion, be complicated by serious allergic reactions, all rescuers giving this treatment also had to be certified in advanced resuscitation. Where these conditions were met, the authors arranged to leave three ampoules of *Chironex* antivenin in each beach clubhouse refrigerator.

By 1989, *Chironex* antivenin had been used in over three hundred patients, but it was not until that year that nonmedical personnel first administered it at the beach. At about ten-thirty a.m., members of the Queensland Ambulance Transport Brigade arrived at a tidal inlet off the Queensland coast to care for an eight-year-old boy who had extensive stings over both legs. A nursing sister had arrived on the scene and doused the patient's legs with vinegar, causing the tentacles to fall off. The skin looked burned but exhibited the characteristic, frosted-ladder pattern of *Chironex fleckeri*.

The victim was in so much agony from the stings that he didn't complain of pain when the ambulance crew gave him three injections of *Chironex fleckeri* antivenin—one ampoule in his arm and two in his thighs. Three minutes after the injection, the child had a low blood pressure but was alert and in less pain from his stings. After several hours of observation in the hospital, he was able to go home the same day. Three days later, the Ambulance Transport Brigade successfully treated another severely stung eight-year-old at the same beach.

The authors noted that the case of the pregnant woman cast serious doubt on the time-honored practice of dousing jellyfish stings with alcohol. Not only did their patient become intoxicated, but also alcohol packs are dangerously flammable. In an article published in the same issue of the *Medical Journal of Australia,* the authors reported their studies of the best method for disarming the box jellyfish.

They captured living specimens of *Chironex fleckeri* at night near Townsville, North Queensland, and took the specimens to the laboratories at James Cook University. By examining the jellyfish tentacles under the microscope, the authors found that rather than inactivating the stinging cells, ethanol caused them to rapidly discharge. Those nematocysts that did not discharge were still fully active. In fact, a piece of tentacle soaked in alcohol and then applied to the skin of one of the authors was still able to deliver a painful sting.

However, when the tentacles were soaked in household white vinegar, which is a five-percent aqueous solution of acetic acid, the stinging cells remained undischarged and were also inactivated. The tentacles treated with white vinegar were not only no longer capable of stinging, but they had also lost their ability to stick to human skin. As a result of these experiments, dousing *Chironex fleckeri* stings with white vinegar is now standard practice.

These researchers were able to tolerate minor *Chironex fleckeri* stings, and subsequent investigations have shown that for every life-threatening box-jelly sting, there are dozens of less severe injuries. In 1995, Drs. Bart Currie and Yvonne Wood reported research carried out on twenty patients who had been stung by jellyfish treated in the Accident and Emergency Department of the Royal Darwin Hospital in the Northern Territory of Australia. After vinegar and ice packs were applied to the stings for analgesia, the investigators scraped the sting site firmly with a sterile scalpel blade, and filtered the debris. They also applied sticky tape to another part of the sting site and then anchored the tape, sticky side up, onto glass slides. Microscopic examination for nematocysts was positive by one method or the other in eighty-five percent of the patients and all of the stinging cells were of the *Chironex fleckeri* type. Only four patients in this series required narcotics for pain control, and none required antivenin.

Jellyfish stings continue to be a serious problem in Australia. *Chironex fleckeri* has caused at least sixty-three recorded deaths since 1884. Stinger-resistant enclosures are erected at very popular beaches during the jellyfish season, and radio announcements and warning signs on beaches alert people when risk is particularly high. But there are hundreds more miles of beaches and tidal estuaries than can be patrolled or enclosed, and none of the enclosures reliably prevent the stings of the little Irukandji jellyfish, *Carukia barnesi*.

One way to prevent jellyfish stings is to create a barrier

between the skin and the water. Elaborate, skintight stinger suits that cover the swimmer from neck to toe are available, but simpler, readily available measures are also effective: The intrepid Australians of the Surf Life Saving Association wear pantyhose when they dash into the water to rescue victims of jellyfish stings.

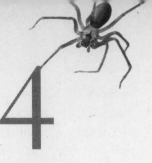

4

Beautiful, Deadly Cones

Of the approximately five hundred species of cone snails that inhabit the oceans of the world, almost all are beautiful and all are venomous. The Glory of the Sea cone (*Conus gloriamaris*), for example, was once so highly prized that it was listed at auctions with paintings by the old masters. Predatory mollusks of warm waters, cone snails immobilize their prey by harpooning it with hollow, venom-filled teeth. One species entices fish to approach with a wormlike proboscis, then kills by shooting the fish in the mouth.

The cone venoms can cause a paralytic syndrome resembling botulism. The following case, the envenomation of a twenty-four-year-old male nurse, reported in the *Medical Journal of Australia,* is typical.

The patient came to the Honiara Central Hospital in the Solomon Islands complaining that he had felt weak and clumsy for the past twelve hours. On the previous night, while collecting seashells, he had suddenly felt a "mild stinging sensation in his right hand." He noticed a small puncture wound on his middle finger. Within thirty minutes, he developed slurred speech, droopy eyelids, and a drunken walk. All of his muscles were weak, including the chest and abdominal muscles used for breathing. The patient's relatives brought the snail in with the victim. It was *Conus geographus,* one of the deadliest known species.

The man was admitted to the hospital for observation. The cone toxin had paralyzed his bladder, so his doctors inserted a temporary rubber catheter to drain his urine. After forty-eight hours, he was still weak but he could walk unaided. After three days, the man's strength was normal, and he was able to go home.

The first reported human fatality from a cone snail sting is the brief report by G. E. Rumphius in 1705. The species was *Conus textile,* the Cloth of Gold cone; the victim was a female slave in Banda, Indonesia. "She kept this shell in her hand after she picked it up when hauling in the seine at sea. As she went to the beach she felt a faint tickling sensation in the hand which crept through her entire body—she died on the spot."

This woman may not have been native to the region, since people indigenous to the natural habitats of these snails often have a healthy respect for them. Mr. B. Hinde of the Royal Navy, while on HMS *Diamond* in 1884, was examining a specimen of *Conus geographus.* He wrote that when a native of Nodup, New Britain, who was on board as an interpreter, saw the writer with the specimen in his hand, he said, "Suppose he bite he kill man."

The author was at first skeptical, thinking the interpreter meant to warn him against being cut by the sharp edge of the shell, but later, on the Island of Matupi, New Britain, he saw a native who had just been stung by a cone snail. The man "at once cut small incisions with a sharp stone all over his arm and shoulder, from which the blood flowed freely, and he explained . . . that if he had not taken these precautions that he would have died." He then showed Hinde a small mark, "about the size of a three-penny piece," where he had been stung. Dr. Hugo Flecker, of later jellyfish fame, described the first well-documented modern fatality.

On June 27, 1935, while on a pleasure cruise off the Great Barrier Reef, Charles Garbutt, a twenty-seven-year-old man, landed at Haymen Island. He picked up a live cone shell and gripped it in the palm of one hand, with the open side downwards, facing his skin. With the other hand he proceeded to clean the shell by scraping it with a knife. "A spike" came out and punctured his palm, leaving only a small mark. Almost at once his hand grew numb. Ten minutes later, according to the victim's mother, who was with him, Garbutt began to feel stiff about the lips. Twenty minutes later his vision blurred, and his mouth burned. At thirty minutes, his legs were paralyzed, and within an hour he lost consciousness. The coma deepened as his pulse became weak and rapid. Garbutt died on the way to the hospital, five hours after he was stung.

The poisonous cones belong to the class of snails in the phylum of mollusks, a group of invertebrate animals that includes both oysters and octopi. The snails, or gastropods, comprise the largest class of mollusks, with approximately 35,000 living and nearly 15,000 extinct species identified. They arose in the late Cambrian period about 500 million years ago, and though many of the Cambrian mollusk families died out, the gastropods are represented in an unbroken line through the fossil record. Today, snails are among the most successful of the invertebrate groups and are said to be at the peak of their evolutionary development.

Although they originally arose in the sea, many have lost their gills, developed a kind of lung, and invaded land to become the escargot of French restaurants—or garden pests, depending on your point of view. Others have lost most or all of their shells and have become the unattractive land slugs and the marine nudibranchs, whose gorgeous, iridescent tentacles rank them among the most beautiful creatures on the earth.

Almost all gastropods have a feeding organ, the radula, armed with specialized teeth. A snail crawling up the side of a glass aquarium is probably feeding on algae, which it scrapes off with these teeth. Cone snails, being predators, have refined this design. In its radula sac, a cone snail carries a quiver of grooved teeth tipped with sharp, barbed points, like harpoons. All cones are armed with a long duct that manufactures venom and has a muscular bulb at the end, which propels the venom into the tooth. The venom-filled tooth is held at the end of a long, nose-like structure, the proboscis, near the mouth. When prey draws near, the snail uses its proboscis to spear it with a harpoon tooth, paralyzing it with venom so that it can be engulfed whole and digested.

At first glance, a slow-moving snail would seem an unlikely predator. Although the proboscis may dart at and harpoon prey very quickly, the cone snail itself is incapable of rapid pursuit of stung victims, whether they are marine worms, other mollusks, or, in the case of the most dangerous cones, small fish. But cone snails are so successful because they have evolved a collection of extremely rapidly acting venoms that can immobilize prey instantly.

The earliest attempt to study cone snail venom was undertaken by Dr. L. C. D. Hermitte in the Seychelles Islands in the Indian Ocean. At nine p.m. one evening in June 1932, a Monsieur Frédérique de Lafontaine, aged thirty-two, arrived at Dr. Hermitte's surgery at Mont Fleuri on the island of Mahé. He had been brought by pirogue and was carried in on a long chair. Monsieur de Lafontaine told the doctor that he had been wading at low tide in the shallow water of a lagoon when he picked up a cone snail. He was holding the snail in the palm of his hand and scraping the shell with a pocketknife when he felt a sharp sting immediately followed by a burning sensation. Turning the shell over he saw the mouth of the animal and, as it retracted into the shell, he saw a "fine sharp needle" protruding from a narrow, tongue-like organ.

The burning sensation soon gave rise to numbness, and spread within a few minutes to involve his entire left arm. He felt his head was getting "queer" and decided to regain the shore. Within an hour his entire body was numb, his sight was impaired, and he became dizzy and nauseated. Paralysis followed, and he could no longer move his limbs or sit up.

After five or six hours, he seemed to improve a little and asked to be taken to the doctor. On examination, nine hours after the accident, Dr. Hermitte found the victim giddy and unable to stand. He tapped de Lafontaine's knees but got no reflex response. At the sting site, there was no abnormality whatsoever. To aid his recovery, he gave the patient a diluted injection of the neural stimulant strychnine and sent him home. It took three more days for the weakness to resolve completely.

Fortunately, Monsieur de Lafontaine had brought in the offending mollusk alive in a vessel containing fresh seawater and sand. Like his patient, the doctor was an avid shell collector and identified the snail as *Conus geographus*. It was a medium-sized specimen, about three and one half inches long.

Dr. Hermitte, who had never seen a living cone snail, was amazed that such a small animal could exert such powerful effects on a human many times its size. He dissected a number of specimens and, after leaving the Seychelles in March 1933, he presented his findings at Edinburgh University. But he still knew nothing about the cone poison, and he had no live specimens on hand. What he needed was an alcohol extract of the crushed venom apparatus.

He decided to write to the patient's sister, Mademoiselle

Agnes de Lafontaine, knowing that she had an interest in shells. He sent her labeled bottles, dissecting instruments, mortar and pestle, and reagents, along with clear illustrations on each step of the dissection and extraction process. After many months, the specimens from the intrepid Agnes arrived. But alas, when he tested the extracts on mice, Dr. Hermitte found that the poison had lost all of its toxicity during extraction and transport.

For the next twenty years, scientific interest in cone snails waned. Though beautiful and of interest to shell collectors, they remained an obscure family of snails living quiet nocturnal lives along tropical reefs in the South Pacific. And, although dangerous, human stings were rare, since cone snails hide during the daytime under rocks and sand, only emerging at night to hunt. But during the 1950s, interest in cone snails was revived by the research of one person, a Yale professor of zoology named, coincidentally, Alan J. Kohn.

Dr. Kohn made a detailed and exhaustive study of the cone snails of Hawaii. His 1959 monograph showed that the forty-five *Conus* species found in Hawaii were among the dominant predators of the coral reefs and marine benches surrounding the islands.

Yet cone snails are evolutionary newcomers. At the end of the Mesozoic era, the dinosaurs dominated the land, and the ammonite mollusks, shelled cousins of the octopi, ruled the oceans. Then, about sixty million years ago, a wave of mass extinctions, probably caused by a meteor impact, claimed the dinosaurs and the ammonites. Into this marine ecological vacuum exploded the cone snails. With over five hundred species, they are the largest single genus of marine animals living today.

Unlocking the secrets of the cone snail's evolutionary success story has been the life work of Dr. Baldomero Olivera, now at the University of Utah. During his youth in the Philippines,

Dr. Olivera learned about the beautiful, deadly cones. But his Ph.D. work at the California Institute of Technology and his postdoctoral research at Stanford seemed to take him in an entirely different direction—toward the molecular biology of ion channels. Ion channels are the protein portals of all cells, by which sodium, potassium, and calcium move in and out.

In 1970, Dr. Olivera found himself back in his homeland, as an assistant professor at the University of the Philippines. In an interview for the journal *Science,* Dr. Olivera recalls, "I ended up in a lab that had essentially no equipment. No ultracentrifuge, no scintillation counters, no cold room." Then Dr. Olivera remembered the cone snail toxins. For many years, molecular biologists had used natural toxic compounds to study ion channels. By binding to specific channel molecules, many toxins exert their effects. Despite the limited equipment, Dr. Olivera had a plentiful supply of living cone snails.

He began studying the venom of local cone species, expecting to find one active ingredient, which he dubbed in advance conotoxin. But there was no single conotoxin. Instead, each species had a unique cocktail of about a dozen small toxic compounds. It became immediately clear why Mademoiselle de Lafontaine and Dr. Hermitte's efforts to isolate the toxin had been doomed from the start. The venoms were small, structurally specific proteins, too delicate to withstand pickling in alcohol.

In any given cone species the venom family is designed to paralyze the nervous system of their prey at multiple sites. Because the venom molecules are small, they move through cell membranes rapidly and are extremely fast-acting. To match the major toxins of a fish-eating species, such as *Conus geographus,* Dr. Olivera writes, "a potion would have to contain curare, the poison arrow ingredient of the Amazonian Indians; tetrodotoxin, the deadly toxin in fugu puffer fish; and . . . botulinum toxin."

This lethal combination of toxins is necessary for a slow-moving snail to capture and engulf fast-moving prey without losing the meal or being injured while feeding. No snail can engulf a human being; however, a cone sting can be deadly if the victim's respiratory functions are not supported until the paralysis wears off, as in the following case.

On August 27, 1954, around noon, a cone snail stung an eight-year-old girl at Manus Island, New Guinea. The wound appeared as a black spot on her palm near the thumb. Soon after being stung, the girl collapsed, and examination showed slurred speech and shallow breathing. She was able to move only her fingers and the muscles of her face. Shortly afterward the victim stopped breathing and lost consciousness.

The child's doctors inserted a tube into her airway and attached her to a portable anesthesia apparatus. Two hours later she awoke, and after two more hours she was able to breathe on her own. By the next day she had recovered without ill effects.

Although paralytic venom is found in all cone snails, one striking finding of Dr. Olivera's research was the unexpected diversity of the toxins. No two species have exactly the same venom proteins. The cone toxins are like molecular snowflakes, with over 25,000 unique small proteins in the various species. For molecular biologists, these compounds are a golden library of new keys with which to study ion channels.

All proteins are composed of specific sequences of small molecules called amino acids. Just as an almost infinite variety of words may be spelled out by the letters of the alphabet, so are all the myriad proteins found in plants and animals defined by their specific sequence of amino acids. These sequences are encoded, in turn, by the organism's genes. Dr. Olivera discovered that all species of cone snails had specific genetic regions that tended to mutate or change at a much higher rate than normal genes. This implies that cone snails frequently manufacture toxin molecules with new amino acid sequences.

Dr. Olivera speculates that the evolutionary success of the cone snails over the last fifty million years derives from their ability to rapidly evolve new toxins to meet changes in their environment. In other words, cone snails have been able to adapt and evolve along with their prey.

The "designer genes" of the cone snails have created a baffling array of toxins whose actions scientists are just beginning to study. What is the purpose, for example, of the King Kong toxin that triggers bizarre aggressive behavior in lobsters? Why does *Conus geographus* produce GIV, a protein that puts mice, but not fish, to sleep?

Dr. Olivera's decision in 1970 to study cones, and his lifetime pursuit of their toxins, may have profound ramifications, not only for biological research but also for the practice of medicine. He has discovered a conotoxin that has the power to alleviate intractable pain. Using the amino acid sequence of this protein as a model, a biopharmaceutical company Neurex has developed a drug that is one hundred to one thousand times more potent than morphine. In a clinical trial at Stanford University, researchers are using a tiny pump to infuse a constant dose of the drug around the spinal cords of seven volunteers with chronic severe pain. Patients report few side effects and none of the lethargy and intellectual dullness they endured with the high doses of narcotics they had to use before.

In 1796, Jan Vermeer's painting "Woman in Blue Reading a Letter" was put up for auction. Also on sale that day was a two-inch specimen of *Conus cedonulli,* the rare "matchless" cone. Vermeer's masterpiece sold for forty-three guilders. A bidder was happy to acquire the rare shell for 273 guilders.

The cone snails are living drug factories that are synthesizing and testing new toxins in the laboratory of the oceans. It will be many years before scientists complete their study of the conotoxins, and cone snails are still creating new ones. If, as a result of this research, patients no longer have to choose between mind-numbing narcotics and agonizing pain, then the cone snail will prove to be a matchless treasure indeed.

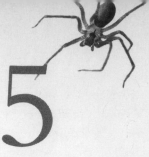

5

The
Limbless
Ones

❝ Arms and legs gone, no ears, only
one functional lung, voiceless, eyelids
missing—a human being in such
condition would be institutionalized
and under constant care. ❞

—JAMES A. PETERS,
the 15th edition of the
Encyclopedia Britannica

A few years ago, on a hot spring afternoon, I was hiking alone in the hills bordering the northern end of the San Fernando Valley, near Los Angeles. The narrow trail I followed skirted Bee Canyon on my right, and on my left, about thirty yards away, were the groomed lawns and glistening swimming pools of the adjacent homes. There was a scent of sagebrush and peaceful stillness everywhere. Suddenly, a loud buzz much like a swarm of bees broke the air around my ears. The vibrating pierced my heart. I jerked backwards. My canteen belt flew off and landed ahead of me, inches from an incredibly irate three- to four-foot long rattlesnake—most likely a western diamondback. It darted into a small bush, setting the leaves in nervous motion with its unmistakable rattling. After about thirty seconds, the rattling died away and, with my heart still pounding, I considered what to do about my belt, which lay near the bush. I had no walking stick and there was none in sight. Foolishly risking the strike of one of the most venomous snakes in North America, I bent over and quickly snatched the belt. Fortunately, the bush remained still. I exhaled, buckled on my belt and retreated down the path, my legs a little wobbly and my pulse subsiding in my throat.

There are approximately 450 species of venomous snakes in the world, and their bites kill thirty to forty thousand people annually. In the United States, with the exception of Alaska, Hawaii, and Maine, which lack at least one venomous species, between seven and eight thousand people annually are bitten—five to six fatally. And within that statistic, eastern and western diamondback rattlesnakes cause the greatest number of deaths.

The rattlers are members of the viper family, which includes cottonmouths and copperheads, as well as the bushmaster, fer-de-lance, puff adder, and gaboon viper. The American coral snakes belong to the Elapidae family of snakes, which includes the cobras, the mambas, and the kraits. The extremely venomous sea snakes make up the third family.

These three families of snakes belong to the reptile suborder Serpentes, a highly evolved, uniquely specialized group of animals. Despite their limbless state, the snakes have become very successful, with representative species in all regions except the poles, and even inhabit the Pacific and Indian Oceans.

The delicate bones of snakes make poor fossils, but there is strong enough evidence that they probably arose from a lizard ancestor in the monitor family during the Upper Cretaceous period, about eighty million years ago. A limbless body may offer a survival advantage in three environments: water, dense grass, and underground. Most paleontologists currently believe that the lizards that became snakes were burrowing animals. About sixty-five million years ago, near the end of the dinosaur era, snakes underwent a spectacular adaptive radiation and expansion, developing over two thousand species and conquering virtually all available environmental niches.

All snakes, which are members of the cold-blooded reptilian order, cannot perspire or pant if they overheat; their body temperature is almost completely dependent on the temperature of their surroundings. Their limbless bodies allow them access to tunnels, crevices, and abandoned burrows, but, once they are asleep or hibernating, if temperatures do not rise above the threshold necessary to rekindle their metabolism, they eventually die.

There are no plant-eating snakes. They are all flesh-eaters, and, depending on the species, they will devour insects, frogs, fish, and small mammals. Some snakes, such as the king cobras, prefer to eat other snakes, while others live entirely upon eggs. For as yet unknown reasons, snakes have never evolved efficient chewing teeth. They swallow their prey whole and must complete the process of digestion before the prey begins to putrefy. To ensure a speedy digestion, snakes have developed specialized salivary glands. About fifteen percent of the species have taken this process a step further: they have developed venomous saliva.

Regardless of species, snake venoms are a complex cocktail of enzymes and small protein molecules. Enzymes are large proteins that function as chemical matchmakers. They bring other molecules in the body together and catalyze rapid chemical reactions between them. Without enzymes, many of the chemical reactions that keep us alive could not take place at our body temperature. But when snake venom enzymes are injected into another animal, the results can be catastrophic.

In 1998, doctors from France reported the case of a ten-year-old boy who was bitten on his left leg by a European viper. The bite occurred on the Island of Oleron off the southwest coast of France, but the boy was admitted within an hour of the bite to the Hôpital Pellegrin-Enfants in Bordeaux. On arrival, the vomiting child was sweating profusely and had a low blood pressure. There was a two-inch area of swelling around the bite; within twenty-four hours of admission it had spread to the left groin and the left side of the chest. Over the next two days the swollen area had become red, tender, and so bloated that the arteries to the boy's leg were compressed, and his doctors could barely feel the pulses in his foot.

Blood tests showed that some of the enzymes in the snake venom were causing both the muscle cells and the red blood cells to disintegrate. The child's doctors gave him two units of transfused blood, but the proteins released by the dying cells were interfering with kidney function. Other enzymes in the snake venom had activated the clotting system, causing depletion of the normal factors. On the third day, the patient was given antivenin to European viper venom, prepared at the Pasteur Institute. After sixteen days in the hospital, including several days in the pediatric intensive care unit, the boy made a gradual and complete recovery.

Although the offending snake was never identified in this case, it was probably either *Vipera aspis* or *Vipera berus,* both of which are members of the viper family. Generally, most people don't associate snakebites with European vacations; however, Europe is home to eleven species of venomous vipers. *Vipera berus* is the world's only cold-weather snake and is active up to altitudes of nine thousand feet, with a range extending across Scandinavia and Northern Russia.

All vipers have two large, needle-sharp fangs, one on each maxillary bone. In order to allow these fangs to fold neatly into the viper's mouth, the maxillary bones have evolved into small, moveable pivots. Unique to the viper's fang is that it is hollow along part of its length. When the viper strikes, the fang flips out of the mouth, penetrates the victim's body, and injects venom through a pore near the tooth tip. The venom, which in vipers contains modified salivary enzymes, pours through the circulation of the still-living prey, beginning the process of digestion. Blood and muscle cells dissolve, the clotting system unravels, and the victim begins to bleed, first from the fang wound, and then elsewhere.

The boy in France had access to immediate, specialized care in the hospital. In remote, rural environments, the outcome of snakebites is often not as favorable. In 1997, doctors at the University Hospital in São Paulo, Brazil, reported their study of twenty-nine cases of bites by the jararacuçu (*Bothrops jararacussu*), a giant semiaquatic pit viper belonging to the rattlesnake family. Pit vipers have deep pits on each side of the head between the eye and the nostril. These temperature-sensing organs help the snake strike warm-blooded prey accurately. All vipers, including the jararacuçu, create venom that causes tissue degeneration and bleeding, digesting prey from within. Normal human blood drawn into a glass tube clots immediately, forming a solid mass of red cells and a layer of amber serum. But it is not unusual for victims of the jararacuçu's bite to have blood that will not clot.

One of the patients in the São Paulo series, a thirty-five-year-old farm laborer, was struck twice on the right forearm by a jararacuçu and was admitted to the Hospital Vital Brazil nine hours later. The admitting doctors found painful swelling that extended from the bite site to the chest wall. The victim had passed no urine since the bite. Despite treatment with specific antivenin, the next day he still had not urinated, the bitten arm and adjacent areas of his neck and chest were massively swollen. His kidneys failed, and he was placed on dialysis. Soon after, he was brought in to the operating room so that his right arm could be surgically explored.

When surgeons incised the victim's arm, they found an abscess caused by bacteria from the snake's mouth. The disintegrating muscle provided a perfect culture medium for these microorganisms, which had been injected along with the venom when the snake's fang penetrated the farmer's arm. The patient's arm eventually healed, but a kidney biopsy performed on his thirtieth day in the hospital showed that his kidneys had been permanently destroyed, necessitating lifelong kidney dialysis treatments.

Every year thousands of people worldwide die from the bites of poisonous snakes, often because they choose to rely on local folk remedies until they are too ill to be saved by conventional medicine, or because they live in areas remote from medical care. The rise in popularity of ecotourism, in which people from the developed world visit remote locations, creates unique problems when medical emergencies arise.

In the late afternoon of July 1, 1995, near the south bank of the Alto Madre de Dios River in Peru, a snake struck the right leg of a thirty-two-year-old man on a bird-watching expedition. The bite occurred near the village of Atalaya in the Manu National Park, at an altitude of 1,450 feet. Cuzco, the nearest city, can only be reached by a single-track road that climbs for miles to an altitude of 11,600 feet.

While one of the excursion leaders ran to summon help, the other leader used the six-foot extended legs of a tripod to find and identify the snake, which had retreated into a thick stand of bamboo. As the snake struck at the tripod, the leader was given a clear view of the massive, nine-foot-long serpent. It was a bushmaster, *Lachesis muta muta,* a member of the viper family. With an average mature length of nine to twelve feet, the bushmaster is the largest pit viper in the world.

The injured man had two fang marks about an inch and a half apart, the deepest two inches below the knee and oozing bright, unclotted blood. The victim was carried piggyback to the lodge, driven a mile to the river, and then taken across by boat to the village of Atalaya. After being loaded onto the floor of a bus, he was transported up the winding Cuzco road to the rural Clínica Médica de Pilcopata, where he arrived five or six hours after the bite.

A doctor promptly examined the patient, who was in severe pain. A nurse inserted an intravenous line and administered the only available vial of antivenin. The patient was then given intravenous fluids and oral Valium and Darvon, as the clinic had no morphine. The next morning the man was transported by truck over rough roads to a semi-abandoned airstrip near the clinic, but the pilot from Cuzco declined to land because of the terrain. He was then returned to the clinic, loaded back on the floor of the bus, and driven for thirteen hours to the outskirts of Cuzco, arriving at one-thirty a.m. on July 3. He was transferred to a car and taken to the Clínica Pardo, which he reached at three a.m. (about thirty-five hours postbite).

He was immediately given more antivenin, and antibiotics were started by vein. By nine a.m., the patient appeared to have improved. His pain was controlled, and he was alert and optimistic. However, at about four p.m. that day "his condition worsened dramatically." The snake venom had been working insidiously inside his leg and had destroyed the walls of the arteries and veins. The physicians could see by ultrasound two quarts of unclotted blood inside his leg, while the vital circulation through the blood vessels had shut down completely.

By nine p.m., the bird-watcher had been stabilized as much as possible, and he was taken to the operating room, where deep exploratory cuts were made down to the bone. The surgeons found "vast areas of gangrene," dead tissue that had to be removed if the patient were to survive. The next morning he was loaded onto the folded rear seats of a Folker 27 and flown to Lima where he was admitted directly to an intensive care unit. The man urgently needed more surgery, but it had to be delayed until enough type-A, Rh-negative blood could be collected. The tour leader and several American and European embassy personnel were donors.

At five p.m., July 4, seventy-two hours postbite, the operation was begun. The surgeons found that despite removal of gangrenous tissue at the first surgery, the internal destruction had continued to progress. In order to save the patient's life, his entire right leg had to be amputated at the hip. On July 22, 1995, the man was sufficiently recovered to return to his home country, where he spent another month in the hospital being treated for a resistant bacterial infection in his amputation site.

These patients illustrate two important principles at work in the treatment of venomous snakebites: bacterial infection can make a bad snake bite even worse; and, in serious cases, early treatment with adequate amounts of specific antivenin may be critical to prevent a dangerous, chemical chain reaction inside the patient. These tissue reactions so disrupt the integrity of muscle tissue and blood vessels that the damage may prove irreversible.

Antivenin is created by inoculating horses with increasing amounts of specific snake venoms until they develop very high levels of antibodies against the venom proteins and become immune to the venom's effects. The horse serum enriched with these antibodies is then harvested and packaged in sterile vials. When administered early and in sufficient doses, antivenin can diminish many, but not all, of the effects of snakebite. The most dramatic effects occur in patients who are bitten by snakes that paralyze the nervous system: coral snakes, kraits, and cobras. But even following bites by pit vipers in the United States, the use of antivenin has contributed to a decline in mortality from up to twenty-five percent in the nineteenth century to less than a half percent today.

Patients who have received antivenin raised in horses run a high risk of serum sickness, a nasty immune reaction in the weeks following treatment. They develop fever, rash, joint pains, and swollen glands. Manufacturers of some antivenins used in the United States have recently switched from horses to sheep and are producing a more refined product that should have fewer side effects.

To deal with the infectious complications of snakebite, it is important to understand the unique mouth flora of snakes. When snakes swallow prey whole, they come into intimate contact with the bacteria that inhabit the intestines of the animals they eat. In one of the best studies of snakemouth bacteria, Dr. Ellie Goldstein and his colleagues in Los Angeles, made meticulous cultures of venom milked from captive rattlesnakes. Dr. Goldstein found that when a snake's fang sheaths are carefully retracted and the fangs swabbed with alcohol, the venom, like most body fluids, is sterile. However, within the snake's mouth, he found a complex mixture of germs of all kinds. Using special techniques, he was able to culture anaerobes, bacteria that die rapidly when exposed to oxygen but which can produce dangerous infections inside the dying tissues of a patient with a viper bite.

Despite the potential for bacterial hitchhikers in snakebite wounds, infection is not an inevitable outcome, especially in the United States where most patients receive prompt medical attention for their injuries. However, there is one germ, *Aeromonas hydrophila,* which can cause life-threatening infections if it finds its way into a bite wound, whether from the snake's mouth or from the environment in which the injury occurred.

Aeromonas hydrophila is a pink-staining, rod-shaped bacterium that inhabits both fresh and brackish water. It causes diseases in fish, amphibians, and reptiles, or in people who have sustained water-related injuries. Surgeons sometimes apply medicinal leeches to reduce swelling in a flap of the patient's skin used in tissue reconstruction. Patients have developed wound infections from the *Aeromonas hydrophila* in the leech's mouth. *Aeromonas hydrophila* infection has also followed bites by piranhas, sharks, alligators, and crocodiles.

In 1998, physicians from Brazil reported three cases of *Aeromonas hydrophila* infection as a complication of snakebite. In one case, a thirty-four-year-old man was bitten on his right ankle, through boot and sock, by a *Bothrops moojeni,* a relative of the jararacuçu. He applied a tourniquet to his leg, sprinkled the bite wound with powdered tobacco, and then headed to the hospital. Despite receiving twelve vials of antivenin and antibiotics by vein he developed an abscess involving most of his leg. Pus drained from the wound grew *Aeromonas hydrophila* in pure culture.

Aeromonas hydrophila is not limited to tropical environments. In a case reported in the *Southern Medical Journal* in 2002, a thirty-eight-year-old man came to the emergency department at the University of Mississippi Medical Center seven hours after being bitten on the top of his left hand by a water moccasin, a cousin of the rattlesnake. On arrival he was in shock, with a blood pressure of 71/30, dangerously below the normal reading of 120/80. His entire left arm was swollen and red up to the shoulder. The emergency room doctors treated the patient with fourteen vials of antivenin and admitted him to the intensive care unit. On the third day after the bite, the man was taken to the operating room where surgeons found gangrene reaching from the skin of his forearm down to the fascia, the connective tissue partitions that separate the muscles. Again, *Aeromonas* was isolated along with a complex mixture of bacteria from the snake's mouth. The victim recovered after a month in the hospital and multiple surgical procedures, including skin grafting.

When people get into trouble with snakes and the bacteria that snakes acquire from their environment, they are in contact with nature, wild and untamed. However successfully they have adapted to varied habitats, snakes have never been successful competitors with man. They do not willingly share living space with us. Outside of the United States, people encounter snakes as a result of their work in forest and field. But in this country, snakebites occur most often as a result of human folly or carelessness. The typical snakebite victim in the United States is young, male, and drunk.

In one study published by emergency medicine physicians in West Virginia, intentional exposure to snakes preceded twenty out of thirty bites. Seven bites occurred in professional snake handlers, eight happened during snake hunts, and five happened as the result of "playing with snakes in the wild." Forty percent of the thirty victims had consumed alcohol before the snakebite incidents.

Intimate contact with venomous snakes is an intrinsic part of two American activities: rattlesnake round-ups and religious snake-handling. Rattlesnake round-ups began in the nineteenth century as a way of controlling the snake population, and they have become an annual commercial activity in several communities. In his book *The Red Hourglass,* Gordon Grice describes a round-up in Waynoka, Oklahoma, in which he observed men working in a twenty-by-ten-foot concrete pit with over two hundred rattlesnakes. Besides long metal rods, called snake hooks, their only protective gear was the leather boots they wore. Grice observed barehanded participants picking up large snakes by the tail.

The connection between religion and reptiles is more ancient, but it continues to the present day. The Aztecs honored Quetzalcoatl, the feathered serpent. The Hopi Indians dance with and handle rattlesnakes in their religious rituals. In India, the worship of cobras has been traced to prehistoric Dravidian times before 1600 BC. In Pakistan, life in the Jogi tribe is centered on the ritual capture and display of snakes.

The first Protestant snake-handling sect was founded in 1908 by George Hensley and was based on the following passages from Mark 16:17–18, "And these signs shall follow them that believe; In my name shall they cast out devils; . . . They shall take up serpents; and if they drink any deadly thing, it shall not hurt them." The cult flourished in Kentucky in the mid-1930s, survived the death of Hensley in 1955 following the bite of an eastern diamondback rattlesnake during a service, and still finds some adherents today.

One of these worshippers, a thirty-five-year-old man from Tennessee, was brought to the Holston Valley Hospital and Medical Center in Kingsport in 1994. The patient had been handling a timber rattlesnake (*Crotalus horridus horridus*) during a religious service and had been bitten on the left cheek. He had at first refused treatment, but had allowed his coreligionists to take him to a local hospital when he developed nausea, vomiting, headache, and shortness of breath. Despite ten vials of antivenin, he was in shock and dependent on a plastic tube and a manual ventilator to breathe when he arrived by ambulance at the Holston Valley Hospital. However, he eventually recovered after several days in the intensive care unit and a bout of serum sickness.

A twenty-one-year-old man in Arizona was not so fortunate; his father found his corpse on the floor of his apartment. His friends and family said that the man had captured a rattlesnake two months earlier at a construction site where he worked, and had kept it as a pet. According to the case report, he was often seen kissing the snake and, on the night of his death, was last seen at midnight, apparently intoxicated, "letting the snake slither around his arms, neck, and head."

When he was found eighteen hours later, the only evidence of trauma was two puncture holes on his right arm. Photographs in the article detailing the case show marked swelling of the neck, face, lips, tongue, and throat. The victim probably asphyxiated, choked to death by his own swollen flesh. Investigators found "many opened beer cans" in the apartment, and small drops of blood near the terrarium where the snake was kept. A trail of blood led to the bathroom, where the patient had vomited. Investigators followed another blood trail back to the living room, where the body had been found.

The patients described thus far have all been bitten by members of the viper family. The second largest family of venomous snakes is the Elapidae, the family of cobras and their kin. Although they are placed in a separate family, the sea snakes share many characteristics of the elapid snakes. Elapids and sea snakes have short, fixed fangs attached to the maxillary bone, with which they tenaciously pump venom into victims by a succession of chewing movements.

There are about 180 species of elapid snakes. In the United States, where they are represented by just two species of coral snake, they are of minor importance. But in Australia, where there is no competition from the viper family, about sixty species of elapid snakes have evolved, ranging in size from tiny burrowers to the eleven-foot taipan.

The most famous elapids are the cobras, which live in India, southern Asia, and Africa. Named after the Portuguese word for "snake," these large serpents are best known for their ability to spread modified ribs in their necks to form a menacing hood. The king cobra, the largest of the group, reaching lengths of twelve or more feet, may rear up four feet when curious or threatened. In addition to biting, some African species can spit venom into a victim's eyes, causing temporary or, in untreated cases, permanent blindness.

Equally dreaded are the four species of African mambas— long, aggressive, whiplike snakes with slender fangs. Of the four species that make up African mambas, three are tree snakes. But the highly venomous black mamba lives on the ground and is famed for its speed, ferocity, and territoriality.

The kraits are South Asian elapids with short fangs but very toxic venom. The bite of one krait can kill an average adult in less than ten minutes. The elapids of Australia, New Guinea, and nearby islands include the black snake, which possesses a cobralike hood, the death adder, the tiger snake, and the brown snake.

In contrast to the members of the viper family, all of these elapids inject venom that targets the victim's nervous system. Severe tissue damage at the site of the bite may not always occur and, in fact, the snakebite may not be suspected in time to save the patient's life with antivenin.

The first reported victim of an elapid-type bite was not a person but the sun god Ra. Ra's "case history" appears in the Eber's Papyrus about 1550 BC and is given by the Mintons in their book *Venomous Reptiles*:

Ra wailed, "I have been stung by a serpent which I could not see. This is not the same as fire; it is not the same as water. But still I am as cold as water and then again as hot as fire. All my body sweats, and I tremble. My eyesight is not steady, and I cannot see, for the sweat pours over my face in spite of the summer's pleasant air."

The accuracy of this ancient text may be appreciated when it is compared to a modern case report of a bite by a black mamba, *Dendroaspis polylepsis,* which was reported in the *Wilderness and Environmental Medicine* journal, in 1996. While attempting to capture a ten-foot black mamba in order to collect venom, a thirty-four-year-old professional snake farmer was bitten through his trousers and socks on his left leg. Within one minute, the patient injected himself with mamba antivenin into the skin and muscle around the bite. Shortly afterwards, his wife injected more antivenin into his buttock. A local doctor administered additional antivenin into a muscle, and the patient was driven 160 miles from his snake farm in northern Transvaal to Johannesburg.

While en route to the hospital, the snake farmer complained of abdominal cramps and vomited several times. He "felt hot and sweated profusely." Upon arrival at the hospital, seven hours after the bite, he was having difficulty swallowing and speaking. The bite site showed only slight redness and swelling, but it was quite tender to the touch. The patient exhibited the typical eye signs of neurotoxic envenomation: droopy lids, dilated pupils, and limited ability to move his eyes.

Eight and a half hours after the bite, the patient's condition worsened, and all of the nerves of the face were involved. He was unable to move his lower jaw, and his mouth hung slackly open. His face frozen in a rigid mask, the restless but fully conscious victim was unable to move his head or neck. Because he was too weak to breathe on his own, his doctors performed a tracheostomy and connected him to a mechanical respirator. After receiving large doses of antivenin by vein, he gradually recovered over the next two days.

The quick administration of antivenin doubtless saved the farmer's life, as mamba venom is extremely fast-acting and potent. Containing proteins that block the transmission of nerve impulses to the muscles, the poison quickly paralyzes and kills. Scientists have also isolated a number of protein fragments from the venom that stimulate the involuntary nervous system to overreact, producing the profuse sweating and chills that patients experience.

Cobras also have potent, neurotoxic venom, and, in addition, their bites cause local tissue swelling and severe pain. They are not aggressive snakes, but people sometimes come upon them accidentally. One patient, whose case was described in 1998, was admitted to the Chulalongkorn University Hospital in Bangkok, Thailand, in severe respiratory distress. He was resuscitated and placed on a ventilator. His doctors found fang marks on his right hand. A hotel bellboy reported that he had been called and told that the man had just been bitten by a cobra. Hotel management searched the patient's room, the hallway, and the air-conditioning ducts and, when they were unable to find the snake, they evacuated that floor of the hotel.

When he was sufficiently recovered, the patient told his doctors that he had been bitten in a grassy spot behind the hotel "when he parted the vegetation to see what was moving there." He then decided to go back to his hotel room for some cigarettes before seeking medical help, and he remembered having trouble focusing his eyes. He made a full recovery, but lost his right index finger.

Cobras often conjure images of snake charmers inducing a cobra to rear up from a basket. The snake follows the charmer's body movements; having no ears, it does not hear the accompanying flute solo. Some charmers insist on additional precautions, clipping the fangs of their performers in order to render them harmless. However, new fangs grow in with the next molt or even sooner. Sometimes the snake charmer will sew the cobra's jaws shut, but the snake eventually dies of starvation. Others, however, use fully venomous snakes, as in the following case reported in 1976.

During a performance at Makarfi, near Zaria, Nigeria, an Egyptian cobra that "had gotten out of control" bit a ten-year-old Hausa boy on the hand. The boy was given herbal medicine to swallow. He began to vomit, and within an hour he was unconscious. Two hours later he was dead. Aside from two fang punctures two centimeters apart on the boy's right middle finger, and some swelling of the hand, the victim's autopsy was normal. The boy most likely died because the cobra's venom paralyzed his ability to breathe. The snake charmer gave the cobra to the authors of the article, who then used it for venom production.

Australia, where some of the deadliest snakes in the world are found, is the only continent that has more species of venomous than nonvenomous snakes. One of the most easily recognized is the death adder, which is not a true viper but a viper look-alike. Unfortunately, many of the roughly sixty other poisonous elapids in Australia resemble harmless species, like racers, rat snakes, or king snakes.

Despite an annual incidence of between one and three thousand snakebites each year, Australia averages only about three deaths. One cause of this low fatality rate is proper education in first aid. Australians are taught to wrap a bitten extremity gently but firmly in a crepe bandage, like those used to immobilize sprained ankles, and then to splint the affected limb. This is the same pressure-immobilization technique that is used in funnel web spider bites, and it is believed to delay absorption of venom long enough for antivenin to take effect.

Much of the credit for Australia's good survival statistics following venomous snakebite is due to the efforts of the Commonwealth Serum Laboratories in Melbourne (CSL). They have developed a sensitive, easy-to-use, snake-venom detection kit. Samples may be taken from the skin in or around a bite wound or from urine in patients showing signs of envenomation.

The kits come with easy-to-follow instructions in which a color change is observed in one or more of five wells. For example, if Well Two turns blue first, the victim has been bitten by a brown snake, but if Well Four changes color first, a death adder is responsible. Prompt treatment with appropriate antivenin is then started.

The kits and antivenins from CSL only cover the major and most dangerous species of venomous snakes on the continent. But Australians, even young ones, seem to view the dozens of other species with curiosity and unruffled aplomb.

In 2002, Dr. Geoffrey Isbister and his colleagues in Newcastle, Australia, reported two cases of bites by the black-bellied swamp snake, *Hemiaspis signata*. The first patient was a twelve-year-old boy who had found a snake by a school building and had carried it by the tail to the principal's office. On the way there, the snake bit him on the right index finger. The live snake was brought with the patient to the emergency department, where it was put in a freezer "to allow safe examination." The boy had some pain around the bite, and mild abnormalities of his clotting system, but did well without specific therapy. Dr. Isbister came over to the hospital, took the snake out of the freezer, and photographed it. (In the picture, it is apparently unfrozen and alive.) He confirmed its identity by describing it over the telephone to herpetologist Ross Sadler of the Australian Museum.

The second patient was a seven-year-old boy who came to the hospital after being bitten on the left thumb by a "white-lipped" snake the previous evening. On arrival, his left index finger was red and swollen, and he had an inflamed gland in his left armpit. The next day, however, he recovered and was able to go home. The authors then add that the snake was "captured *by the patient* [italics mine] and formally identified at the Australian Reptile Park as *H. signata*," the black-bellied swamp snake.

. . .

Sea snakes generally inhabit tropical and subtropical coastal waters of the Indian and Pacific Oceans, but are also found in such freshwater lakes as Lake Taal in the Philippines. All of the fifty species of sea snakes are venomous, and they are not rare; in 1975 alone, fifty thousand sea snakes per month were killed for their skins in the Philippines. Although they are classified as a separate family, sea snakes are actually closely related to the elapids. They have vertically flattened tails to facilitate swimming and possess exceedingly potent neurotoxic venom. Besides causing paralysis, sea snake venom may lead to muscle destruction and kidney failure due to the excretion of muscle proteins in the urine.

Sea snakes are not aggressive. The usual bite victim is a fisherman who accidentally catches one in a net, as in the following case reported in the *Journal of Tropical Medicine and Hygiene* in 1994. The victim, a twenty-four-year-old fisherman, was admitted to the General Hospital in Colombo, Sri Lanka. He had been fishing two miles off the coast when, at about six a.m., he noticed that a sea snake had become entangled in the net that he had just hauled into his boat. He freed the snake, let it lie in the bottom of the boat, and began sorting out the fish. However, the snake was within striking distance and promptly bit him on the left foot. He killed it and returned to his task, noting only a pricking pain in his foot. By the time he reached home at nine a.m., he was having trouble keeping his eyes open and had double vision. He was experiencing "moderately severe pain" in his left groin. At ten-thirty that morning he consulted a family physician because of increasing weakness in his legs. The doctor gave him penicillin and a tetanus shot and arranged for his admission to the hospital.

When the fisherman was examined eight and a half hours after the bite, he couldn't walk or even sit up unaided. His eyelids drooped, and his pupils were abnormally dilated. Two rows of puncture wounds marked the bite site. There were tender, swollen glands in the left groin. The doctors gave the patient an intra-venous cocktail of land-snake antivenins, and he made a gradual, complete recovery in four days.

In his review of sea snake bites, Dr. Charles M. Phillips rec-ommends the use of Sutherland's compression-immobilization technique. If a sea snake bites through a wet suit, as occasionally happens, the wet suit is left in place during transport to the hos-pital, as it provides a good compressive dressing. Early signs of en-venomation include muscle aches and pains, and swollen glands. Dark urine three to six hours after a bite is a particularly ominous sign, suggesting severe muscle damage and potential kidney failure.

Dr. Philips recommends treatment with the sea snake antivenin cocktail available through the Commonwealth Serum Laborato-ries. In a pinch, tiger snake antivenin can be used, but large doses may be required. Signs of life-threatening envenomation include multiple teeth marks, vomiting, inability to move the eyes, droopy eyelids, and pupils that react abnormally to light. The fisherman from Sri Lanka had several of these signs and was therefore lucky to have survived his bite.

Many reasons have been proposed for the snake's endur-ing hold on human imagination. They were considered phallic symbols long before Freud. Because snakes are in intimate contact with the earth, the Greeks thought they possessed special knowl-edge. The priests of Asclepius kept them in their temples, so that this knowledge could find its way into the dream cures of their sleeping patients.

But the snake also derives its symbolic power from the very

real power the venomous ones have over all animal life. No doubt our fascination with snakes stems from a combination of dread and respect.

According to the ancient Egyptians, the sun god Ra, after suffering his terrible snakebite, was determined to protect gods and men from the serpent tribe. First he drew up a treaty, but the snakes would not abide by its terms. So he decided to give earth dwellers powerful magic words that could ward off snakes. These magic words were supposed to have been communicated to the Psylli of North Africa, who have been snake shamans since at least 1500 BC. Pliny the Elder knew of them and described their pungent, snaky smell.

In time, the Psylli forsook their ancient Egyptian religion and found new holy words, so by the time Napoleon summoned them to evict a cobra from his quarters, they had forgotten the incantations of Ra.

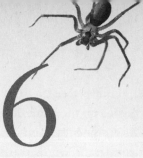

6

Silent
Stowaways

The six-year-old girl who was being wheeled in for a brain scan was not alone. She unknowingly carried a silent passenger, its mouthparts embedded in her scalp, its swelling body hidden by her long, brown hair. Doctors helped the limp child roll on to her side so that a spinal tap could be performed. Meanwhile the girl became weaker and weaker. Though she seemed fully aware of her surroundings, her speech was slurred, and she could no longer raise her eyelids. The paralysis that had started in her feet crept up to her breathing muscles. Concerned that she might suffocate without the support of a mechanical ventilator, doctors transferred her to intensive care.

The girl seemed to have all of the signs and symptoms of Guillain-Barré syndrome, a paralytic condition in which the immune system turns against itself. Her physicians made preparations to give plasmapheresis treatments for this disease. In this procedure, a large needle is placed in the big vein in the groin; a machine pumps the patient's blood plasma through special filters to remove proteins and returns the plasma to the circulatory system.

But before the intravenous needle was inserted, the youngest doctor on the team decided to perform one more test. The pediatric resident passed a fine-toothed comb through the girl's long hair. In the words of the *New England Journal of Medicine* report, "To the surprise of the three pediatricians, the pediatric neurologist, and the pediatric intensive care specialist who were caring for the child, an engorged tick, fifteen millimeters in diameter, was embedded in . . . the scalp." A photograph in the article shows the engorged and attached tick. A second photograph shows the little girl twenty-four hours after the tick was removed, fully recovered and standing next to her hospital bed, holding her teddy bear.

In 1912, Dr. John L. Todd, a professor at McGill University in Montreal, Canada, mailed two hundred letters to practicing physicians in Southern British Columbia, asking them if they had any experience with patients becoming ill after being bitten by ticks. Dr. Todd, a parasitologist, had learned that the tick *Dermacenter* had been found in this region; he wanted to find out if it was transmitting Rocky Mountain spotted fever in Canada, as it did in the United States.

To his surprise, Dr. Todd received six letters from physicians describing not spotted fever but paralysis following tick bite. One doctor in Creston, British Columbia, wrote about a four-year-old girl who had over two or three days gradually lost the use of her legs, until she was unable to stand. A tick was removed from the nape of her neck, and within three days she was well again. A doctor from Fernie, British Columbia, wrote that, in about 1898, he lost two infants to convulsions, both of whom were found to have wood ticks on their necks. A third physician in Nelson, British Columbia, lost one child in 1900 and another in 1901; engorged ticks clung to both bodies. Then, in early 1912, a three-year-old girl became paralyzed. This time the physician looked for and found three ticks on the nape of the child's neck, removed them, and saved her life.

Dr. Todd wrote a brief report about the disease in the *Canadian Medical Journal* later in 1912, with the hope that physicians might come forward with additional cases—and also that someone might mail him a live tick removed from such a patient, for study.

One year later, in April 1913, the Canadian Department of Agriculture dispatched a young veterinary pathologist named Seymour Hadwen to the farm of a shepherd in British Columbia. Over three successive spring seasons, the shepherd had lost large numbers of sheep to a mysterious paralytic illness, which had baffled local veterinarians. On one affected sheep that had just been shorn, Hadwen found a large tick cut in half by the shears. It is not unusual to find ticks on sheep, and the significance of this finding might easily have been overlooked, but Hadwen had read Todd's 1912 account. So, instead of mailing live ticks to Dr. Todd, Hadwen took them back to his own laboratory in Agassiz, British Columbia.

Hadwen allowed the toxic ticks to feed on three lambs, a dog, and several guinea pigs. All of the animals became paralyzed. At death, he found nothing unusual about the victims' tissues, nor could he transmit the paralysis from one animal to a second one by injecting it with blood from the paralyzed subject. Dr. Hadwen deduced that the saliva of the tick contained a potent toxin of some sort, rather than an infectious agent that would have been passed from animal to animal.

In the same year as Dr. Todd's paper appeared, a physician in

Oregon independently published a report of twelve cases of tick paralysis, three of which were fatal. However, neither of these investigators could claim to have published the first words on the subject. That posthumous honor falls to the Australian explorer William Hovell, who in 1824 wrote of a "tick, which buried itself in the flesh and would in the end destroy man or beast if not removed in time." In fact, accounts of tick-paralyzed livestock appeared in the veterinary literature of Australia and South Africa in the late nineteenth century, but apparently went unnoticed in Canada and the United States.

Although tick paralysis is most common in the areas where it was first reported—Canada, the United States, and Australia—it is likely that the syndrome occurs everywhere ticks are found. It has been reported in Europe, Greece, Israel, Mexico, and Russia. It's not a new disease, but whether it is as ancient as the tick family itself is unknown.

Ticks are arachnids, eight-legged cousins of spiders and scorpions. In the late Paleozoic or early Mesozoic era, about 225 million years ago, their ancestors gave up an independent existence and evolved into bloodsucking parasites. Ticks probably fed on the first reptiles and, as the birds and mammals evolved, ticks evolved along with them. There are three families of ticks, of which two contain species that cause human illness. The smaller group (170 species) contains the soft-bodied or leathery ticks, and the larger group (650 species) the hard ticks. Members of both families may transmit infections to people, but paralysis is limited to 40 species of the hard ticks.

Hard ticks have complex life cycles that usually take from two to three years to complete. The female lays 400–20,000 eggs (depending on the species) in a mass in the leaf litter from which six-legged larvae hatch. Ticks lack antennae and have only rudimentary eyes or none at all. However, on the top of the first leg, they have a sensory complex called Haller's organ. The larvae move up blades of grass and wait with their front legs uplifted and waving until they detect body heat, vibration, carbon dioxide, and various other chemicals emanating from a suitable host. The larvae scramble onto the host and remain attached for three to nine days until they are swollen with blood, then drop off and molt within a week to several months into an eight-legged nymph. A nymph has the same round flat body and small head as the adult, but lacks a genital aperture. Both nymphs and adults have fully-formed mouthparts, which include two saw-like blades for puncturing the skin and a hollow tooth for attachment to the host and for feeding. During attachment, hard ticks secrete anticoagulants, enzymes, painkillers, and, in most species, cement to stick to the host. While feeding, the tick will alternately suck blood and regurgitate saliva into the host's body.

After feeding for between three and eleven days, nymphs detach and then molt, usually within a month, and assume the adult male or female form. Adult ticks range in girth from less than a sixteenth of an inch to marble-size, depending on the species and the state of engorgement with blood. After finding a suitable host, adult females attach for about a week and feed, during which time mating takes place. In most species, the males feed sparingly at this stage or not at all. In Australian paralysis ticks, the males feed parasitically off the females by puncturing their bodies and sucking blood and lymph. Toxin production, when it occurs, begins in the female tick at the end of the engorgement period as the eggs are beginning to form inside her ovaries. After mating and egg laying, adult hard ticks die within a few weeks.

Tick paralysis is an enormous veterinary problem, particularly in Australia where twenty thousand domestic animals are affected each year. In northern New South Wales alone, it kills ten thousand calves annually. In a recent epidemic in North Queensland, hundreds of the large fruit bats known as spectacled flying foxes died, and many more were incapacitated. Local volunteers even set up a bat hospital to deal with the problem.

Between 1958 and 1994, U.S. wildlife veterinarians tabulated numerous cases of tick paralysis among ten species of wild birds from five southeastern states. There are also reports of paralysis of a red wolf in North Carolina and of a gray fox in California.

In a remarkable case reported in 1980, wildlife researchers in northern California inspecting live traps found an engorged hard tick attached to the base of the skull of a paralyzed harvest mouse. The tick toxin made the mouse so sensitive to sound that each time the camera shutter clicked, the animal went into convulsions. The mouse began to recover as soon as the tick was removed, and within twenty-five minutes it tried to bite one of the investigators.

The human cases in North America usually follow the same pattern of recovery once the offending tick is removed, as in one adult patient reported in 1938 by Dr. J. Heyward Gibbes. According to Dr. Gibbes, Mrs. H.E.T. of Columbia, South Carolina, went to inspect some prize pigs in a nearby town. Four days later she began to have tingling and numbness in her legs. Later that day her legs felt weak and she said she "did not know just where they were going." The next morning she could not stand. The numbness and tingling had spread to her arms. She was brought to the hospital by ambulance.

On arrival she was "in a semi-hysterical condition." She appeared entirely well on careful physical examination, but her neurological examination showed some loss of strength in her legs and clumsiness in her movements. Dr. Gibbes tapped on her knees and the backs of her ankles, but there was no answering reflex jerk. He was able, however, to obtain the normal muscle jerk reflexes in the arms.

By her sixth day in the hospital, the woman's legs were worse, and her arms and hands were becoming weak and clumsy as well. By the seventh day, she could no longer feed herself. On the eighth day her speech had become thick, though she thought her legs were a little better. Later that day the cause of the condition became clear. A nurse who was combing the patient's hair told the doctor she had found a "tumor on the scalp." It turned out to be a half-inch-wide wood tick, fully distended with blood. Dr. Gibbes promptly removed it.

By the next day the patient said she felt "better all over." Her reflexes returned by the following day, and the day after that she went home. When Dr. Gibbes examined her two weeks later in his office, she "seemed none the worse for her experience" with tick paralysis.

Although disorders of sensation, like numbness and tingling, are not supposed to be an important part of the syndrome of tick paralysis, these sensations may be underreported because young victims may not describe their symptoms as well as adults do. However, in the case of Mrs. H.E.T. and in the following patient, abnormal sensations were clearly described.

In July 1923, Dr. Peter Bassoe visited a forty-nine-year-old university professor at his cottage in Rocky Mountain National Park. The professor had just recovered from a "curious illness," which he described to his friend.

In the early afternoon of the first of July, the man went out for a walk, and although he had felt fine all day, he noticed that his gait was slightly unsteady. That evening his fingers were "numb and prickling." When he got up during the night he staggered badly, and by the next morning he could walk only by holding on to a chair. He told Dr. Bassoe that the palms of his hands were now numb and that his toes tingled. He had some blurry vision and felt nauseated when his eyes were open. On the third day, the professor was unable to empty his bladder completely, and he lost control of his bowels. He felt a little short of breath and his hands and feet were cold. When he tried to touch his finger to his nose, he banged his face.

Then, at six p.m., the professor found an engorged tick in his left groin. A local doctor came to the cottage and removed the tick through a small incision. Over the next six days the man made a gradual but complete recovery.

During the 1940s and 1950s, summer epidemics of the viral disease poliomyelitis were paralyzing children around the world. Since tick paralysis is also a summer disease, there was a real danger that physicians could mistake it for polio. In 1946, two doctors in Australia described an infant who was thought to have died of poliomyelitis. When the child was examined after death, an engorged tick was found under a piece of adhesive plaster that had been applied by the first doctor who examined the child.

In 1952, Dr. Joseph A. Costa of Bedford Hills, New York, published a cautionary article in a pediatric journal. He described the typical American case of tick paralysis as a girl aged three to ten who falls getting out of bed one morning, or who, if she makes it to the table, can't feed herself because her hands are clumsy. In the doctor's office, she is often quiet, passive, and apathetic. She may not be able to sit up unsupported, collapsing "in the same fashion as a 'rag doll.' " Dr. Costa then offered important clues to differentiate the syndrome from polio. In tick paralysis there is no fever, the spinal fluid is normal, the knee jerk and other reflexes are lost early, the patient is passive and apathetic, and, of course, the child has had a recent tick bite, or an attached tick is found.

Although the early cases of tick paralysis collected by Dr. Todd in Montreal often ended in death, the case fatality rate from tick paralysis in this country since 1946 has usually been under ten percent. However, in Australia, where it seems that all toxic animals are more toxic, tick paralysis is often lethal. In 1983, Dr. Struan

Sutherland reported twenty fatal human cases there between 1904 and 1947. Most of the patients were infants and children. The youngest was a two-month-old baby girl who died in 1939, but of the three adults, two were in their thirties. The oldest victim was a seventy-five-year-old man who died in 1939. In fact, tick paralysis has killed more people in Australia than either the red back spider or the funnel web spider. The following case occurred in about 1904 in Mullumbimby, New South Wales, and was reported by Dr. Leighton Kesteven:

> The mother brought the child (aged about thirteen or fourteen) to me one morning to 'see if there was not something in her ear.' On examination I found the tick, fully distended, fastened on the *membrana tympani* (eardrum). The child was in a semi-comatose state and only made to give unintelligible answers with difficulty (sic). I filled the ear with carbolic oil—1 in 40—and the beastie floated up, sting and all, intact. I administered brandy and strychnine freely, but the patient gradually sank and died about eighteen hours after.

One species of tick, the bush tick *Ixodes holocyclus,* is responsible for all deaths due to tick paralysis in mainland Australia. The species is restricted to scrub and brush areas on the eastern coast of the country. Man is an incidental host of the scrub tick; in nature it relies on the blood of the long-nose bandicoot, a rat-sized marsupial insect-eater. Bandicoots and the other marsupial hosts of the bush tick build up a natural immunity to tick toxin by constant exposure to tick bites. However, a captured bandicoot, after being confined in a tick-free environment for several months, may be fatally paralyzed by the bite of a single adult female tick.

The incidence of tick paralysis in people and animals in Australia parallels fluctuations in the bandicoot population. A brush fire that destroys the bandicoot's habitat may render an area tick-free for up to five years. But when ranchers poison predators, like dingoes and foxes, the bandicoot population rises, and so do cases of tick paralysis.

Tick paralysis in Australia, as in North America, begins with unsteady walking and with paralysis that moves from the toes up the legs. But rather than improving after the tick is removed, the patient's condition will often worsen in the next forty-eight hours. There may be paralysis of the muscles moving the eyes, and the pupils may fail to react to light. In surviving patients, recovery is slow, with strength returning only after several weeks.

The Commonwealth Serum Laboratory developed an anti-toxin for tick paralysis in 1935, even before the chemical nature and mode of action of the toxin were known. Using dogs as an-tibody factories, they allowed toxic ticks to feed on the animals in gradually increasing numbers, enabling the dogs to build up im-munity. They then harvested the dog serum for use in paralyzed animals and people. Patients may develop serum sickness from this tick antivenin, like that following the use of snake antivenin raised in horses. But in severe cases of tick paralysis, the antivenin, combined with ventilator support in the intensive care unit, can mean the difference between life and death.

In April 1993, a twenty-three-month-old girl was brought to Westmead Hospital in Sydney with a twenty-four-hour history of lethargy, vomiting, and poor eating and drinking. She had stopped talking, had become unsteady, and could no longer walk by her-self. The examining doctors found a drowsy, irritable child whose right pupil was dilated, compared with the left. Her blood tests showed signs of dehydration and muscle breakdown.

At first the hospital staff thought that she might have been poisoned, but the next morning a nurse discovered a tick behind her right ear, which was removed. During the day the patient deteriorated. She could not move her eyes; her eyelids drooped, and neither of her pupils reacted to light. The rest of the muscles of her face became weak, she lost the gag reflex when the back of her throat was touched, and she was in danger of choking on her own secretions. There was no reflex response when her tendons were struck with a rubber hammer, and her arms and legs were limp.

The toddler was transferred to intensive care, and her doctors put a small plastic tube in her airway to protect her breathing. She was given half an ampoule of tick antivenin by vein and a whole ampoule the following day. That evening, her pupils began to react to light, and her gag reflex returned. On the fourth day she was able to move her arms and legs, and on the sixth the plastic tube was removed. However, it was almost three weeks after her admission to the hospital before she could walk unaided, and full recovery was not reached until four months later.

Dangerous cases of tick paralysis occur most often in infants and toddlers, probably because they weigh less than adults. But it's still remarkable that a creature no larger than a garbanzo bean can paralyze a child many thousands of times its size and weight. Tick toxin is so potent, causing paralysis in such minute quantities, that it has been difficult to collect and analyze.

In 1926, Dr. I. C. Ross paralyzed mice by injecting them with an extract of tick salivary glands, proving that the syndrome was caused by a toxin secreted by the tick. However, it wasn't until 1966 that a partially purified sample of the toxin was prepared. To accomplish this, Dr. G. H. Kaire of the Commonwealth Serum Laboratories in Melbourne homogenized almost four hundred replete ticks. The toxin samples he obtained paralyzed dogs forty-eight hours after injection, and he could prevent the symptoms by treating the animals in advance with serum from immune dogs.

Subsequent studies showed that the toxin is a medium-sized protein whose action is more potent at higher temperatures than at lower, cooler ones. Exploiting this property, the volunteers at the bat hospital on the Atherton Tablelands in Queensland sometimes place ice packs around tick-paralyzed bats to speed their recovery.

Although not all of the actions of the toxin have yet been explained, the principal effect is on the nerve endings. Like the toxin of botulism, tick toxin blocks the chemical signal that nerves send to muscle fibers, thus paralyzing muscle contraction.

Research has also been done on the more mundane question: What is the best method for removing an attached tick? Dr. Glen R. Needham, a tick specialist at Ohio State University, allowed dog ticks to attach to the back of a sheared female Dorset sheep for up to four days. The following traditional methods of tick removal were then attempted: (1) petroleum jelly applied to the tick; (2) clear fingernail polish similarly applied; (3) 70-percent isopropyl alcohol application; and (4) holding a red-hot kitchen match to the tick's back immediately after blowing the match out.

None of these techniques induced ticks to detach. Ticks breathe too slowly to be suffocated by methods one or two in any reasonable length of time. In addition, ticks coated with nail polish couldn't move at all once the polish hardened, which would impede their ability to back out of the host. Isopropyl alcohol had little effect on the ticks. Even hot matches didn't induce the ticks to detach and seemed dangerous to use on a squirming child or pet. In addition, heated and exploding ticks could spread infectious diseases.

The authors then experimented with several mechanical methods for tick removal, with the goal of removing the tick with mouthparts intact. The following recommended procedure, which also minimizes transmission of tick-borne diseases, is now standard practice for both health professionals and laypersons. It can be used for removing ticks either from pets or from people.

1. Blunt curved forceps or tweezers should be used. If fingers are used, shield them with a tissue, paper towel, or rubber gloves.
2. Grasp the tick as close to the skin surface as possible and pull upward with steady, even pressure. Do not twist or jerk the tick, as this may cause the mouth parts to break off.
3. Take care not to squeeze, crush, or puncture the body of the tick, as its fluids may contain infective agents.
4. Do not handle the tick with bare hands, as infectious agents may enter via mucous membranes or breaks in the skin.
5. After removing the tick, thoroughly disinfect the bite site and wash hands with soap and water.
6. Ticks can be safely disposed of by being placed in a container of alcohol or flushed down the toilet.

We have learned a great deal about tick paralysis since Dr. Todd received those six letters from the physicians of British Columbia. We know how to recognize the illness and support the patients until they recover. We understand something about how the paralytic toxin works, and we have an antivenin for the Australian form of the disease.

But the most fundamental question about tick paralysis has never been answered. Why do some ticks paralyze their hosts? Why does it happen at the end of a blood meal, when the tick has already evaded all of the host's defenses? Of what use to a tick is a host that dies after the tick has detached?

Some authorities have suggested that tick paralysis is an accident of nature, and that the paralyzing effect of the toxin is an unexpected by-product of some necessary action, like the anesthesia or anticoagulation that allows the tick to feed. But could it be that in their evolutionary past, ticks were once predators, like their cousins, the spiders, and that they used toxins to capture prey? If so, then paralyzing the host may be just a bad habit that some ticks never gave up.

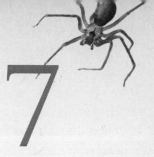

7

Nightmare

In 1998, during a period of civil war, a French human rights leader in the Democratic Republic of Congo was taken prisoner and tortured. The man escaped and spent a year hiding in the bush. About two years later, he was able to emigrate with his wife and four children to Canada. Shortly thereafter the man began having religious delusions. He heard voices. In his hallucinations, people were trying to kill him.

At first his physicians considered posttraumatic stress disorder, though he was able to describe his harrowing experiences in Africa without discomfort. His doctors gave him medicine for depression and paranoia, but the man's psychiatric symptoms did not resolve, and, after a few weeks, he lost his appetite, became weak and dizzy, and began having headaches. Following a minor injury at work that resulted in severe back pain, he sank into a deep depression and talked of committing suicide.

The émigré's doctors admitted him to the hospital, where an x-ray scan of his chest revealed enlarged lymph nodes. More tellingly, magnetic resonance imaging showed subtle abnormalities deep in his brain. The cause of this physical and mental illness remained a mystery until, during a lucid interval, he consented to a spinal tap. The cerebrospinal fluid was wildly abnormal with over nine thousand white blood cells per cubic millimeter (up to two thousand is normal). A second tap was done, and there, under the microscope, the doctors saw the eel-like protozoa called trypanosomes. During his year in the bush the professor had contracted sleeping sickness. Long latent in his body, it had finally reached his brain.

Sleeping sickness—or, more properly, human African trypanosomiasis—is a protozoan disease, similar to malaria. But while malaria is transmitted by the bites of mosquitoes, it is the tsetse fly that spreads sleeping sickness. The tsetse gets its name from the sound of its buzz, rendered onomatopoeically by the Tswana people living along the border of the Kalahari Desert in South Africa. Large, brown flies with evil-looking reddish eyes, tsetse flies live only in equatorial Africa, that broad zone lying between the Sahara and Kalahari deserts. When a tsetse fly alights upon a host, its closed wings criss-cross over each other like scissors. With long, tubular mouth parts, it then pierces the skin and probes for blood vessels.

The first descriptions of sleeping sickness are also accounts of European oppression of the Africans. John Atkins, a British naval surgeon, visited the Guinea coast in 1721 and wrote:

The sleepy Distemper gives no other previous notice than a Want of Appetite two or three Days before; their

Sleeps are sound and Sense of Feeling very little; for pulling, drubbing or whipping, will scarce stir up sense and Power enough to move; and the Moment you cease beating, the Smart is forgot, and down they fall again into a state of Insensibility; driveling constantly from the Mouth . . .

Thomas Masterman Winterbottom observed the disease in Sierra Leone and on the Gulf of Benin, and wrote in 1803:

The disposition to sleep is so strong, as scarcely to leave a sufficient respite for the taking of food; even the repeated application of a whip, a remedy which has been frequently used, is hardly sufficient to keep the poor wretch awake.

Winterbottom described the swollen lymph glands that appear on the back of the neck during the incubation period, when the patient may still appear well. He remarked that slave traders, understanding their significance, either avoided buying slaves with these swellings or got rid of any slaves that developed them as soon as possible.

Some of the native people of Africa recognized that the bite of the tsetse caused "fly disease," a fatal, wasting illness of cattle and horses. The Zulus called the wasting disease nagana, the name adopted by Europeans. Because of nagana, neither the Portuguese in the sixteenth century nor the Moslem cavalry in the nineteenth were able to penetrate central Africa. In the 1830s, attempts by the Boers to settle Northern Transvaal ended with the death of all their livestock. And twenty years later, the celebrated missionary explorer Dr. David Livingston recorded in the region between Lake Ngami and the Zambezi River "the presence of a biting fly called tsetse." A few days after the bite of this fly "the eye and nose [of an ox] begin to run, the coat stares [sic] as if the animal were cold—emaciation commences accompanied by a peculiar flaccidity of the muscles and this proceeds unchecked until the animal perishes in a state of extreme exhaustion." Because of na-gana, much of equatorial Africa remained limited to "the hoe and the head load" until the advent of the internal combustion engine and the railway.

Of course the real culprit was not the tsetse fly, however painful and irritating its bites often were. The fly was only the ac-complice; the perpetrator of the disease is a parasitic protozoan, a one-celled microscopic animal called a trypanosome.

The first person to see a trypanosome was Professor Gabriel Valentin of Berne, who in 1841, while examining the blood of a trout under the microscope, noticed a dark, oval object moving between the blood cells. The next year the Hungarian micro-scopist, David Gruby, observed similar organisms in the blood of frogs. He described the undulating membrane that runs the length of the protozoan and likened it to the blade of a saw. Be-cause the motion of the organism resembled a corkscrew, Gruby named it *Trypanosoma,* from the Greek *trupanon*—"an auger or corkscrew"—plus *soma,* "body."

Although trypanosomes were found in a variety of warm and cold-blooded animals, they remained zoological curiosities until 1880, when Griffith Evans, a veterinary officer working in the Punjab in India, found them in the blood of horses, mules, and camels dying of the febrile disease surra. Evans was able to trans-mit the disease to a healthy dog and a horse by inoculating them with the trypanosome. Native lore held that bloodsucking horse-flies spread surra, and this was later proved to be the case.

At this point the history of African trypanosomiasis intersects the life and career of one of the giants of medical microbiology, Sir David Bruce. In 1894, Surgeon-Captain David Bruce was posted to Pietermaritzburg, Natal, South Africa, to investigate an outbreak of nagana that was destroying the cattle of British colonial farmers of Zululand. Students of Robert Koch's laboratory in Berlin, both Dr. Bruce and his wife were accomplished bacteriologists. During his previous posting on the island of Malta, Dr. Bruce had discovered and described the cause of a dangerous fever that was decimating British troops there. He christened the new organism *Micrococcus melitensis*. (The name of the bacterium was later changed in his honor to *Brucella melitensis,* and the disease became known as brucellosis.)

After their arrival in Natal, the Bruces set off on a cross-country trek for Zululand. On November 24, 1884, they set up housekeeping and a rudimentary laboratory in a wattle-and-mud hut on Ubombo Hill, altitude two thousand feet. Although the hill was tsetse fly free, it was surrounded on all sides by fly country.

At the beginning of his research, Dr. Bruce believed nagana was a bacterial disease, like Malta fever, but his cultures of blood and tissue from nagana victims gave negative or inconsistent results. In addition, although he did not know about Gruby's trypanosomes, when he microscopically examined blood from sick animals, he saw living protozoa, which he called *Haematozoa,* or "blood animals."

Dr. Bruce found that if he took healthy calves into the low country, they developed nagana, and their blood teemed with up to ten thousand Haematozoa per cubic millimeter. Two of the Bruces' pet dogs developed fatal nagana, and in one, a pointer named John Keats, Dr. Bruce saw one Haematozoan for every four red blood cells, an enormously high parasite load. He noted the creatures "wriggling about like little snakes" and "moving from point to point . . . thin end foremost."

In fact, trypanosomes belong to a highly motile group of protozoa called the flagellates, which move by means of a whiplike tail, the flagellum. In the trypanosomes, the flagellum starts at the back of the tiny animal, is anchored to the undulating membrane, turning it into a kind of fin, and then ends by projecting for a short distance from the thin front end of the cell.

These preliminary studies seemed to point to the protozoan as the causative agent in nagana, a theory supported by the absence of the parasites in the blood of healthy cattle. At this point, Dr. Bruce's research was interrupted when he was recalled to military duty in Natal, but seven months later, in September 1885, he and his wife were back at Ubombo with permission from the war office to continue their work on nagana.

Assisted by his wife, Dr. Bruce next produced the disease in healthy animals by inoculating them with the blood of infected ones. He fed tsetse flies on sick cattle and noted the retention of the trypanosomes in their gut. Satisfying himself that tsetse flies fed on diseased animals could transmit nagana to healthy ones, Bruce became the first investigator to demonstrate transmission of a protozoan parasite by an insect bite.

Dr. Bruce was aware that although Europeans, like Livingston, thought that nagana came from tsetse fly bites, the Zulus believed that their cattle were being poisoned by something from wild game. He conducted a survey of the Zulu cattle kraals over many miles of territory, and found that animals kept in open country, away from wild game, were indeed more likely to be free of nagana than those kept near wild animal habitats. He succeeded in infecting a dog with nagana by inoculating it with the blood of an antelope, even though the antelope did not appear to be ill. He concluded that about one fourth of the local game animals harbored the *Haematozoa* in their blood without ill effects.

So both the Europeans and the Zulus had been correct. Nagana required the tsetse fly to transmit infection, but the reservoir host was wild game that could harbor the parasite without ill effects. No doubt cattle, dogs, and horses brought from Europe died because, unlike the native animals, they had not evolved to live in balance with the African trypanosome.

Happily, human beings are not susceptible to the trypanosome of nagana, and, in fact, Dr. Livingston wrote a description of the feeding habits of the tsetse after observing a fly taking a blood meal from his own hand.

It wasn't until 1901 that the first piece of the human African trypanosomiasis puzzle fell into place. On May 10 of that year, a forty-two-year-old Englishman named Kelly was admitted with a fever to the hospital in Bathurst, in the British colony of the Gambia on the west coast of Africa. The Gambia is a narrow strip of land on either bank of the Gambia River. Except at its coastal capital, Banjul, the former Bathurst, it is surrounded on all sides by the former French colony of Senegal.

Mr. Kelly was master of a government steam launch on the Gambia River, whose health "broke down after especially heavy duty occasioned by a punitive expedition up the river." Dr. R. M. Forde, the attending physician, made a fresh preparation of Kelly's blood, suspecting malaria, but was surprised to see many "actively moving, worm-like bodies" that he could not identify. On June 1 the patient was homebound, and on August 12 he was admitted to the Royal Southern Hospital in Liverpool.

During his hospital stay, Kelly had intermittent fevers. His liver was enlarged, as eventually was his spleen, which could be felt as a tender mass below his left ribs. The patient also complained of shortness of breath when he exerted himself. However, over the next four months, the pain in his spleen disappeared, and he felt well enough to return to the Gambia. But on the return voyage, in December 1901, he was attacked by pneumonia, and on arrival in Bathurst he was thin and easily fatigued. The shortness of breath had returned, and he now had weakness in his legs, loss of appetite, and intermittent insomnia. On December 16, he had a slight nosebleed—a subtle but ominous symptom of the disease to come.

At this point, Dr. Forde consulted a young colleague, Dr. J. Everett Dutton, who had just arrived in the Gambia on a scientific mission. Dr. Dutton, then about twenty-five, was a recent graduate of the Liverpool Medical School. On December 18, the two doctors examined Mr. Kelly.

The man had a "distinctly puffy and flushed" face; "the eyes appeared sunken" and watery; "there was a distinct fullness of the lower eyelids." Drs. Dutton and Forde found that Mr. Kelly's skin was congested and doughy, especially on the chest, thighs, and ankles. Irregular purplish blotches spotted his body.

Next the two physicians made a fresh preparation of Mr. Kelly's blood. Although there were now only a few protozoa moving between the red blood cells, Dr. Dutton recognized them as trypanosomes.

In his report in the *British Medical Journal* of September 1902, Dr. Dutton summarized what was then known about trypanosomal illness. Trypanosomes were responsible for nagana in Central Africa (Dr. Bruce's *Haematozoa* had since been identified), as well as for surra in India, and two other veterinary diseases, not tsetse-transmitted (*mal de caderas* and *dourine*). The affected animals had fever, swelling, red patches on the skin, and bleeding from the nose, just as Mr. Kelly did.

After a partial remission of his symptoms in January 1902, Kelly made his last voyage up the Gambia. Shortly thereafter, his sickness returned with full force, and he sailed home to England, where he died a few months later.

Not long after Dutton described this unfortunate patient, another case report appeared. The eminent Dr. Patrick Manson and his colleague Dr. C. W. Daniels published a detailed description of African trypanosomiasis in a forty-year-old white woman. While spending fifteen months at Monsembe, a mission station on the Upper Congo, she had suffered a painful bite by an unknown insect on her left leg. Two weeks later, on August 28, 1901, she began to have fever. She took quinine tablets for malaria, without benefit.

The woman returned home, and in September sought treatment at the London School of Tropical Medicine. Dr. Manson wrote that she was "a fair-skinned woman, having a somewhat plump and fictitiously healthy appearance," which he ascribed to the pink flushing and puffy swelling of her face. Like Mr. Kelly, the patient had an enlarged spleen. Later she developed the same patches of skin redness as well. Examination of her blood under the microscope showed trypanosomes and, like Kelly, she died after several months of debilitating illness.

The story of African trypanosomiasis now becomes intertwined with the career of one of the most colorful characters of the nineteenth century, Sir Henry Morton Stanley. Sir Henry began life in 1841 in Denbign, Wales, as John Rowlands, an illegitimate son whose mother abandoned him to the St. Asaph Workhouse. At fifteen he ran away, and at eighteen he sailed from Liverpool to New Orleans as a cabin boy. A kindly merchant, Henry Morton Stanley, adopted him there and gave him his name.

Stanley fought in the American Civil War, and worked on ships before becoming a journalist. In 1871, the *New York Herald* commissioned him to go to Africa. His mission was twofold; he was to write a report on the recently opened Suez Canal and then to find David Livingston, from whom there had been no news in five years. Stanley found the missionary explorer on Lake Tanganyika on November 10, 1871, addressing him with the immortal words, "Dr. Livingston, I presume?"

Between 1879 and 1884, Stanley explored the entire length

of the Congo River and helped King Leopold II of Belgium organize the Congo Free State. In 1887, funded by a British steamship company, Stanley set out to find and rescue Emin Pasha. Emin, a German explorer and physician whose original name was Eduard Schnitzer, had succeeded General Charles Gordon as governor of the Equatorial Province of Egypt, but the Mahdist revolt of 1882 had cut him off in the neighborhood of Lake Albert. Although it would never gain as much fame as his search for Livingston, Stanley's journey to rescue Emin Pasha would have a terrible impact on public health in Africa.

Stanley left England in January and reached Zanzibar on the East African coast (in present-day Tanzania) by way of the Suez Canal. After recruiting men there, he continued his voyage around the continent, arriving in March at the mouth of the Congo River, on the west coast of Africa at the northern border of present-day Angola. By June, Stanley and his men had reached the navigable head of the river at Yambuya, now in Zaire. He then set out with an advance guard and, after a grueling march through dense forest, reached Lake Albert five months later. It was another five months before Stanley made contact with Emin in April 1888.

The two men then traveled together around Lake Albert and Lake Victoria. Near Dar-es-Salaam, in present-day Tanzania, Stanley almost lost Emin Pasha for good, when Emin, his vision impaired by cataracts, fell off a second-floor balcony, breaking several ribs and fracturing his skull.

Although it helped to put Uganda into the British sphere of influence, this last expedition was, for Stanley, ill-fated in many ways. Emin Pasha did not return home with him but remained in Africa, only to be murdered three years later in the Congo. Stanley lost all of his officers in the rear guard when his friend, the Arab trader Tippu Tib, failed to send promised porters and supplies. Of the 646 men who started the trek in 1887, only 246 remained alive a year later. But the worst misfortune resulting from the expedition was only gradually revealed.

Toward the end of 1900, two brothers, Drs. Albert and Jack Cook, pioneer missionaries who had set up a bush hospital in Mengo, Uganda, began to see large numbers of patients with a virulent and fatal disease, previously unknown in the region. The patients had a bizarre sensitivity to cold, often setting huts on fire to warm themselves, and such a morbid craving for meat that they sometimes ate the dead bodies of their companions. This abnormally increased appetite, which has been linked to early stages of sleeping sickness, was succeeded by the classic symptoms of the disease.

Word of the epidemic reached London, and Sir Patrick Manson and Sir Ray Lankester arranged for a commission to send three investigating physicians to Uganda—Dr. G. C. Low, Dr. Cuthbert Christy, and Dr. Aldo Castellani. Theirs was not a congenial party; Drs. Low and Christy actually came to blows over precedence. Shortly after their arrival at Lake Victoria, Christy, the field man, went off into the bush to study the local distribution of sleeping sickness. (He was later killed by a rhinoceros.) Dr. Low stayed only a few weeks and then returned home, leaving the twenty-three-year-old Castellani on his own.

Castellani, who was not aware of Bruce's work with nagana, began performing spinal taps on patients sick with sleeping sickness. He found trypanosomes in the cerebrospinal fluids of seven of them, but he failed to grasp the significance of his findings, because he had a preconceived theory that sleeping sickness was caused by a bacterium. But on March 16, 1903, Dr. and Mrs. Bruce arrived at Entebbe. After a long discussion in which he was promised sole credit for his discovery, Dr. Castellani shared his findings with Dr. Bruce, who understood their significance immediately. Experiments on monkeys then demonstrated that the trypanosome of human sleeping sickness, like that of nagana, is transmitted by the bite of the tsetse fly.

By 1910, the sleeping sickness epidemic in Uganda had claimed over 200,000 lives, representing two thirds of the area's population. Experts now believe that this may have been the direct result of Henry Morton Stanley's last expedition. Of the native porters that Stanley had brought east along the Congo to central Africa, one or more had probably carried what became known as the West African form of trypanosomiasis in his bloodstream. The tsetse flies were already present along the Lake Victoria shores; once the trypanosomes were introduced, sleeping sickness spread rapidly through the human population with deadly results.

Caused by *Trypanosoma brucei gambiense,* West African or Gambian sleeping sickness is transmitted by the *Glossina palpalis* group of tsetse flies, which live in forests and wooded areas along rivers. Man is the favorite host of this fly, and human beings are the principal reservoir of the disease, although pigs may also play a role. Since West African sleeping sickness is primarily a human disease, the trypanosome and its human host have adapted to each other over the years to some extent. Many people infected with *T. brucei gambiense* may, like Stanley's porters, remain without symptoms for years and thus act as inadvertent natural reservoirs of infection.

In many patients, the disease begins with a painful sore at the site of the tsetse's bite. However, even without treatment, this trypanosomal chancre will heal in a few weeks. In the next stage, which occurs anywhere from weeks to many months following infection, the trypanosomes find their way into the lymph nodes and thence to the blood stream. It is in this stage that the victim may develop swollen glands in the neck, as Winterbottom had observed in slaves.

Patients in this stage of sleeping sickness often have swellings in the hands, feet, and face, and the red rash that Dutton and

Manson described in the case reports of the riverboat captain and the woman from the mission station. The patients may itch and complain of fever, headache, flulike symptoms with muscle aches and fatigue, weight loss, joint pains, and a racing pulse. In young women, the menstrual cycle ceases, and in men there is impotence.

In the final phase of West African sleeping sickness, the trypanosome invades the brain. This may not occur for months and even years after infection, but it is the inevitable fatal outcome in all untreated patients. The victim becomes indifferent and sleepy during the daytime, but may suffer from restlessness and insomnia at night. There is a loss of spontaneity and initiative, and the patient develops a listless stare. They may tremble and walk unsteadily, with odd movements of the °, neck, tongue, and extremities. Advanced sleeping sickness may mimic Parkinson's disease as a shuffling gait, muscle stiffness, tremors, and slurred speech develop. Joseph Conrad vividly describes the final phase, in which the patient stops eating, shrinks to cadaverous thinness, and finally slips into coma, in the following passage from *Heart of Darkness:*

> Black shapes crouched, lay, sat between the trees leaning against the trunks, clinging to the earth, half coming out, half effaced within the dim light, in all the attitudes of pain, abandonment, and despair . . . they were nothing earthly now—nothing but black shadows of disease and starvation, lying confusedly . . . the sunken eyes looked up at me, enormous and vacant, a kind of blind, white flicker in the depths of the orbs, which died out slowly.

However, as horrific as West African sleeping sickness is, it is not the most severe form of the disease. In 1910, Dr. J. W. Stephens of the Liverpool School of Tropical Medicine diagnosed African trypanosomiasis in a European hunter named William Armstrong. The patient had never traveled in any areas where Gambian sleeping sickness was known to occur, limiting his safari to Northern Rhodesia (present-day Zimbabwe). His trypanosomes, when inoculated into rats, killed quickly.

The agent of Rhodesian or East African sleeping sickness, as this virulent illness came to be called, is *Trypanosoma brucei rhodesiense,* and it is transmitted to man by tsetse flies of the *Glossina morsitans* group. The first epidemics of East African sleeping sickness occurred in the Luangwa Valley in Northern Rhodesia, and succeeding epidemics up to 1946 killed at least twenty thousand people in eastern Africa.

Similar to rabies, Rhodesian sleeping sickness is a zoonosis, an animal infection that finds its way into a human host, usually with dire results. In general, microorganisms and the animals that they infect evolve together, so that the host animal adapts over time to the presence of the microbial parasite. Bats, for example, carry the rabies virus without apparent ill effects, but the virus produces rapidly fatal infection if it finds its way into a human host.

The natural hosts of *Trypanosoma brucei rhodesiense* are wild animals, primarily the bushbuck and the hartebeest. Unless weakened by other diseases, these animals tolerate infection with this trypanosome quite well. But in cattle and people, *T. brucei rhodesiense* produces fatal infection. The tsetse flies that transmit this form of sleeping sickness inhabit dry, thorny scrub away from water. However, like all tsetses, they require shade and disappear during the hottest hours of the day.

Unfortunately, since Rhodesian sleeping sickness occurs in game parks, it is the form of the disease most often contracted by tourists visiting Africa. In 2001 alone, there were nine cases contracted in East African game parks. Patients often become ill within a few days of being bitten by an infected fly. Before the end of their trip or shortly after returning home, they may have fever, muscle aches, fatigue, and headache. Most patients develop a rash, but swollen lymph nodes are unusual in East African trypanosomiasis. A telltale trypanosomal sore or chancre may be present. One of the hallmarks of this infection is a racing pulse, as the trypanosomes cause severe and sometimes fatal inflammation of the heart.

Once infection reaches the brain, both forms of human African trypanosomiasis are uniformly fatal if not treated. The duration of the disease from tsetse bite to death ranges from about eight months to several years in West African sleeping sickness, but in the East African form, untreated patients die within a few weeks to months following infection.

Human African trypanosomiasis is therefore a disease that mandates swift treatment in all patients. However, therapy is difficult, dangerous, and expensive. The first drug developed for sleeping sickness, suramin, is still the most widely used. It is a complex synthetic organic compound that was developed by Bayer in Germany in 1920, based on the observation by Paul Ehrlich that certain dyes, like trypan red and blue, not only stained trypanosomes but also killed them. While sharing some of the structural features of the synthetic dyes, suramin is actually a white powder.

When the newly synthesized compound was ready for clinical trials, Bayer Pharmaceuticals petitioned the British government to allow tests of suramin to proceed in Northern Rhodesia. But, in the aftermath of World War I, there was considerable reluctance. However, Winston Churchill, then colonial secretary, overruled officials, and the first patients were successfully treated.

No one is exactly sure how suramin works, but it is active against the early stages of both West and East African sleeping sickness. Suramin should only be administered under close medical supervision, because, in rare patients, it may precipitate shock and death within minutes. It can also be quite toxic to the kidneys.

A complete course of therapy is given intravenously and is spread out over twenty-one days.

Another drug that is effective against the early stages of both types of human African trypanosomiasis is pentamidine. Introduced in 1939, pentamidine is given over ten days. It may cause vomiting, a racing heart, and a dangerous drop or climb in blood sugar. It can also damage the pancreas and kidneys, but it is less toxic than suramin. However, the drug is too expensive to use in most African hospitals and clinics. Another problem with pentamidine is that the trypanosome of East African sleeping sickness is developing resistance to its effects.

Neither suramin nor pentamidine penetrate the central nervous system well enough to cure sleeping sickness once the trypanosomes reach the brain. At this point, very dangerous treatment is necessary. For over fifty years there has been only one drug that can cure late-stage East African sleeping sickness, the arsenic compound melarsoprol, introduced in 1949. Melarsoprol is a terrifying drug to administer, because it is only slightly less toxic to people than it is to trypanosomes. The drug is dissolved in propylene glycol—an intense irritant—and it must be given very slowly, through a fine needle placed in a secure intravenous line. If any of it leaks into the flesh, it can cause a deep, destructive wound, on rare occasions forcing amputation of an arm. And since propylene glycol dissolves ordinary intravenous tubing, it has to be administered through special coated tubing.

In up to eighteen percent of patients, melarsoprol causes a severe, often fatal brain reaction within the first four days of treatment. The drug may also damage the heart or the liver. Treatment consists of at least three courses of three days each, with one-week rest periods in between. For obvious reasons, melarsoprol should only be given in the hospital.

The only new drug for human African trypanosomiasis is

eflornithine, the so-called resurrection drug. Eflornithine was initially developed in the 1970s as a possible cancer-fighting medicine, but was found to have more activity against the trypanosomes. In 1983, Belgian physician Henri Taelman used eflornithine to successfully treat a comatose woman in Antwerp.

Eflornithine is active only against West African sleeping sickness, but, as its name suggests, it is often miraculously effective even in cases where the infection has reached the brain. The drug selectively poisons a vital enzyme in the parasite, called ornithine decarboxylase. Of four hundred patients with West African sleeping sickness treated with the drug in 1988, only twenty-eight died. For the six percent of Gambian sleeping sickness patients whose infection relapses after melarsoprol therapy, eflornithine is the only chance of survival. Eflornithine is relatively nontoxic, with diarrhea, seizures, and hair loss being its major side effects. Doctors in Canada used eflornithine to cure the delusional French human rights worker whose case history opened this chapter. The following report shows the life-saving actions of the drug in children.

In January 1985, the parents of a three-and-a-half-year-old girl brought her to the Children's Hospital of Oakland, California, with a two- to three-month history of unsteady walking and frequent fevers. The child, who had been speaking in full sentences, was now uttering only single words.

The patient was the twelfth child in her family and was born prematurely, at seven months. Delivered at a hospital in Kinshasa, Congo, she weighed less than five pounds at birth. Despite her small size, she was hospitalized only one day. When she was four months old, the family left Kinshasa. Shortly after arrival in the United States at the age of seventeen months, the girl was hospitalized with fever and swollen lymph nodes. Her doctors noted that she was underweight, anemic, and had "gross motor dysfunction."

Between eighteen and thirty-six months of age, the child was seen thirteen times in the clinics and emergency rooms for various complaints, among which three were classic for human African trypanosomiasis: fever, hand swelling, and rashes. Despite this, the diagnosis was never considered.

In January 1985, however, the child's symptoms and signs clearly pointed to a serious disorder affecting her brain. Her physicians performed a lumbar puncture (spinal tap), and when the cerebrospinal fluid was spun in a centrifuge, they saw a large number of trypanosomes under the microscope. Based on her country of origin, the diagnosis was West African sleeping sickness.

The child's treatment was delayed, because her parents refused to consent to any form of treatment. After ten days, a judge granted permission through the courts. Eflornithine was administered by vein for two weeks and then by mouth for another four. By the time the therapy was completed, the child was able to walk without support, though she was still unsteady. Her language recovery was dramatic; she progressed from single words in Lingala and French, her native languages, to short sentences in her new language, English. Over the next three months, the child continued to improve, and seven months after discharge from the hospital she was almost completely normal. Two years later she was ready to begin kindergarten with her peers.

Despite the fact that the incidence of sleeping sickness has increased nearly a hundredfold in the last forty years, returning to levels as high as those of the 1950s, eflornithine was never a profitable venture for its manufacturer, Aventis. It requires intravenous administration in the hospital for the first two weeks, which is not feasible for poor patients in Central Africa. So, in 1995, Aventis halted its production, along with that of melarsoprol and pentamidine. Simultaneously, Bayer AG threatened to stop making suramin.

Jean Jannin at the World Health Organization (WHO) and the group Médecins Sans Frontières worked frantically to try to stave off disaster. But it was hairy women in rich countries who provided at least a temporary reprieve. Exploiting the eflornithine side effect of hair loss, Bristol Myers Squibb in North America had formulated a topical preparation of the drug, which they called Vaniqua, to eliminate facial hair. Jannin's group at WHO persuaded Bristol Myers Squibb to donate eflornithine for five years, starting in 2001. Additional lobbying induced Aventis and Bayer to continue to produce the other drugs for sleeping sickness, also for five years, and to donate five million dollars a year during that time to the fight against human African trypanosomiasis.

The threat of catastrophic shortages of antitrypanosomal drugs comes at a time when efforts to control sleeping sickness are failing all over Africa. In Tambura County in southern Sudan, twenty percent of the population is infected with either East or West African sleeping sickness in an epidemic that is sweeping the region and merging with another epidemic in the adjoining Central African Republic. This Sudan outbreak has its roots in a civil war in which the southern-led rebel force, the Sudanese People's Liberation Army, is battling the government in Khartoum. War, famine, the movement of refugees, and the breakdown of the rural health system have contributed to perhaps hundreds of thousands of new sleeping sickness cases. Most of these will remain untreated and end tragically in death.

Ironically, it is not only the disruptions of war that lead to sleeping sickness outbreaks, but the very efforts being made for economic recovery. The Soroti District in east-central Uganda, an area previously free of sleeping sickness, suffered an outbreak between December 1998 and June 2000. Although only about sixty cases were recorded annually, the patients all had the rapidly lethal East African form of the disease.

The roots of this outbreak can be traced to the Ugandan civil war in the late 1970s, during the mass movement of people and livestock out of Soroti. After the area was depopulated and left uncultivated, it reverted to bush habitat suitable for the tsetse fly. As people started to return in the 1990s, the Soroti could not reestablish herds, because of cattle rustling by hostile members of the Karimojong ethnic group.

In 2000, when the political situation finally stabilized, the national government helped the Soroti to buy cattle from southeastern Uganda. Unfortunately, eight percent of the imported cattle were carrying *Trypanosoma brucei rhodesiense,* and a human outbreak began, centered around the Brookes Corner cattle market, where the imported cattle were being sold.

Our failure to devise human and veterinary vaccines has resulted in our inability to control human African trypanosomiasis. Unfortunately, it is unlikely that a vaccine will ever be developed in the future, as trypanosomes have evolved a powerful mechanism for eluding the host's immune defenses.

The trypanosome carries on its surface a protective coat of variable surface glycoproteins, which are proteins to which sugars are attached. Early in the course of infection, animals and human beings generate antibodies that are able to kill 99 percent of the trypanosomes carrying a given glycoprotein coat. However, a few of the protozoa always escape, as they are able to synthesize a different variable surface glycoprotein to which the host is not immune. Hidden by this new mask, these trypanosomes multiply and again fill the bloodstream. If the patient has enjoyed a fever-free interval, the appearance of the new clone of parasites causes a relapse. The process continues twenty times or more until the trypanosome invades the patient's central nervous system and escapes circulating blood antibodies altogether. In this way, the trypanosome is like the much smaller human immunodeficiency virus. Both have frustrated all attempts to create protective vaccines because of their ability to change their outer membrane proteins.

Since the colonial period, there have been repeated efforts to control sleeping sickness by eliminating the tsetse fly or restricting its reservoir hosts, wild game. In 1945, after the end of World War II, returning South African Air Force pilots and their ground crews were recruited to perform aerial spraying of DDT over game parks. By 1954, they had successfully eradicated tsetse flies from Zululand, and cattle can now be raised there. However, a downside is that long-acting insecticides are too toxic to the environment and too expensive to apply in most areas in Africa.

The most draconian and controversial method of sleeping sickness control is the destruction of wild game. It was first attempted in 1911 in Nyasaland (in present-day Malawi) by a commission headed by Dr. David Bruce. A second extermination campaign was also carried out in East Africa in the 1950s.

In addition to being repugnant to practically everyone, these efforts were ultimately doomed to failure for two reasons. The tsetse flies, deprived of the hartebeest, the lion, and the bushbuck, turned to smaller mammals that had not been targeted for destruction. Herdsmen and their livestock moving into the cleared areas became new hosts to the tsetse and the trypanosome. Wildlife elimination programs were then abandoned.

In his essay on sleeping sickness, "The Fly Who Would Be King," Dr. Robert Desowitz points out the ironic truth that, by preventing overexploitation of enormous areas of Africa, "the tsetse and the trypanosome are the most stalwart guardians of the African ecosystem and its magnificent wild fauna."

In Africa today there are at least three epidemics of human trypanosomiasis in progress. The largest epidemic is centered in the Democratic Republic of Congo, affecting also the Central

African Republic and southern Sudan, with approximately a hundred thousand cases of West and East African sleeping sickness. The cause is recurrent civil war, and the final effects will depend in part on the attitude of international donors toward the new regime in the Congo.

In a review of the problem in the *British Medical Bulletin,* the authors wrote that, despite the presence of twenty-five mobile teams in the Congo, the "ridiculous salaries, poorly motivated staff, dismal road conditions, recurrent petrol shortages and widespread corruption all damaged the efficacy of mobile teams" in controlling the epidemic.

The second epidemic is in Angola, where Gambian (West African) sleeping sickness, which had been under control up to 1974, has been resurfacing since the civil war began in 1976. Contributing factors are continued tension between warring factions and the complete collapse of the health system. In some northern districts, sleeping sickness is now a major cause of adult mortality. Villages are abandoned as their dying inhabitants lie helpless along the roadsides in the glaring sun.

Finally, an epidemic of East African trypanosomiasis caused forty thousand confirmed cases between 1976 and 1990 and is still continuing. Again, according to the *British Medical Bulletin,* "war, insecurity, civil unrest, and deteriorating economic circumstances led to a breakdown of health service and disease control." Political turmoil brought ecological disaster. As crop cultivation declined, large tracts of intensively cultivated land fell into disuse and were replaced by the scrub and brush habitat of *Glossina morsitans,* the tsetse of East African sleeping sickness.

Victims of this epidemic arrive at medical clinics with irreversible advanced disease. If they are treated at all, they still frequently die in coma, of toxic brain reactions to melarsoprol, of secondary infections, or of heart failure. In some villages, more than 25 percent of the population has contracted trypanosomiasis.

The three regional epidemics of sleeping sickness, combined with some two hundred microfoci—areas where trypanosomes, suitable tsetse flies, and human beings exist in close proximity—place some sixty million Africans at risk for the disease. Approximately half a million people already carry the parasite and will eventually die if left untreated.

Although human African trypanosomiasis has existed on the continent since prehistoric times, wide dissemination of the parasite only began to occur during the colonial period, when Africans infected with the disease left their ancient homelands at the behest of the Europeans, made long journeys, and worked far from their villages. Roads and railways helped diseases to disseminate widely, and ecological disruptions caused by European influences had unexpected effects. Despite this, some measure of disease control was maintained as long as the colonial empires held sway. But as the Europeans left Africa, civil wars unraveled control efforts and health services.

None of these remote consequences were foreseen in the nineteenth century by Europeans who came to Africa as missionaries, explorers, and exploiters. Young doctors came simply to test themselves against new diseases whose infectious agents and modes of transmission lay open to discovery. But Africa is not a sanctuary for the intellect or a place to test one's ideals. It is a vast unknown, impartially dangerous to the unwary.

In 1903, Lieutenant Forbes Tulloch, a medical officer with the sleeping sickness commission in Entebbe, Uganda, began having unexplained fevers. On March 12, his colleagues found trypanosomes in his blood. Knowing that there was no treatment for sleeping sickness, Tulloch, accompanied by his colleague Lieutenant Gray, left Uganda in April and traveled down the Nile. He died in June of that year, at the age of twenty-seven.

Dr. Tulloch was not the only researcher to fall to disease. Between 1899 and 1914, the Liverpool School of Tropical Medicine sent out thirty-two expeditions to equatorial Africa. Drs. John Lancelot Todd and Joseph Everett Dutton were companions on two of the expeditions. Dr. Dutton, it will be remembered, had already established his reputation by identifying trypanosomes in the blood of a human case for the first time—that of the boat captain Kelly, who had contracted sleeping sickness on the Gambia River.

On August 21, 1902, the two young men set sail for the Gambia as part of the society's tenth expedition. Dr. Todd, a twenty-six-year-old from Canada, wrote a series of enraptured letters home. In their dispensary and laboratory at Cape St. Mary, near Bathurst, the two doctors worked long hours seeing patients and conducting research. They dissected a horse that had died of trypanosomiasis. They even once rowed all night to attend to a trader with the disease, only to arrive shortly after the trader had died.

Two years later in 1903, the young men again set out together, this time to the Congo territory as part of the twelfth expedition of the Liverpool School of Tropical Medicine. By the end of 1904, they had reached Stanley Falls, in the interior of present-day Zaire. It was here that their luck ran out.

Dr. Dutton's last letter home was dated February 9. Illustrated with drawings, it was full of details about their most recent work on tick fever. Shortly afterward, he accidentally pricked himself while conducting a postmortem examination on a patient, and contracted the disease. He died of tick-borne relapsing fever at the age of twenty-nine and was buried at Kosongo, Congo. The causative organism, *Borrelia duttoni,* was later named in his honor.

Dr. John L. Todd also fell ill with tick fever, but he recovered. In 1907 he returned to Canada, where he became professor of parasitology at McGill University. It was about five years after his return that he mailed his letters to the physicians of British Columbia asking about adverse effects following tick bite, and so learned about tick paralysis. Dr. Todd had a long and distinguished career and died in 1949.

Nowadays we are barraged with reports about the African epidemic of human immunodeficiency virus infection. But outside the urban centers in South Africa, Rwanda, and Uganda, lethal outbreaks of sleeping sickness continue to kill the world's poorest and most isolated people. It is no longer politically correct to call Africa the Dark Continent, as Sir Henry Morton Stanley did in 1878. But if there is a heart of darkness beating there, it's the trypanosome—flickering behind the vacant stare of an African dying along a river or a road.

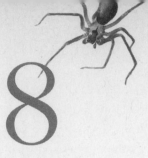

8

Sponge Face
and
Black Fever

Peru, the third largest country in South America, had
its beginnings in the ancient Andean cities of the Inca. Today, the
country could not function without a twentieth-century inven-
tion, the airplane. Before air travel, the preferred route from Iquitos
on the upper Amazon to the capital, Lima, six hundred miles away,
was a seven-thousand-mile detour down the Amazon to the Atlantic, over the Isthmus of Panama to the Pacific, and thence
down the coast. The Andes, towering over fifteen thousand feet,
formed an impenetrable north-south barrier.

The dense tropical rain forests that comprise over half the
area of present-day Peru are also arduous to traverse. Puerto Maldonado, a jungle frontier town on the Madre de Dios River in
southeastern Peru, can be reached by ground transportation from
Cusco only during the dry season. Even then it's a treacherous
three-day trip over the Andes on mostly unpaved road. By air it's
a one-hour flight, weather permitting.

On November 9, 2002, a group of professional biologists from

Earthwatch, accompanied by volunteer research assistants, arrived at Puerto Maldonado. They drove down the unpaved main street with its motorbike taxis, passing wooden and cement-block houses, a school, and a small hospital, to the Central Research Office, where they registered their expedition. From Puerto Maldonado the group continued two hours southeast by bus and boat to the Posadas Amazonas Lodge on the Tambopata River, near the Bolivian border.

Although there is no electricity, and light is produced by oil lamp and candles, the Posada Amazonas is said to be one of the best jungle lodges in the world. The group listened to orientation lectures and reviewed important tropical hazards to avoid, such as malaria, venomous snakes, and the parasite *Leishmania*.

The next day the group made the six-hour river trip to the Tambopata Research Center, located in the heart of the Tambopata Candano National Reserve. The Research Center includes a kitchen, dining area, bathrooms, and living quarters for twenty-five people. It is built on four-foot stilts and connected by thatch-covered causeways. Living quarters consist of three closed walls, with the fourth open to the jungle. Mosquito netting envelops each bed.

The kitchen and dining room are open patios with overhanging thatched roofs. The macaws, which were the subjects of the group's research project, do not confine themselves to their jungle habitat but frequently fly into the rooms and dining area, foraging for forbidden handouts. Visitors learn to avoid sitting under macaws perched on the rafters.

The Tambopata Candano National Reserve is home to seven percent of the world's bird species (about six hundred) and four percent of the earth's mammal species, including thirteen endangered species, such as the great anteater and the jaguar. The habitat near the station is waterlogged swamp forest, dominated by palms and bamboo, and clay forest with broadleaf trees.

A volunteer research assistant I'll call Alfred Eliah, a seventy-two-year-old retired chemistry professor, and his wife, Helene, had previously worked as volunteers in central Mexico on a fossil dig. On another trip further south, Alfred had contracted dengue fever. The couple had survived bouts of turista, and Alfred had a scar on his left arm, a souvenir from Costa Rica, when an octopus bit him. This, however, was their first trip to the tropical forests of Peru.

Alfred and Helene completed a week of six- to seven-hour shifts, either under a nest tree recording the movements of macaws or observing the birds visiting a clay lick. The lick was located fifteen minutes by boat down the river, and, on one of her shifts, Helene had to be rescued and moved to higher ground because of heavy rains.

For protection against the insect swarms, Alfred and his wife wore long-sleeved shirts, pants tucked into rubber boots, gloves, and mosquito head nets. They sprayed themselves and their clothing with DEET insect repellant. Despite these measures, Alfred said that when they returned to their quarters at the end of their shifts they looked "like pin cushions."

The volunteer research assistants, when not on duty, photographed the wildlife, including six species of monkeys, many exotic birds, butterflies, and flowers. They hiked through the jungle with local guides. One of the guides had two peculiar ulcers on his arm, leishmania sores, they told Alfred.

The week of Thanksgiving, the Eliahs returned to the United States and settled into the holiday season, shuttling between their cabin in the snowy San Gabriel Mountains near Los Angeles and their home in Port Hueneme north of the city. They showed friends and relatives photographs of their trip, red and green macaws, their rustic room with its open wall, the dining patio, but tropical Peru seemed far away now.

It was at the end of December that Alfred first noticed one and then two red bumps under the right side of his chin. He gave them little thought at first. They seemed like pimples from shaving irritation, or maybe ingrown hairs.

But the bumps didn't go away. Instead, though painless, they got gradually larger. Their tops broke open to form shallow ulcers, which drained a small amount of yellow fluid. Alfred dabbed them with an antibiotic ointment, without effect. At the end of January, he became aware of a vague swelling just under the point of his chin, also painless. Over the next week it slowly enlarged to the size and the firmness of a hard-boiled egg yolk. The ulcers had also gotten bigger; each was now about a quarter-inch across.

It was at this point that Alfred realized that the ulcers under his chin and the lesion on the guide's arm looked disturbingly similar. He tried to remember what he had been told at the orientation lectures in the jungle lodge. Leishmania was a one-celled protozoan parasite, transmitted, like malaria, by the bite of an insect, not a mosquito but a midget-sized fly.

On February 1, 2003, Alfred Eliah came to the walk-in clinic at my hospital, which is part of his health maintenance organization. He showed the ulcers and the swelling under his chin to a physician on duty, and told him about his tropical exposure and about the warnings he had received. The doctor took one look at Alfred's sores and decided to consult a specialist in infectious diseases.

It was mid-Friday afternoon at the end of a rather routine week on call. I was in my office when my beeper went off. The doctor who answered the phone didn't mince words.

"I've got a seventy-two-year-old guy down here who was in a jungle in Peru and now has a weird ulcer. He says he thinks it might be leishmaniasis."

I had never seen a case of leishmaniasis, but I knew that the

American form, untreated, could eat up the middle of a person's face, starting with his nose. The Portuguese in Brazil call the condition *espundia,* or sponge, because that's what the patient's face becomes—a ragged, porous hole, like a sea sponge.

"I'll be right down," I said.

Leishmania belongs to the same family of protozoans as the trypanosomes of sleeping sickness. Both of these groups of one-celled animals are hemoflagellates. They live in the blood streams of their hosts and, during at least part of their life cycles, they have a whiplike structure, the flagellum.

Credit for the first description of a protozoan in a chronic ulcer is usually given to Dr. D. D. Cunningham, a British medical officer in India, who made microscopic sections of flesh snipped from a skin lesion called Delhi boil. Cunningham published a description in 1885 of "nucleoid bodies," but he mistook the host cell engulfing the parasite for the parasite itself. Nor did he understand the protozoan nature of the creature, pronouncing it a fungus.

The true discoverer of the organism we now call *Leishmania* was Dr. Alfred Borovsky, a medical officer with the Imperial Russian Army. In 1892, aged twenty-nine, he was appointed to Turkestan, in central Asia, to take charge of the Surgical Department and Bacteriological Laboratory of the Tashkent Military Hospital. The most valuable piece of equipment in Dr. Borovsky's simple laboratory was a Zeiss microscope, which he brought with him from Saint Petersburg.

Dr. Borovsky became interested in a chronic skin ulcer called, after a local tribe, Sart sore. Borovsky believed that Sart sore was identical to similar, slowly healing and sometimes disfiguring skin conditions in the Middle East, called, variously, oriental sore, Aleppo boil, and Pendeh sore. Although he was unfamiliar with Cunningham's work, Borovsky had read papers on this condition, in which the authors had advanced various species of bacteria as the causative agent. But, based on his own inconclusive bacteriological results, he was skeptical and reluctant to believe these theories.

Under the microscope, Borovsky examined fluid and tissue scrapings from the sores. He took biopsy specimens from patients and prepared stained-tissue sections on glass slides. After a prolonged search, Borovsky found cells in the tissues, which he correctly identified as belonging to the patient's own immune system. Today we would call these cells that gobble up invaders macrophages. The cells were stuffed with many small, round bodies, like beads of tapioca. Using the highest power of his microscope, he could see within the small bodies a nucleus. In some cases, he could just make out a second, smaller, dark-staining knob, now called a kinetoplast, which he knew to be found in protozoa that have a flagellum. Based on these findings, Borovsky wrote, in the journalistic plural, "we are inclined to refer the parasites described by us to the class of protozoa."

In 1898, Dr. Borovsky published his findings in Russian in a journal with limited circulation. The international medical community remained ignorant of his discoveries for many years. In fact, they might never have come to light if, in the late 1920s, certain Russian doctors had not brought them to the attention of Dr. C. M. Hoare, of the Wellcome Bureau of Scientific Research in London. Not until 1938, six years after Borovsky died, was his paper published in its entirety in English. Unrecognized in major textbooks even today, Borovsky was a meticulous and insightful microscopist who deserves his place in history.

However, the physician after whom the protozoan was named, Major W. B. Leishman, was directly inspired not by work on oriental sore but by Dutton and Forde's description of the riverboat captain with sleeping sickness and of the parasite they found in his blood. Like Dutton and Forde, Dr. Leishman was struggling to help patients with another chronic tropical fever that did not respond to malaria treatment.

The disease first appeared in epidemic form around 1887 in Southern Assam, in eastern India. The patients had fever, an enlarged spleen, and a peculiar, black skin color that gave the illness its native name kala azar—black fever. Kala azar spread gradually along the lines of communication, clinging to the cultivated valleys where it wiped out whole villages. In some areas, cultivated lands fell back into jungle. The disease moved through the region at a rate of about five miles per year. In each affected village, the earliest cases usually began after the arrival of people from an affected locality.

Soon cases began to appear among the colonial population in and around the Dum Dum military station near Calcutta in nearby Bengal State. Doctors there called the illness "Dum Dum fever" and thought at first that it was an atypical form of malaria, because, as in malaria, the spleen was always enlarged. Thinking the hot Indian climate was impeding their recoveries, the afflicted English colonists usually returned home. In a 1905 lecture given in San Francisco, Dr. Patrick Manson described the thwarted hopes of these invalids:

> . . . in spite of quinine, in spite of aperients, in spite of tonics, in spite of change, in spite of the many therapeutic measures friends and physicians suggest, the case goes slowly to the bad, and the patient, after a few months or even a year or two, dies.

One such patient was J.B., a twenty-three-year-old private with the Royal Irish Rifles, who had served in India and, in April 1900, was an invalid with Dum Dum fever in the military hospital in Netley, England. When he died seven months later, Dr. Leishman made stained smears of the pulp of his grossly enlarged spleen and examined them under the microscope. The report of his findings appeared in a paper published in the *British Medical Journal* of May 30, 1903. "I was struck," he wrote, "by the curious appearance . . . of enormous numbers of small round or oval bodies . . . which corresponded with nothing I had previously met with or had seen figured or described."

However, on closer examination, Dr. Leishman observed within the little cells the two pigmented knobs, one large and the other small, found in all members of the trypanosome family. Because of their resemblance to some of the microscopic bodies seen in animals with nagana and in Dutton and Forde's patient with sleeping sickness, Leishman thought he had discovered a variation of these African diseases in India.

Just two months later, Captain C. Donovan, Second Physician at the Government General Hospital in Madras, India, hurried into print a preliminary report of his observations of the same organism. Not only had he observed the protozoa in the spleens of three patients who had succumbed to "chronic Malaria," but he had also obtained them from a living twelve-year-old boy by splenic puncture. In this audacious procedure, still used in India today, the physician introduces a large hollow needle through the left side of the patient's abdominal wall into the spleen to capture a long plug of the living tissue.

The two nearly simultaneous reports set off an immediate scramble for precedence, which was effectively settled by the eminent Dr. R. Ross, one of the discoverers of the malarial parasite. He validated the equality and simultaneity of the two reports and dubbed the parasitized cells Leishman-Donovan bodies. The infecting protozoan was ultimately named *Leishmania donovani.*

Although the causative organism is a cousin of the trypanosomes of sleeping sickness, kala azar or Dum Dum fever was a separate and distinct disease. Within the next few years the Leishman-Donovan bodies were found in patients suffering from an identical illness in China, Africa, the Assam region of India, and in southern Italy. Regardless of where they contracted the disease, all the patients eventually died. Dr. Manson vividly described the appearance of the sufferers at the end:

> . . . the spleen and liver are enlarged, the anaemia is pronounced, the physical weakness is marked, and there is generally progressive emaciation: so that the penultimate clinical outcome is the production of a big-bellied, emaciated, sallow, dirty skinned, anaemic, fever-stricken patient . . .

But kala azar—or visceral leishmaniasis, as it is known today—while the most dangerous, is not the only form the disease takes. Alfred Borovsky, the forgotten Russian microscopist, had already observed the protozoan in patients with oriental sore in 1898. But it wasn't until 1903 that an American pathologist Dr. James Homer Wright rediscovered the organism in the chronic ulcer of an Armenian patient at the Massachusetts General Hospital in Boston. Dr. Wright christened the protozoan of oriental sore *Leishmania tropica.* We now know that *Leishmania tropica* is one of several species that primarily infects the skin—and sometimes the moist membranes of the face—rather than the liver and spleen.

But how do patients become infected with *Leishmania*? In oriental sore there is a striking predilection for lesions to occur on the exposed parts of the body—face, legs, and arms. Skin covered by clothing is rarely affected. It seemed reasonable to assume that oriental sore and kala azar were contracted from the bite of some insect, just as sleeping sickness had been shown to be.

An astounding discovery in 1904 added weight to the insect theory of transmission. In that year, Sir Leonard Rogers, working in Calcutta, placed a tiny piece of *Leishmania*-infected spleen into a solution of nutrient salts. When he examined the culture fluid a week later, Rogers found that his small round Leishman-Donovan bodies had given rise to large numbers of motile, eel-like protozoa equipped with whiplike flagella. This is exactly the form a trypanosome takes in the body of a tsetse fly, suggesting that Dr. Rogers had discovered the insect phase of leishmaniasis.

But it was at this point in the investigation of kala azar that researchers stumbled into one of the most unfortunate blind alleys in the history of science. In 1907, Dr. W. S. Patton, working in Madras, India, fed bedbugs on kala azar patients and succeeded in transforming Leishman-Donovan bodies from the patients' blood into flagellated bodies in the insect's intestine. As Dr. Robert Desowitz observed in his essay "In Search of Kala Azar,"

> The bedbug, even when dignified by its Latin name of *Cimex lectularius,* is a loathsome creature. During the depth of night it creeps from its hiding places—whether the cracks of mud-walled hovels in the tropics or the steam pipes and crannies of North American's tenements—to feed on its sleeping blood supply.

It seemed likely that the despicable bedbug was the perpetrator of kala azar, but there were problems with the theory from the outset. In five years of experiments from 1907 to 1912, Dr. Patton was able to infect only a few of the many bedbugs that feasted on his patients. In addition, he was never able to demonstrate migration of flagellates to the bug's salivary glands, as happened in the insect vector in both malaria and sleeping sickness. Although there are some insects that transmit protozoan parasites directly through the feces, this did not seem possible in the bedbug because the flagellates did not flourish in the insect's gut, but died out after a few days.

Despite a lack of supportive evidence, medical protozoologists were reluctant to abandon the bedbug theory. As late as 1922, Mrs. Helen Adie, a kala azar researcher working in Calcutta, claimed to have found the elusive trypanosome in the saliva of the insect at last. On closer examination, however, the organism turned out to be *Nosema,* a bedbug parasite, and not a trypanosome after all.

The first real breakthrough in the search for the insect transmitter of leishmaniasis came not by observations made through a microscope but by deductive reasoning. Major John Sinton of the Indian Medical Service compared the geographic distribution of kala azar in eastern India with maps showing the habitats of various bloodsucking insects there. Based on the areas of overlap, Sinton wrote in 1924 and 1925 that the best candidate insect was the sandfly, *Phlebotomus argentipes.*

Major Sinton's theory was absolutely correct. Regardless of what form it takes or on what continent it occurs, leishmaniasis is always contracted from the bite of the unobtrusive sandfly. However, it took almost fifteen years of frustrating research to confirm the chain of transmission in the laboratory.

By 1925, Dr. Robert Knowles of the Calcutta School of Tropical Medicine had accomplished the essential first step. He had established a colony of sandflies in the laboratory, a difficult feat, as the flies are finicky in their requirements. He then fed these leishmania-free flies on kala azar patients and was gratified to find that even twelve days later the flagellate forms of the leishmania parasite were alive and well in the sandflies' intestines. The next step, however, was the crucial one. As Dr. Desowitz aptly puts it, "an infected sandfly had to bite a human 'guinea pig,' and that human had to come down with kala azar."

For the next fourteen years, scientists of the Indian Kala Azar Commission performed experiments that would be impossible to carry out under modern standards governing research on human subjects. By feeding infected sandflies on people, they tried to infect them with kala azar. However, all attempts to transmit the disease through the bites of infected sandflies failed.

Finally, in 1939, Dr. R. O. Smith, a medical entomologist working in Bihar, India, discovered that if he gave leishmania-infected sandflies a fruit meal (raisins worked well), the flagellates multiplied to enormous numbers, plugging the sandflies' throats. Unlike the malaria parasite and the trypanosome, sandflies don't inject the parasitic protozoan into their victim with their saliva. They vomit it into the wound from their obstructed and over-flowing gullets. In 1940, Drs. C. S. Swaminath and Henry Edward Shortt allowed infected, raisin-fed sandflies to feed on six Indian volunteers. Three of them came down with kala azar.

Sandflies are mosquito-shaped insects, only a tenth of an inch long. Weak fliers, they tend to hover near their abodes in the cracks of walls of houses, in rubbish, or in rodent burrows. In the forest, sandflies are abundant in tree holes, near pools of water, and around clearings and farms. Females of the genus *Phlebotomas* in the Old World and *Lutzomyia* in the Americas are the vectors of leishmaniasis.

Sandflies are intolerant of cold climates, which explains why leishmaniasis is only contracted in tropical and subtropical regions. Despite these limitations, the World Health Organization reports that leishmaniasis is currently endemic in eighty-eight countries on five continents—Africa, Asia, Europe, North America, and

South America. They estimate that twelve million people are infected with the parasite worldwide.

Every year about a half million people contract the visceral form of leishmaniasis, kala azar. Ninety percent of these cases occur in Bangladesh, Brazil, India, Nepal, and Sudan. Visceral leishmaniasis also occurs in countries bordering the Mediterranean (Spain, France, and Italy) and in Portugal. In this region, the disease often occurs in people infected with the human immunodeficiency virus (HIV). These patients are not only highly susceptible to leishmaniasis, but the parasite multiplies in them exuberantly and teems in their bloodstream, making them walking incubators of infection for others. Coinfection with *Leishmania* and HIV also occurs in Africa and in South America, as in the following patient reported in the *New England Journal of Medicine*.

A fifty-five-year-old HIV-positive man from Guyana was hospitalized in Toronto with a history of low-grade fevers for one week and diarrhea for two months. Despite taking a cocktail of powerful antiviral drugs, the patient had advanced acquired immunodeficiency syndrome (AIDS).

Tests of the man's blood showed anemia and a diminished number of the blood-clotting bodies called platelets. His liver was moderately enlarged, but the most remarkable finding on examination was a massively swollen spleen. A normal spleen is tucked up under the left ribs and just out of reach of the doctor's probing fingertips. This man's spleen was felt below the level of his belly button.

A physician performed a bone marrow biopsy. In this procedure, a large, hollow needle is forced, under local anesthesia, into the center of a bone, usually the hip or the sternum. The doctor then attaches a syringe to the end of the needle, and aspirates a sample of bone marrow. A drop is then smeared on a glass slide, which is treated with a sequence of special stains.

In addition to being the body's blood-making factory, the bone marrow is richly endowed with macrophages, which gobble up *Leishmania*. Unable to kill and digest the parasites, they become the microscopic mobile nurseries Drs. Borovsky, Leishman, and Donovan first described—and the hallmark of the disease.

This patient's bone marrow showed abundant macrophages crammed with leishmania parasites. A culture confirmed the diagnosis, and the patient showed some improvement with antiparasitic therapy, though in his state of advanced immunodeficiency, the illness is usually ultimately incurable.

Even before the days of HIV, epidemic waves of visceral leishmaniasis swept over wide areas. From 1890 through 1937, there were three such epidemics in northeastern India. Bihar State in the same region is currently battling an epidemic that began in the 1970s when insecticide spraying for malaria ceased. Up to 1999, there were approximately two hundred thousand new cases annually.

Kala azar can also invade new regions when the conditions are right. Refugee populations resulting from a civil war introduced *Leishmania donovani* into southern Sudan where the illness had been previously unknown. Despite the heroic efforts of Médicins Sans Frontières, more than ten percent of the population succumbed to what came to be known as "the killing disease."

Not only war, but also changes associated with social progress have expanded the habitat of the sandfly and the *Leishmania* protozoa. Migration of infected rural people to cities—and, conversely, rural agro-industrial projects that attract nonimmune urban dwellers into the country—have increased the prevalence of kala azar worldwide. Dams, irrigation systems, wells, and even deforestation have all contributed to its spread.

The cutaneous (skin) and mucocutaneous (skin and moist membrane) forms of leishmaniasis, while usually not fatal, cause disfigurement and disability over wide areas of the world. *Leish-mania tropica,* the agent of oriental sore, infects a million to a million and a half people in Afghanistan, Brazil, Iran, Iraq, Peru, Saudi Arabia, and Syria. In these countries it is a common sight to see young children, usually under three years old, with one or more ulcerating sores on exposed parts of their bodies, upon which swarms of flies are feeding. "Since one attack usually confers immunity," wrote Dr. Asa Chandler in the 1930s, "oriental sores appearing on an adult person in Baghdad brands him as probably a new arrival." Oriental sore usually heals without treatment after a few months to a year, though it leaves a pale, puckered scar for life. In a practice that was formerly widespread in the Middle East, mothers of girls introduced infectious matter, obtained from another child with oriental sore, under the skin of a part of the body normally covered. When this procedure, called scarification, was successful, the resulting sore produced immunity and prevented disfiguring ulcers from developing elsewhere.

During Operation Desert Storm in 1990, a half million soldiers were deployed into an area endemic for *Leishmania tropica.* Not unexpectedly, there were twenty cases of cutaneous leishmaniasis among this large group of people with no prior immunity to the parasite.

However, within a year of returning home, eight Gulf War veterans sought treatment for chronic illnesses consisting of various combinations of fever, abdominal pain, weight loss, fatigue, diarrhea, and swollen glands. Not one of these patients had had oriental sore and none fit the textbook descriptions of kala azar. But when the doctors at Walter Reed Army Medical Center examined stained smears of bone marrow or lymph node tissue, they saw the telltale amastigotes of leishmaniasis. In six, the organisms were definitely identified as *Leishmania tropica,* a species that is almost always limited to the skin. The previous textbook descriptions did not take into account the effects of mass movements of people into parasite habitats that were not just geographically but also genetically remote from the areas of origin of most of the soldiers. Between 2002 and 2003 there were twenty-two reported cases of cutaneous leishmaniasis in soldiers serving in Afghanistan, Iraq, and Kuwait. Patients with kala azar will probably be diagnosed, as well.

Perhaps the most dreaded complication of infection involving these parasites is *espundia,* or mucocutaneous leishmaniasis. The disease begins with the usual skin ulcers of cutaneous leishmaniasis. While the ulcers are still present, for months or years after they are healed and forgotten, the infected person notices tiny, itchy spots or a bump, usually inside the nose. The lymph glands in the neck swell, and the bump turns into a spreading ulcer that slowly but relentlessly consumes the nasal septum. Infected fluid pours out of the nose and infects the upper lip, which swells to grotesque size. The mucus, teeming with leishmania parasites, drips down the back of the throat and infects the palate. The nostrils become clogged; the mouth must remain permanently open—day and night. The nose may collapse into the face or turn into a dangling tube (tapir nose). In the most extreme cases, the nose may be totally lost, and the person is left with a circular hole where the nasal passages and the mouth become one common cavity. Long before this stage, the person's repulsive appearance and fetid breath often make the sufferer a social outcast. Unable to eat, the victim weakens and usually succumbs to pneumonia or another infection, such as tuberculosis.

Any one of the many *Leishmania* species infecting humans can cause *espundia,* but it most commonly follows infection with *Leishmania braziliensis,* the dominant species in the Peruvian jungle. *Espundia* develops in less than ten percent of patients who get a skin ulcer due to this species, but once it develops, it may resist all treatment.

· · ·

As I rode the elevator down to the walk-in clinic, I had the not-unfamiliar feeling of insecurity I get when confronting an infection I have never seen before. I knocked on the door of the exam room and went in.

"I'm Dr. Nagami," I said, shaking Alfred's hand. "I'm an infectious diseases specialist."

Alfred Eliah was a tall, elderly man with a straight back and a strong handshake. I asked him to tell me his story. Some of the place names sounded familiar: Madre de Dios River, Tambopata.

Thinking of the bird-watcher who lost his leg from snakebite, I asked him, "Were you near Manu Park?"

"Not far from there," he replied.

Next I asked Alfred to look up so I could get a good look at his skin ulcers. They were nickel-sized, shallow craters, with a crusted scab in the center and round, pink edges. Under the point of Alfred's chin I felt a rubbery lymph node the size of a jacks ball. They were not tender, foul smelling, or running with pus, but in these chronic ulcers and the swollen lymph node a battle was nonetheless taking place. Macrophages residing in the skin were fighting an invader, and, judging by the enlarging lymph node, they were in retreat, carrying the engulfed, but still-multiplying parasites within them. And if the parasites were *Leishmania braziliensis,* they had the power to escape the confines of the skin and invade and destroy Alfred's mucous membranes from his nose to his larynx.

I took Alfred up to my office to complete the preliminary examination and order laboratory tests. Although he looked and acted like a man ten years younger than his seventy-two years, Alfred had had a heart attack at the age of forty and had a coronary bypass operation at age sixty-eight.

I was walking Alfred out to the nursing station, when he said, "You know, there were about thirty of us on the trip, all working under the same conditions as I was. Do you think any of the others could come down with this thing?"

"I think it's not unlikely someone else will," I replied, remembering the reports I had read of large outbreaks of leishmaniasis among American soldiers during jungle training in Panama.

"Our group included people from all over the United States and Europe. I think I'll send out an e-mail and tell them to be on the alert."

As my nurse ordered Alfred's laboratory tests in the computer, I told him that on Monday I would talk to some leishmaniasis specialists and find out what our next step would be.

"They'll probably recommend biopsies and special cultures. In the meantime, don't worry, this is a slow-moving infection and we have plenty of time to take care of it." I said good-bye to my new patient, giving him a confident handshake, masking my worry, not so much about Alfred's nose falling off—I figured I could prevent that—but about the ability of a seventy-two-year-old cardiac patient to withstand leishmaniasis treatment.

On Monday morning I called Susan Novak, associate director of microbiology at the Regional Reference Laboratory for the Southern California Permanente Medical Group. She put me in touch with Frank Steurer of the Parasitology Branch of the Centers for Disease Control and Prevention in Atlanta.

"We're getting quite a lot of these leishmaniasis cases," Steurer said after he heard Alfred's story. "We've got about five patients that we're evaluating or treating now. I'm going to send you some special culture media for leishmaniasis. When it arrives, put it in the refrigerator and don't let it dry out. You'll need to take biopsies of the ulcers, make touch preps on slides, and do an aspirate from the lymph node. Pack them up according to the instructions and send them back to me at room temperature by overnight air."

Two days later I received a cardboard-and-metal cylinder, labeled with an orange biohazard insignia. Inside this outer mailing tube, I found a second cylinder, similarly labeled. It held two carefully padded screw-top plastic tubes. Each tube contained beige agar layered along one side, and some pink liquid. I replaced the plastic tubes in the inner cylinder, dropped it back into the larger container, sealed them in their Ziploc bag and carefully placed the container on its side in the clinic refrigerator with the solid media on the bottom, so that it would stay moist.

After a series of telephone calls, I arranged for Alfred to come in the following Tuesday to collect the required specimens. First, Dr. Paul Wolfish in the dermatology department performed a punch biopsy of the larger of Alfred's ulcers. He divided the piece of flesh in half, using one part to inoculate the culture tubes and leaving the other part for staining.

Dr. Wolfish's nurse Linda then walked Alfred, his precious media, and his biopsy specimen down to the pathology department in the basement of the hospital. In pathology, Dr. Jeffrey Shiffer inserted a needle several times into the swollen lymph node under Alfred's chin, each time aspirating a small amount of fluid into a syringe. He smeared some of this fluid on glass slides and also lightly pressed Alfred's biopsy specimen against other slides, to make "touch preps" for later staining by Frank Steurer. Then he dropped the biopsy specimen in formalin preservative for staining.

Finally, the specimens were packed in the CDC mailing tubes and taken to the laboratory where I had made arrangements through the director, Michael Collier, to have them picked up and shipped by air to CDC. It was a carefully coordinated team effort, and I was relieved it had gone smoothly.

Just forty-eight hours later I received a call from Frank Steurer. The touch preps were positive for *Leishmania* organisms. The written report I eventually received noted "very few amastigotes, in very bad shape, but nucleus and kinetoplast present." Remarkably, more than a hundred years after Borovsky's report, it was still the combination of the dark staining knob of nucleus and the little spot of the kinetoplast that had given the parasites away.

"I put the cultures you sent me on my 'supermedia.' If they grow, I can do special tests to tell you the exact species, but judging from where this patient got infected, it's probably going be *Leishmania braziliensis.*"

At that point, I had done enough reading to know what that meant. Alfred was at significant risk for *espundia,* and there was only one drug that could reliably prevent it.

"Do you recommend treatment with Pentostam?" I asked.

"I'm going to put you in touch with James Mcguire, who is in charge of our drug division."

A few minutes later I was speaking with Mcguire. He confirmed what I had read, that Alfred should have Pentostam treatment.

"I'll send you the relevant literature and drug information. You'll need to get consent through your IRB and fax it back to me, but I can have the Pentostam out to you by Thursday. How much does your patient weigh?"

"I'm not sure. I'll find out and call you back." Worried about the medicine arriving after hours, I asked him if it had to be refrigerated on arrival. No, it was stable at room temperature, he told me.

The Centers for Disease Control maintains a supply of vaccines, anti-sera, and drugs, which are either in short supply or whose use is in some way restricted. The antimony compound Pentostam is one such drug. It has never been released by the Federal Drug Administration (FDA) for use in this country; the manufacturer did not wish to go through the expense of obtaining approval for a drug that is both toxic and rarely used here. As a result, every physician who needs Pentostam has to apply through the CDC for an investigational new drug permit for the patient they are treating. All this has to go through the hospital IRB, the institutional review board. The drug is then sent, free of charge, from Atlanta, for use in that one patient, who must sign an informed consent document after reviewing the medicine's side effects.

Antimony, the active ingredient in Pentostam, is a bright, silvery metal in the nitrogen family. When heated in air, it burns with a brilliant-blue flame. As with water, it expands when it solidifies, which makes it a valuable ingredient in alloys used in casting, because it swells to fill the small crevices in molds. Antimony sulfide imparts a vermilion color to fireworks and is used in tracer bullets.

It was antimony's property of forming bright red compounds that brought the element to the attention of alchemists, one in particular, John of Rupescissa. He wrote around 1350: "Pulverize the mineral antimony until it is imperceptible to the touch and put it in the best distilled vinegar until the vinegar is colored red." After a series of steps in which more vinegar is added and heated, Rupescissa directs the alchemist to heat the mixture in a still:

> Then you will see a stupendous miracle, because through the beak of the alembic, you will see as it were a thousand particles of the blessed mineral descend in ruby drops like blood. Which blessed liquor keep by itself in a strong glass bottle tightly sealed, because it is a treasure which the whole world cannot equal! . . . For it takes away pain from wounds and heals marvelously. Its virtue is incorruptible, miraculous, and useful beyond measure.

In the sixteenth century, the alchemist and physician Paracelsus popularized the use of medicinal cordials containing antimony combined with iron, tin, or copper. However, in 1566, physicians of the Parisian school, who advocated the used of botanical remedies over metals and who were concerned about the toxic effects of antimony, succeeded in getting its use as a drug banned by royal decree. But a hundred years later, antimony was reinstated when Louis XIV believed that a large dose of it had cured him of typhoid fever. In the eighteenth century, the antimony-based Dr. James's Powders were patented as a fever remedy. As a component of Feltz's solution, antimony was used against syphilis in the 1900s. Into the 1940s, doctors used antimony potassium tartrate, or tartar emetic, in patients with acute bronchitis and laryngitis to increase secretion and to facilitate the coughing up of sputum.

It seemed, however, that antimony was destined to join the list of toxic and obsolete remedies, like the mercury compounds that were once the mainstay of treatment for syphilis. Then, in 1912, doctors discovered that intravenous tartar emetic could cure some patients with oriental sore and kala azar. By the 1940s, chemists had at their disposal, less toxic antimony compounds for treatment of these diseases; however, as late as 1973, Dr. Bryce Walton of the U.S. Army Medical Research Unit in Panama wrote that the use of the cheap but toxic tartar emetic was still widespread. In discussing an ultimately fatal case of *espundia* in a thirty-four-year-old Bolivian man in whom the disease had destroyed his upper lip, soft palate, and larynx, he noted that the patient had received sporadic injections of an unknown drug, which he believed was most likely sodium antimony tartrate, known locally as "tartaro." He described the drug as being "widely available without prescription and frequently used without benefit of medical supervision by *espundia* sufferers. Injections are available in many pharmacies or from 'curanderos' whose only qualification is possession of a syringe and needle."

The pentavalent antimonials have been mainstays in the treatment of leishmaniasis for over half a century. They are complex organic molecules built around two antimony atoms linked by oxygen. Neither their exact structure, nor their mechanism of action is known with certainty. (Alfred Eliah, a retired chemist, made me a diagram of one possible structure.) The compound, Glucantime, is favored in French-speaking countries, while Pentostam is used everywhere else.

Alfred's Pentostam arrived two days later, two vials of colorless liquid, enough for a course of twenty consecutive days. Dr. Maguire included an information sheet listing the principal toxic effects and an informed consent sheet. Half or more of patients could expect to have muscle and joint aches, often severe. Nausea and vomiting were common, sometimes accompanied by elevation of amylase and lipase, enzymes released into the bloodstream when the pancreas is damaged. One- to two-thirds of patients have abnormal blood tests for liver enzymes. Depression of one or more of the blood elements—red cells, white cells, and platelets—occur in a third.

Cancer specialists may administer drugs with side effect profiles like these, but for an infectious disease doctor, this stuff was pretty toxic. And as bad as these problems were, what worried me most in Alfred's case was the drug's effect on his heart. In some patients, Pentostam slowed the conduction of the electrical impulses that controlled the heartbeat and prolonged the phase of the electrocardiogram called the QT interval. The drug information sheets noted that "occasional deaths that may have been due to cardiotoxicity have been reported," though at higher doses than Alfred would be receiving. But Alfred already had a problem with his cardiac wiring, called left bundle branch block. I decided to call his cardiologist, Dr. Jocelyn Turnier, for advice.

After I explained his predicament, she said, "Well, if the treatment's necessary, it will most likely be okay. Alfred's condition has been stable for a long time. But you'll need to get an EKG before each dose and measure the QT interval; if it increases by a half a second, hold the treatment and call me."

The next step was for the nurse in charge of the hospital out-patient infusion center to set up a protocol with the hospital pharmacists for Alfred's Pentostam treatment. On Monday, February 11, Alfred came in with Helene and received his first intravenous drip of the drug. Other than bloodshot eyes and an intense flushing reaction in his face and scalp he had no untoward effects.

About three days into his treatment I brought my team of interns and residents to the infusion center to see him. The ulcers under Alfred's chin were now quarter-sized and were covered with a thin, maroon scab.

It was during the second week, as the drug started to accumulate in his body, that Alfred began having fatigue, headache, loss of appetite, and pains in his muscles. By now his face remained red between treatments. On the plus side, his electrocardiogram had not changed, and, best of all, his lesions had become slightly smaller, and the swollen lymph node under his chin had started to recede.

By the end of that week, Alfred's blood tests showed significant abnormalities. He was mildly anemic, and his liver enzyme tests had risen to between two and three times normal. Most alarming was his pancreas test, the amylase, which had tripled. That Thursday, although Alfred did not have the abdominal pain of pancreatitis, I decided to send him home without his dose of Pentostam while I considered what to do.

According to the treatment guidelines, I was to order another test of the pancreas, called a lipase level. If the lipase level was under a thousand units per liter (normal is under twenty-three in our lab), I could continue treatment if the patient remained well. Alfred's level was 515. On Saturday, I resumed therapy, and he continued it without interruption to the end. His skin ulcers healed completely, and he was apparently cured, though, for the rest of his life, there will always be a risk of relapse in the skin or in the nasal membranes.

On March 3, I received Frank Steurer's final report. Alfred's cultures had grown *Leishmania braziliensis*.

Because of increasing resistance to antimony compounds worldwide, "cure" has become a provisional term in leishmaniasis treatment. Incomplete courses of treatment and sporadic injections of "tartaro" select for resistant organisms, not only in South America, but also in India, where kala azar is now often incurable with antimony.

One of the most promising new drugs for treating leishmaniasis is liposomal amphotericin B. Long used to treat fungal infections, amphotericin is also active against some protozoa. When molecules of amphotericin are packaged inside a fatty or lipid coat, they find their way into the macrophages of the liver, killing the leishmania of kala azar. The drug is extremely expensive, but a five-day course of therapy will cure many patients with visceral leishmaniasis. Unfortunately, it is still less effective than Pentostam in preventing *espundia* in patients like Alfred, who have the *Leishmania braziliensis* form of skin infection.

Alfred Eliah was not the only member of his group to contract leishmaniasis. A few weeks after he sent out his e-mail, he learned that after his return to San Diego, a filmmaker in his thirties had broken out with leishmaniasis ulcers on one arm. His doctor called the CDC and, with their help, he treated the patient with Pentostam, also with good results.

On April 4, Alfred came to my office for a follow-up appointment. The ulcers under his chin had healed completely, leaving pink, puckered scars. The lymph node swelling had subsided. However, his left eye was red, irritated, and teary. It looked uncomfortable to me, but Alfred insisted it was getting gradually better.

After I finished checking his skin, Alfred sat on the edge of the examination table holding some papers in his right hand. I noticed a slight movement and a rustling sound. Alfred's hand was shaking.

"You have a tremor?" I asked.

Alfred gave me a look of pained embarrassment. "I noticed it toward the end of treatment. It got worse over the next week, but it seems to be stabilizing now," he said.

I asked Alfred to hold his hands up in front of him with the palms up, and then to touch the end of his nose first with his right index finger and then with his left. His outstretched hands trembled slightly, and, as each finger approached his nose, the shaking became more severe.

"I have trouble drinking coffee sometimes," he said.

"This is terrible, Alfred," I said.

I went to my office and looked through my Pentostam materials to see if intention tremor was a known side effect. It was not listed. The young doctor in the office next to mine ran a quick Internet search but found nothing.

Alfred and I walked sadly out to the nurse's station.

"It's got to be the Pentostam. Maybe it will get better with time," I said, feeling faint hope. Alfred had been off treatment for a month already, without improvement. Of course, I would report his problem to the CDC.

Alfred sat down at the nurse's station. I asked him to write down the telephone numbers of his two homes. I looked at the slip he handed me. The effort of writing had brought out the tremor, and the letters were cramped and shaky.

Two weeks later I called Alfred at home. "How's the tremor?" I asked.

"You know, doctor, I think it's a little better."

This was very good news. "And your eye?"

"A funny thing happened with my eye. About a week ago, I felt something under the lid, so I lifted it and saw a dark red scab there. It fell off and now my eye's fine."

"Great," I said, wondering what was in that scab. Thinking I should make a follow-up appointment for him in my clinic, I asked, "Will you be in town for the next several weeks?"

"Yes," he said. "We were supposed to go to Africa to do some work on a rhinoceros project."

"Sounds interesting," I said.

"Actually, we've had second thoughts. The trip's off."

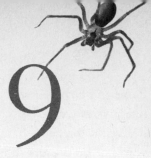

9

New York,
Summer 1999

In late July 1999, Dr. Tracey S. McNamara, head of the veterinary pathology department at the Bronx Zoo, realized that crows were dying in the neighborhood around the zoo grounds. Dr. McNamara's crow count had reached forty in August, about the same time that an infectious diseases specialist, Dr. Deborah S. Asnis, began caring for two elderly patients at the Flushing Hospital, across the East River in Queens.

The first patient, a sixty-year-old man, had been admitted to the hospital on August 12 complaining of three days of fever, weakness, and nausea. On admission, he had a temperature of 103°F and was thought to be suffering from pneumonia. However, on the fourth day he became confused and developed weakness in his limbs. His deep tendon reflexes, like the knee jerk, were feeble, his bladder stopped functioning, and his doctors had to insert a catheter to drain his urine.

Three days later, on August 15, an eighty-year-old man came to the same hospital with fever and weakness. He had collapsed at home and had been resuscitated in the field. On admission to the intensive care unit, he was already being supported by a mechanical ventilator, had a fever of 104°F, and barely responded to the voices of his doctors. Then, on his third day in the hospital, sudden, total paralysis struck.

Laboratory tests suggested that the patients were suffering from viral encephalitis, and that the weakness was due to some kind of nerve damage, perhaps the Guillain-Barré syndrome. Unlike meningitis, which starts with inflammation limited to the membranes lining the outside of the brain, encephalitis affects the deep brain tissues immediately. Permanent neurological damage or death may result.

One of the most common causes of viral encephalitis is *Herpes simplex,* the same virus that causes cold sores. But faced with cases of viral encephalitis during the summer, Dr. Asnis also had to consider infections contracted from the bite of a mosquito. The viruses that cause these arthropod-borne infections are called arboviruses, for short. Arboviruses in the United States include eastern equine encephalitis and St. Louis encephalitis. However, these two patients had a striking clinical feature in common that was not typical of any arbovirus with which Dr. Asnis was familiar. They had both been stricken with paralyzing weakness. Dr. Asnis wondered if she were dealing with an entirely new and very dangerous infection.

On Monday, August 23, she telephoned the New York City Health Department. She was put through to Dr. Marcelle Layton, the head of the department's Bureau of Communicable Diseases. Dr. Layton asked Dr. Asnis to submit samples of blood and of cerebrospinal fluid (the liquid that surrounds the brain, obtained by doing a spinal tap) to the New York State Health Department laboratory in Albany. Dr. Layton then dispatched an epidemiologist to Flushing Hospital to study the background of the two patients in order to determine whether they were linked by any common factors.

On Friday, August 27, Dr. Asnis called Dr. Layton to discuss a third possible case, and, while they were on the telephone, another doctor interrupted the call to tell Dr. Asnis about a fourth case. On Saturday, August 28, a fifth case was reported, this time from another hospital in North Queens. Rather than a few sporadic cases, this was beginning to look like a true outbreak.

In addition to looking for clinical clues in the patients' histories, health department investigators sent samples of blood and cerebrospinal fluid from suspected encephalitis patients to the state laboratory for analysis. On August 31, the eighty-year-old man who had collapsed at home died in the intensive care unit at Flushing hospital. On September 2, one of the second group of patients Dr. Asnis had discussed with Dr. Layton also died. This victim, an eighty-seven-year-old woman, had been admitted to the hospital on August 20 with headache, loose stools, fever, and weakness. The health department obtained fresh brain samples from both of these fatalities and sent them to the state lab.

The first apparent breakthrough in the encephalitis outbreak came from tests of blood and cerebrospinal fluid of this second fatality. While no specific virus had been isolated on culture, the specimens from the eighty-seven-year-old woman did contain a type of antibody suggestive of infection by the St. Louis encephalitis virus, a mosquito-borne arbovirus in the yellow fever family. Though it had never been reported in New York City, cases did occur during the summer months in rural and suburban areas in the southeast. Carried by birds and transmitted by mosquitoes, St. Louis encephalitis is known to cause very severe illness in patients over the age of fifty.

Based on these preliminary test results, Mayor Rudolph W. Giuliani called a news conference in Whitestone, Queens, on

September 4 and informed the public of the death of the eighty-seven-year-old woman from St. Louis encephalitis. He noted that it was likely, though not yet confirmed, that an eighty-year-old man who died at Flushing Hospital on August 31 had fallen to the same illness. While there is no specific treatment for St. Louis encephalitis, explained the mayor, the public needed to be informed and familiar with the symptoms of the illness. Mayor Giuliani suggested that New Yorkers remain indoors in the evening and use insect repellent whenever they had to go outside. Finally, the mayor reluctantly declared that the city would need to begin a limited program of nocturnal aerial spraying in northern Queens with the insecticide Malathion. This was a delicate issue; not only would he have to reassure people of the safety of the insecticide, but he would also have to convince everybody in the neighborhoods being sprayed to shut their windows tightly and keep air conditioners off all night despite the heat.

While the public was trying to adjust to the first outbreak of St. Louis encephalitis, the crow epidemic spread over the fence and began killing birds inside the Bronx Zoo. By September 9, Dr. McNamara's zoo refrigerator contained a dead Guanay cormorant, five Chilean flamingos, a pheasant, and a bald eagle. Upon performing autopsies on the dead birds, she found that they had all died of encephalitis and severe inflammation of the heart. The forty-five-year-old pathologist felt certain that the bird and human encephalitis outbreaks were linked. However, she was not convinced that the infectious agent was St. Louis encephalitis, because birds infected with that virus typically don't die. On the other hand, she doubted that it was an equine agent, such as eastern equine encephalitis, because her emus were healthy, and emus are highly sensitive to equine encephalitis viruses. Furthermore, Dr. McNamara noticed that only birds native to North and South

America were affected. Like Dr. Asnis, Dr. McNamara suspected an unusual infectious agent, perhaps one that was newly evolved or recently introduced to this hemisphere. Undeterred by the official announcement, she decided to look further.

On September 9, Dr. McNamara called the Centers for Disease Control and Prevention in Atlanta (CDC) to alert them to a possible link between the avian outbreak and the human cases. She voiced her doubts about the diagnosis of St. Louis encephalitis and arranged to send them samples of bird tissue.

The next day Dr. McNamara also sent tissue samples from two flamingos to the United States Department of Agriculture National Veterinary Services Laboratory in Ames, Iowa. By Monday, September 13, cell cultures in Ames showed that the zoo birds and the wild crows appeared to be dying of the same virus. Although they could not tell exactly what it was, electron microscopy showed it to be the size of a flavivirus, the yellow fever group. Because the Ames laboratory lacked the necessary containment facilities to handle an uncharacterized virus that was potentially dangerous to human beings, they notified the CDC.

Meanwhile, Dr. McNamara's inquiries had led her to Dr. Daniel J. Gubler, head of the CDC's arbovirus field station in Fort Collins, Colorado. She sent more specimens and made frequent telephone calls to the Fort Collins laboratory. Later, when asked by the *New York Times* if it was "persistent sleuthing or persistent pestering" that solved the encephalitis mystery, she replied, "Let's say the secretaries recognize my voice."

On September 19, after a week without an answer from the CDC, Dr. McNamara decided to telephone the United States Army Medical Research Institute for Infectious Diseases (USAMRIID) in Maryland. USAMRIID took over the functions of the old biological warfare labs at Fort Detrick, and is now in charge of national defense against biological agents. When she told the army about a possible new virus pathogenic for human beings as well as for birds, they expressed alarm for her safety and asked her to send samples to them immediately. By September 21, USAMRIID had confirmed the presence of a flavivirus in the bird samples and had notified the CDC.

While Dr. McNamara was pursuing a diagnosis of her avian cases, the scientists from the New York State Health Department were following a separate but ultimately converging trail of investigation. During the New York outbreak some of these scientists happened to be attending a conference in Albany, New York. In Albany, they had the opportunity to confer with a group from the Emerging Disease Lab at the University of California at Irvine. The head of the lab, Dr. W. Ian Lipkin, agreed to take brain samples from the fatal encephalitis cases to California and test them using advanced equipment for the study of rare viruses.

In mid-September, Dr. Lipkin began studying the brain samples in his Irvine lab using molecular probes to test the virus's genetic structure. By September 23, when the human toll had reached nine deaths, he had narrowed his search down to two flaviviruses, one native to Australia, called Kunjin, and West Nile virus. The next day both USAMRIID and his laboratories had completed their tests. The virus was West Nile.

West Nile virus was first isolated in 1937 from the blood of a feverish woman in the West Nile district of Uganda. It is in the yellow fever family, the flaviviruses (*flavi* means yellow in Latin)—a group of RNA viruses that also includes Japanese and St. Louis encephalitis, and Dengue fever. It is transmitted by the bite of the female mosquito to its bird host. Humans, horses, and domestic animals may also be infected, but are not important in perpetuating the virus in nature. Found throughout Africa and the Middle East and, less commonly, in Europe, Russia, India, and

Indonesia, West Nile encephalitis caused an outbreak in Romania in 1996, in which there were approximately ninety thousand human cases with seventeen deaths. The strain of West Nile that the two labs isolated closely matched a virus found in a sick goose in Israel in 1998. Since West Nile is not generally lethal to its bird hosts, scientists speculate that the Israeli strain that found its way into the United States may have been particularly virulent. Alternatively, birds in the Western Hemisphere, being evolutionary strangers to the virus, may have been more sensitive to its effects.

In human beings, West Nile infection starts out like the flu, with fever and body aches. Patients may then develop some swollen glands, and about half will have a transient rash. Illness is usually mild, either because in areas where the disease is common, people, like birds, have become adapted to it over time, or because infection in these areas occurs in youth, when serious complications are unusual. In some parts of the Nile Delta in Egypt, for example, 40 percent of young adults show evidence on blood tests of past exposure to West Nile, and most do not recall a specific illness.

However, a fascinating experiment conducted in the early 1950s showed that West Nile could produce severe disease in some patients. Researchers working with cancer in laboratory animals had observed that certain viruses seemed to cause animal tumors to regress. In a desperate attempt to help patients with advanced malignancy, researchers injected them with massive doses of West Nile virus. Most of these patients developed only mild illness, despite their weakened state, but eleven percent of the inoculated patients came down with encephalitis, and one of the patients became paralyzed. Happily, they all recovered from their experimental infection.

We will probably never know how West Nile virus first arrived in the United States in 1999. That the epidemic started in the New York metropolitan area suggests that it was brought to this country by air or ship, rather than as a result of any natural bird migration. The three most likely sources were a recently infected airline passenger from the Near East, who still had the virus circulating in his bloodstream, an infected bird brought into the United States legally or illegally, or an infected mosquito brought by ship or airplane.

The New York patients were not suffering from a new disease then, but were the first cases of an old disease occurring in a new place. Based on past experience with West Nile, the investigators suspected that a wider outbreak of the disease was going on. Therefore, public health authorities asked all the hospitals in New York City and neighboring counties to report any suspected cases of viral infections of the central nervous system, including patients hospitalized back to August 1, 1999. They devised tests for West Nile antibodies in serum and cerebrospinal fluid. In that first year of the epidemic, the investigation identified fifty-nine patients hospitalized with West Nile infection in the New York metropolitan area, with seven fatalities. The median age of hospitalized patients was seventy-one years, but patients as young as five and as old as ninety were also affected. The risk of death was especially high in patients seventy-five years of age or older. In the first outbreak, thirty-two of the fifty-nine patients lived in the New York borough of Queens, and none of the cases occurred outside New York State. An ominous finding, however, was that infected birds were found in three nearby states—Connecticut, Maryland, and New Jersey.

Most North American birds proved more resistant to the virus than the crow; house sparrows and other migratory species can live with West Nile multiplying in their blood streams. Even as scientists were struggling to identify the virus during the fall of 1999, the bird migration season had already begun. West Nile was winging its way in a thousand birds to a thousand destinations.

The last recorded patient that first year fell ill on September 22, and the human epidemic ended when the weather turned cold and the mosquitoes stopped biting. But it was already clear that West Nile could not be contained by spraying affected neighborhoods, or even by spraying whole states. West Nile was sure to return with each summer's birds and mosquitoes. Scientists only hoped that it would be confined to a few states and that its spread through the human population would be slow.

In preparation for the 2000 West Nile season, seventeen eastern states along the Atlantic and Gulf coasts, New York City, and the District of Columbia began West Nile surveillance. Beginning in the winter they collected mosquitoes, set up sentinel chicken flocks, sampled wild birds, and collected serum from horses and other mammals. In 2000, West Nile was found in twelve states, with human cases occurring in three. There were twenty-one cases of acute West Nile infection, with nineteen patients hospitalized, one death, and one patient left in a "vegetative state." Although the number of people identified with severe disease was less than in 1999, CDC estimated that approximately two thousand people had milder forms of the disease. Ominously, animal surveillance found over four thousand dead birds with West Nile, and, in addition, sixty-five horses were identified with severe neurological diseases. West Nile was detected in fourteen bats, four rodents, three rabbits, two cats, and two raccoons in New York, and in a skunk in Connecticut. During this outbreak, the CDC noted that severe disease in people in any given county was always preceded by fatal cases in birds, confirming the value of avian surveillance.

By the end of the next West Nile season in 2001, sixty-six patients with central nervous system disease had been identified over an expanding geographical area of ten states, but the disease was still limited to the eastern half of the United States. By the end of the 2002 season it was clear that neither the Great Plains nor the Rocky Mountains were a geographical barrier to the spread of the West Nile virus within its avian hosts. In that year there were over four thousand cases of human infection reported from forty states, and 284 people died, making this the largest reported West Nile outbreak in the world. A wide range of animal species also proved susceptible to the infection. In Illinois the virus was detected in a squirrel, a wolf, and a dog. In Nebraska, where the most equine cases occurred, mountain goats and sheep fell ill. In many states the virus appeared in nearly all counties, pointing to a pervasive infection in birds rather than a spotty or sporadic outbreak.

The 2003 West Nile season has resulted in over eight thousand documented infections with over 180 deaths and has involved the entire continental United States except Washington, Oregon, and Maine. The epicenter of the disease shifted west, to Colorado, which had over two thousand cases, including that of Dr. Lyle Peterson, director of CDC's division of vector-borne infectious diseases, based in Fort Collins. Although his was a mild form of the illness, he told a reporter from the *New York Times,* "I felt like I was 80 years old."

By the Labor Day weekend of the 2002 season, it had become apparent that West Nile had breached the defenses guarding the nation's blood and organ supply. On September 5, the CDC confirmed West Nile in four organ recipients from an infected donor, a previously healthy accident victim who had received several units of transfused blood prior to her death on August 1. Thirteen days after receiving one of her kidneys, the recipient developed a fever and progressed to encephalitis, requiring support on a mechanical ventilator. His condition improved, but the recipient of the second kidney developed fatal encephalitis seventeen days after transplant. At autopsy, his brain tested positive for West Nile.

A third patient received the donor's heart and he, too, required ventilator support, but recovered. The donor's liver went to a fourth patient, who became only mildly ill with West Nile. The donor's serum was then recovered and tested positive for the virus. The CDC suspected that the donor herself had become infected from one of many units of transfused blood she had received just before her death.

To prevent rejection, patients who receive organ transplants take medications to suppress their immune reaction to foreign tissue. They are susceptible to infections of all kinds, so it is not surprising that three out of four recipients of West Nile–tainted organs became seriously ill. But, like the susceptible crow population, they were sentinels of a wider problem among blood donors and recipients. For every one patient with severe West Nile disease, between a hundred and a hundred and fifty patients suffer only mild infections. During a West Nile outbreak, therefore, it is probable that there will be some mildly ill patients, or patients in the incubation period of the disease, among blood and platelet donors.

On September 20, the CDC reported the case of a twenty-four-year-old woman who received eighteen units of blood products after delivering a baby. She was discharged five days after giving birth, but twenty-two days later she returned to the hospital with headache and fever. Tests on the patient and on one of the units of blood plasma she received were positive for West Nile. This woman recovered, but a second new mother with West Nile transmitted the disease to her baby.

This patient, described on October 4, was a forty-year-old woman who had required two units of transfused blood following the birth of a healthy child. According to the report, the second transfusion was derived from the same donation as a unit of platelets given to a liver transplant recipient who developed confirmed West Nile. Eight days after receiving the tainted blood, the new mother developed a severe headache. Four days later she was admitted to the hospital with a temperature of almost 103°F. Her doctors performed a spinal tap; tests of the fluid done after her recovery confirmed West Nile infection.

Unaware that she was incubating the disease, the new mother began to breastfeed her child on the day of delivery and continued to do so for six days after she developed symptoms. Although her baby seemed healthy, and no further symptoms appeared, blood tests revealed that the infant had been infected with the virus, almost certainly through breastfeeding.

In all there were twenty-three confirmed cases of West Nile infection transmitted through blood transfusion in 2002 and over half of the transfused patients developed encephalitis. The risk of developing severe West Nile disease seems to be higher following exposure through blood products than via mosquito bites. Perhaps the weakened condition of patients requiring blood makes them more susceptible, or the dose of virus delivered by this route is higher.

West Nile infection constitutes a serious threat to the safety of the nation's blood supply, because most of the infected donors are in the incubation phase of the disease and are not yet ill when they donate blood. Researchers rushed to develop a screening test for West Nile, and on July 14, 2003, blood banks in the United States and Canada began testing all donated units for West Nile RNA using an investigational nucleic acid probe. As of early August 2003, 163 blood donations tested positive for the virus and were discarded.

We now know that the muscular weakness that Dr. Asnis found in her first patients at Flushing Hospital was probably not a form of the Guillain-Barré syndrome, as had been previously thought. In Guillain-Barré, an infection triggers an immune reaction in the human body that destroys the insulation around the nerve fibers. Usually the nerve cells themselves are not damaged, and if the process can be stopped, the insulating cells may regenerate. But in West Nile patients, the Guillain-Barré treatments are usually ineffective, because the attack is not on the nerve cell insulation.

The kind of muscular weakness caused by West Nile most closely resembles a disease almost forgotten in the United States, poliomyelitis. Polio, like West Nile, is caused by a small RNA virus that, in severe cases, invades the central nervous system and attacks the nerve cells in the spinal cord, which allow us to use our muscles to move. Even the muscles controlling breathing may be paralyzed. In the dark days of polio in the 1950s, many patients spent months inside the iron lung, the ancestor of our modern ventilator machines.

Poliomyelitis terrorized the United States every summer until Jonas Salk pioneered his vaccine in the mid-1950s. Now a worldwide campaign is underway to eliminate paralytic polio from the face of the earth. But the new summer disease, West Nile, may have taken its place.

In the September 20, 2002, edition of the *Morbidity and Mortality Weekly Reports,* CDC doctors reported six patients with a poliolike syndrome caused by West Nile infection. The first patient was a previously healthy fifty-six-year-old man from Mississippi, who was admitted to a local hospital in July 2002 with fever, chills, confusion, and painless weakness of his arms and legs. Doctors could barely elicit a knee jerk and other tendon reflexes. The patient was thought to have Guillain-Barré syndrome and was given one of the usual treatments: immune globulins by vein. However, his physicians ran further tests. They inserted needles into many muscle groups and tested their ability to contract (electromyography). They sent mild electric shocks along the large nerves in the arms and legs to test their ability to conduct nerve impulses (nerve conduction studies). Both of these tests showed that the patient had suffered damage to the nerve cell bodies in the spinal cord and to their long axon tails.

The second patient, a fifty-seven-year-old man, also from Mississippi, was much like the first, except that his muscle weakness was so profound that he couldn't breathe on his own and had to be supported by a mechanical ventilator. Each of the remaining four patients suffered an attack on the nerve cells in only part of the spinal cord, so they were left with a paralyzed arm or leg, usually with lesser degrees of weakness in the other extremities. The extent of recovery of these patients was not reported, but as other reports were filed, it became apparent that much of the nerve damage in these patients, as in polio, was irreversible.

With human help, West Nile has crossed the Atlantic and established itself in our hemisphere, and is here to stay. In future summers we will hear more about mosquito abatement and control. The backyard birdbath and the decorative pool may disappear. The comparative decline in the number of cases in New York State in 2003 (sixty-seven) probably reflects the success of measures to control mosquito populations and greater care taken by New Yorkers to avoid mosquito bites.

Experimental vaccines for West Nile do exist and, in fact, they are being administered to certain rare birds, like the California condor, a species thought to be very susceptible to infection. A vaccine that uses a harmless strain of yellow fever virus loaded with some of West Nile's genes has protected rhesus macaques from virulent West Nile virus injected directly in their brains. Human trials of this vaccine will begin this year.

Meanwhile, the West Nile survivors struggle to regain their

lost lives. Dr. Asnis's first patient, the sixty-year-old man who was admitted to Flushing Hospital on August 12, 1999, needed a cane to walk five months later and was still having "episodes of recent memory loss." A fifty-year-old woman in Louisiana who had the West Nile polio syndrome eventually left the hospital, but two months later she was still in a rehabilitation facility with weakness and inability to breathe on her own. Another patient, a fifty-six-year-old woman from Poland profiled in the *New York Times,* was still unable to walk after almost a year in the hospital. In a survey conducted by the New York Department of Health, also covered in the *Times,* over half of the patients who were over sixty when they were hospitalized with West Nile were still incapacitated a year later. They reported "serious difficulties with fatigue and muscle weakness" and had "been unable to perform basic tasks like driving, riding the subway, or doing household chores."

With each succeeding year, the West Nile epidemic will extend its range. It has already appeared in five provinces in Canada and will undoubtedly spread north to Alaska. Southern extension through Mexico to Central and South America is also possible. The virus, once introduced, can never be eradicated as long as there are birds to carry it and mosquitoes to bite them.

Before 1999, most people in the United States thought of mosquitoes as annoying insects that spread diseases in the tropics. But throughout our history they have been important transmitters of disease in the United States. In 1878, there were 100,000 cases of mosquito-borne yellow fever in the United States. And, as recently as 1940, approximately 150,000 people in the southern states were reported to have contracted malaria from the bites of this insect.

Humans are not safe from mosquito borne infections, because these illnesses occur wherever there is a summer breeding season and suitable, warm-blooded hosts. Despite our technological sophistication and urban sprawl, we can never isolate ourselves from the natural world. We are always in contact with it, whether it is as invisible as the flyway of a migrating bird or as obvious as a swarm of mosquitoes.

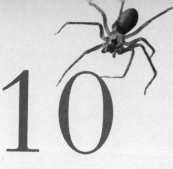

10

"The Jaws That Bite"

The Pulitzer Prize–Winning Foot

It took a piece of the top of his foot off completely, like probably a 4-inch long by an inch and a half, maybe two inches wide, all the flesh. It severed the main tendon to the next toe, crushed the casing to the joints that join the big toe to the foot. So its bacteria was [sic] then inside the bone. This thing carries 22 deadly bacteria in its mouth. His toe was completely hanging off . . .

In June 2001, actress Sharon Stone, who is quoted above, arranged a special tour of the Los Angeles Zoo as a Father's Day present for her then-husband, Phil Bronstein, the Pulitzer Prize–winning executive editor of the *San Francisco Chronicle*. The highlight of the tour was a visit to the Komodo dragon exhibit. The zookeeper invited Bronstein into the cage of one of the zoo's two dragons, a four-year-old named Komo, then about six feet long.

In an interview she gave to *Time Magazine,* Stone described what happened next:

> So he went in and started petting the dragon. The thing has a long, skinny forked tongue with yellow stripes. It started darting out at Phil's shoes. The zookeeper said, "I'm sure he thinks it's the white rats that we feed him. You'd probably be better off without your shoes."

There was a sudden lunge, and the dragon grabbed most of Bronstein's foot, clamping down with a terrible crunching sound. The editor, who had worked as a war correspondent, had the presence of mind to pin the dragon's jaw down with the heel of the bitten foot, prize the lizard's jaws off, and dive through the feeding door with the dragon in hot pursuit. Even after he and the zookeeper were safely through, and the door was secured, the dragon continued to slam its body against the metal grill, trying to get to its prey.

The Komodo dragon, *Varanus komodoensis,* is the world's largest lizard. Adult males are often over ten feet long and weigh two hundred pounds. An endangered species numbering no more than five thousand, the Komodo dragon is found in the wild only on the four Indonesian islands of the Lesser Sunda Group, three hundred miles east of Bali.

These giant monitor lizards are meat-eating predators, attacking deer, goats, wild boar, and smaller Komodos. (Young dragons live in trees to avoid being cannibalized.) They attack by ambush and will spend hours hidden near a trail, smelling the air with their yellow, foot-long, forked tongues, waiting for game. Komodos can run twenty kilometers per hour over short distances. When an animal passes close enough, they rush out of hiding and seize their prey in powerful jaws lined with serrated teeth.

Komodo dragons will often attack two-hundred-pound deer, which they then may not immediately overpower. Instead, they have evolved a unique method of killing prey by inoculating it with a lethal cocktail of bacteria living between their teeth. They track bitten animals up to four miles during the one to two days it takes for the wounds to fester; when infection or bleeding overwhelms their prey, they devour it.

Komodo dragons are members of an ancient family of lizards called the monitors. Their name probably derives from the old belief that the Nile monitor watched, or "monitored," crocodiles. In fact, the Nile monitor, a six-foot lizard, is frequently found in association with the Nile crocodile, because it eats crocodile eggs.

The monitors, family Varanidae, contain forty-four species within its one genus, *Varanus*. Twenty-two of these species live in Australia, where they are called goannas. All the monitors have exactly the same form, but they vary in size from a juvenile pigmy monitor, weighing about half an ounce, to the giant Komodo. When a Komodo dragon is threatened, it inflates its throat, hisses, and lunges. Threaten the little pigmy, and it will behave in exactly the same way.

The genus *Varanus* originated between twenty-five and forty million years ago. One extinct form, roughly the size of a small elephant, would have dwarfed the present-day Komodo. Since this giant monitor did not die out until twenty-five thousand years ago, human beings living in Australia may well have encountered it.

Although monitor lizards are not found in the Western Hemisphere, they share a common remote ancestor with the North American Gila monster. Snakes are also their distant cousins. In fact, the monitor exhibits very snakelike characteristics: it uses its darting, forked tongue and the Jacobson's organ on the roof of its mouth to taste the environment, and swallows its prey almost whole. Its serrated teeth slash off large pieces of flesh without chewing. In one meal it can eat an animal that increases its body weight by over 40 percent.

The western world remained ignorant of the Komodo until 1910, when the Dutch colonial administrator of Indonesia, Lieutenant Steyn van Hensbroek, heard stories of a giant "land crocodile." Van Hensbroek went to the islands of the Komodo group and succeeded in killing a seven-and-a-half-foot specimen. He sent a photograph of the dragon, and its skin, to the Zoological Museum in Java. A 1912 paper by the museum director, Peter A. Ouwens, introduced the Komodo monitor to the world, and, in 1915, under a plan by the Dutch colonial government, it became one of the world's first protected animals.

Komodo monitors are well-adapted diurnal (daytime) predators. In good light they can see objects over a thousand feet away and are particularly adept at picking out movement. Although at first thought deaf, they hear well in a restricted middle range.

Their most important and useful sense, however, is the sense of smell. Each time the monitor darts out its long, forked tongue, it samples the air for the telltale molecules given off by its prey. The Jacobson's organ inside a dragon's mouth is so sensitive that it can tell the direction from which an animal is approaching by simply tasting the different concentrations of the molecules on one forked tip compared with the other. By swinging its head from side to side as it walks, it continuously samples the air in different directions. Given the sensitivity and discrimination of this sense, it is likely that the monitor that attacked Phil Bronstein had obtained two correct readings on his foot before biting it: first "shoe," then "flesh."

Dr. Walter Auffenberg, one of the world's leading authorities on the Komodo dragon, completed a total of thirteen months of field study on the Komodo Island group. He and his associates spent many hours crouched in blinds, observing the lizards. Sometimes, though, they became the object of study:

> October 1 (1972), size 1.2 meters. Came into blind. I hit it on head 3 times with my pencil, but it was not frightened off. It remained and flicked my tape recorder and my knife with its tongue. It then left the blind and climbed a tree to a height of 2.5 m. Approximately 1 hr later it descended the tree and again came into the blind, but this time walked straight through, smelling my bare foot with its tongue as it passed by.
>
> November 7 (1972), size 1.4 meters. Green blotch entered the blind on three different occasions this morning. . . . At one point, he even stretched out in the shade of the blind, with his front leg draped over mine as he lay there half asleep.

The Komodo's habitat islands may be remote, but they are not uninhabited. In fact, the Sultan of Bima established a penal colony there in 1915. Today the villagers on these islands often live in close proximity to the monitors and may lose dogs, goats, and other livestock to dragons. Attacks on humans are rare, however, numbering perhaps twelve in the last sixty-five years.

In 1931 a father and his two sons sat in a clearing in the forest on Komodo Island, cutting and trimming wood. Suddenly a dragon about seven feet long started to move toward the seated men. When the dragon was fifteen feet away, they jumped up and started to flee. The dragon charged the fourteen-year-old boy and bit him severely in the buttocks, tearing away his flesh. The boy bled to death in under a half hour.

In 1987 on the island of Rinca, just east of Komodo, a six-year-old boy living in a stilt house climbed down the ladder and was attacked by a dragon. Hearing his screams, his parents rushed to the rescue. They were able to pull their son away from the dragon, but he was severely bitten in the legs, groin, and shoulder, and died in his mother's arms.

In another attack on Komodo that occurred in the 1950s, four men were hunting water buffalo near the territory of a very aggressive dragon designated 34W. One of the men became ill and was left behind. When the hunters returned with some villagers the next day, they found the man dead. His internal organs had been eaten by dragons, and his limbs had been stripped of flesh. In this case, it is uncertain whether the man was killed by the lizards or only eaten after he died.

A similar case occurred in 1989, when an elderly Swiss man landed on a remote area of Komodo Island with a tour group. After feeding the resident Komodos with goat meat, the group settled down for lunch. The Swiss man, however, decided that he wanted to go back to the boat, and set off alone.

Several hours later the main group returned to the boat, but there was no sign of the man, even after as extensive a search as was possible, given their limited food and water supply. The next day, one hundred searchers returned, but all they were able to find were his glasses and his camera. Komodo dragons eat most of the tissues of their kills, including bone, hide, and hoofs. It seems likely that Komodos had eaten the man, but whether he was attacked and killed or only eaten after having died or fainted is a mystery that will never be solved.

In fact, Komodo dragons are notorious scavengers of dead bodies; inhabitants of the islands have to seal graves with hard clay to prevent the remains from being dug up and devoured.

In addition to these cases, there are two unconfirmed deaths due to dragon attacks. According to villagers, in 1947 a police-man from the island of Flores, one of the Komodo Group, was petting a seven-foot dragon when the lizard apparently lunged up-ward and tore out the man's right biceps muscle. One week later the victim died as a result of infection.

In another dragon attack in Flores, villagers told Dr. Auffen-berg that a man had been bitten on his calf by a five-foot dragon that had been chasing his chickens. This patient healed, but an-other villager, also bitten in the calf, seemed never to have fully recovered. He became pallid and sickly and died two years later.

Although Komodo dragons have a reputation for nasty, infection-prone bites, research on the bacterial flora living in their saliva has been, understandably, limited. However, a paper pub-lished in 2002 reports the findings of a collaborative study by in-vestigators working in Texas and in Bali. The scientists from Bali used nylon rope and tape to restrain smaller dragons, and wooden or metal crate traps for the larger specimens. The Bali team sam-pled saliva from between the teeth and the palate of twenty-six wild and thirteen captive dragons and then froze the samples and sent them back to Texas. Unfortunately, the technique did not allow the investigators to preserve some of the most malignant bite-wound bacteria, the anaerobic germs that die in the presence of oxygen.

Despite these limitations, the microbiologists at the Univer-sity of Texas isolated fifty-seven different species of bacteria from the Komodo saliva. Interestingly, the average number of bacterial species was forty-six percent greater in the samples from the wild dragons compared with the captives. Apparently, wild dragons are able to maintain the diversity of their oral bacteria by picking up new germs from the intestines of their kills, especially as they feed on putrefying carcasses.

The Komodo dragons themselves seem to be highly resistant

to infection from the bacteria from their own saliva and that of other dragons. Large adult dragons usually have numerous scars on their bodies inflicted by other Komodos in disputes over carcasses and territory. Investigators would like to know what substances in their blood afford such a high level of protection, since, if they could be characterized, these antibodies or other compounds might be useful to treat infections.

In the meantime, doctors will continue to rely on massive doses of antibiotics to prevent infection following Komodo attacks. Though bitten by a captive specimen, Phil Bronstein, the newspaper editor, was still at high risk of infection. Without potent intravenous antibiotics, his reconstructive foot surgery would not have been possible. Fortunately, the brave patient was able to quip from his hospital bed a few days later, "It's L.A., I was just taking a meeting."

Saved by the Bible

Alligators and crocodiles belong to the order Crocodilia and are the largest and heaviest present-day reptiles. The Nile crocodile of Africa and Australia's estuarine crocodile may reach a length of twenty feet, and the largest alligators may weigh up to a thousand pounds. Alligators and crocodiles are the sole living representatives of the Archosauria, the ancient reptile group that included the dinosaurs.

The crocodilian ancestors appear in fossil sediments dating back nearly two hundred million years, but certain features of the skull continued to evolve through the upper Jurassic period, about 136 million years ago, when the true crocodiles appeared. The crocodilians and dinosaurs were contemporaries. But three out of the four original suborders of the crocodile group did not survive.

The twenty species that remain today are our last living link with the dinosaurs, and are also the nearest living relatives of the birds.

Crocodiles are limited to the tropical and subtropical zones, while alligators are more tolerant of the cold. The American alligator, *Alligator mississippiensis,* lives throughout the Southeast, in coastal swamps from the Carolinas to Texas and as far north as the flatlands of Arkansas. There is also a small species of alligator that lives in China, but it has not been reported to attack people.

The name alligator derives from the Spanish *al lagarto,* meaning "the lizard." In 1614 Sir Walter Raleigh wrote of "the Crocodiles (now called Alegartos)" and Ben Jonson asked, "Who can tell, if . . . the Alligarta hath not piss'd thereon?" But already in 1623 *Romeo and Juliet* contained the phrase "an Alligater stuft."

An alligator can be distinguished from a crocodile by its broader snout and a fourth tooth that fits into a socket in the upper jaw when its mouth is closed. In crocodiles this tooth juts up along the outside of the jaw. The American alligator, *Alligator mississippiensis,* grows to a maximum length of nineteen feet, but adult specimens usually average six to ten feet in length. Young alligators are black with yellow bands, while adults are black, blending in with the dark mud of their surroundings.

Alligators, like crocodiles, are strictly carnivorous. Young alligators catch crayfish, snails, insects, and spiders, while the adults eat fish and other aquatic animals, including other alligators, snakes, birds, small mammals, and sometimes deer. Alligators have acute senses of sight and hearing and are also very sensitive to vibrations produced when small animals jump into the water. Using their strong jaws and teeth to break the bones of their prey, they shake and slap large animals against the water to rip off pieces they can swallow. When attacking a very large animal, such as a deer or a human, an alligator whirls under the water, drowning and rending the victim.

Alligators are powerful swimmers and can swiftly jump out of the water up to five feet. On land they can run up to thirty miles per hour for very short distances. Like the Komodo dragon, alligators lie quietly camouflaged against their surroundings and capture prey by a sudden, high-speed attack.

Since alligators are cold-blooded and have slow metabolic rates, they can go many months without food. But when water temperatures drop below about 60 degrees Fahrenheit, they will not eat, because at lower temperatures they are unable to digest food in their gut before it putrefies. During the cold months of the year, alligators hibernate in burrows.

Following an elaborate courtship in which the male makes the water dance with an infrasonic signal and then utters a long B-flat bellow, the female lays twenty to forty eggs in a nest mound. The mound functions like a compost heap, keeping the eggs warm for the sixty-five-day incubation period, while the mother stands guard. At hatching time, the baby alligators make chirping sounds inside their shells, and the female digs them out and helps them into the water. They will stay in her vicinity for about two years. Although much smaller than male alligators, females may be dangerous when they perceive a threat to their eggs or hatchlings.

Alligators have been attacking people since the first Native Americans settled in their habitats. Early explorers to Florida wrote that the indigenous inhabitants considered alligators a threat and took precautions to avoid attack. However, by the 1960s, the population of American alligators had been so reduced by the trade in skins that the 'gators were confined to remote swamps, where they rarely encountered humans.

Despite their diminished numbers, alligator attacks did occur. In 1952, a nine-year-old girl was fishing for minnows in a flooded rock pit in southeastern Florida. An alligator, which had grown up in the pit and was well known to local residents, seized her by the arm, but then let her go. As the alligator returned to attack again, a ten-year-old boy dragged the girl to safety. Her arm had been mangled from wrist to shoulder, and both bones below the elbow had been broken. However, the girl survived, and President Harry S. Truman presented her rescuer with an award for his bravery.

By the 1960s it seemed that *Alligator mississippiensis* would not survive the twentieth century, but in 1970 the Lacey Act curtailed the interstate shipment of alligator hides, and in 1973 the Endangered Species Act provided effective protection. Today there are approximately one million alligators in Florida alone, but by 1993, 129 attacks in that state had left us with seven fewer people.

A serious attack was reported in the *Journal of the American Medical Association* in 1971. The victim, a forty-nine-year-old farmer on his way home from a rural prayer meeting, was walking on a path that led through a swamp. There was a hissing and scuffling sound and then he was suddenly attacked "either by the devil or an alligator." The farmer felt his right thigh locked in the animal's jaws but was able to extricate himself by beating the alligator over the head with his Bible.

The physicians in the emergency room removed dead tissue and irrigated the wound with saline solution. Although the patient made an uncomplicated recovery, they decided to embark on "courageous bacteriological studies," because there was little information available on what infections might follow alligator bites.

Armed with culture media for sampling bacteria, the team of doctors went to a nearby wildlife exhibit housing a twelve-foot and a four-foot alligator. The tasks were assigned by rank: those lower on the academic ladder found themselves prying open alligator jaws while the senior investigators swabbed the animals' mouths. The resulting cultures showed abundant growth of both oxygen-tolerant and oxygen-sensitive bacteria (anaerobes), any one of which could cause a dangerous bite-wound infection.

Although the authors of the farmer's case presented their findings with considerable levity, other attacks have been horrific. In 1973, an eleven-foot alligator attacked a sixteen-year-old girl who was swimming with her father in Sarasota County, Florida. The alligator was shot, and parts of the girl's body were found in its stomach.

Another well-documented attack occurred on June 16, 1975, in Polk County, Florida. The victim, a forty-five-year-old man named Thomas Chickene, was swimming in a rock pit in Saddle Creek Park. While underwater, he bumped into what he thought was a log. As Mr. Chickene emerged, a large alligator seized him by the chest and pulled him under. The victim struggled to the surface twice, and was about to be pulled down for a third time when he rammed his hand down the alligator's throat, causing it to release its grip on his chest. After wrenching his wrist free of the animal's mouth, he escaped with a fractured breastbone, collar bone, scapula, and ribs as well as multiple deep lacerations on his body.

An article published in 1997 summarizes alligator attacks in the United States from 1948 through the end of 1995. In all there were two hundred and thirty-six attacks, eight of them fatal. Two hundred and eighteen of the attacks occurred in Florida. Thirty-four percent of the victims were totally immersed in the water when attacked, 17 percent were wading, and a surprising 38 percent were on shore. In Florida, golf seems to be a more dangerous sport than skydiving—twenty-four people were attacked while playing golf or retrieving golf balls. Other ill-advised activities included "pulling alligator from road [two], rescuing alligator in traffic, moving alligator from pool filter, moving alligator from utility room, and removing alligator from pipe [one each]."

For every instance of alligator attack, there are hundreds of complaints of "nuisance alligators." By 1975, the Florida Game and Fresh Water Fish Commission was responding to about five thousand complaints annually, and was capturing and translocating two thousand alligators to more remote habitats. Some of the alligators proved great travelers, moving unerringly over incredible distances back to their original homes. In addition, the human population of the state was growing at a rate of 6 percent a year, limiting the number of remote locations available for settling troublesome alligators. Finally, in 1978, the Florida Game Commission largely replaced the translocation effort with a program of culling nuisance alligators. Licensed hunters are allowed to sell the skins and meat of the alligators they are assigned to kill, and take the profit as their payment.

The program continues to this day, as do the attacks. By 2001 the death toll in Florida had reached thirteen and included an eighty-one-year-old man and a two-year-old girl. The Florida Fish and Wildlife Conservation Commission has published guidelines to help people live with alligators. At the top of the list is a prohibition against feeding them or disposing of fish scraps into the water or along shorelines. Feeding these animals is dangerous, because, as one authority says, "they may not know where the handout ends and the hand begins." In addition, many nuisance alligators were formerly well-mannered creatures who lost their fear of humans as a result of feeding. These animals often become unmanageable and have to be destroyed. The Conservation Commission has posted signs in 'gator territories throughout the state, featuring a picture of an alligator and the following warning: "I Bite the Hand That Feeds Me."

There are a dozen species of crocodiles living in Africa, the Australia region, Asia, and the Americas, and their attacks have killed a thousandfold more people than the Komodo dragon and the alligator combined.

Herodotus devotes a long passage in his *Histories* to the *crocodeilos,* mixing fact and fancy in his description of the animal. He writes that in Lake Moeris, near Thebes, the crocodile is considered sacred, and that the Thebans keep "one particular crocodile, which they tame, putting rings made of glass or gold into its ears and bracelets round its front feet." This description may not be entirely accurate, since crocodiles lack external ears, but Herodotus was correct when he wrote that the animals were embalmed. Archeologists have found the mummified bodies of crocodiles large and small.

Later generations did not share the Egyptian veneration for these animals. A Renaissance bestiary of Edward Topsell contains this entry:

The nature of this beast is to be fearefull, ravening, malitious, and treacherous . . . The males of this kind do love their females above all measure, yea even to jealousie. And it is no wonder if they made much of one another, for beside themselves they have few friends in the world.

Such criticisms not withstanding, crocodiles have the most highly developed brain of any living reptile. They show curiosity, and Herodotus was correct in writing that they can be tamed (to some extent). While alligators rarely live more than forty years, authorities believe that some twenty-foot specimens of the Nile crocodile, *Crocodylus niloticus,* are well over a hundred years old.

Crocodiles have narrower snouts than alligators and are said to be the more active and aggressive of the two. They hunt at night, which is when most attacks on humans occur. Crocodiles live only in tropical and subtropical waters. The American crocodile, *Crocodylus acutus,* is the only crocodile native to the United States, and its habitat in South Florida is the one place in the world where crocodiles and alligators naturally coexist.

Crocodiles are found over much of Africa: along the Nile, throughout the lakes and waterways of most of the continent south of the Sahara, and on the island of Madagascar. Because of the coexistence of dense crocodile and human populations there, Africa leads the world in the number of attacks on humans. But crocodiles have been a threat to humankind since they first began to evolve in Africa. A hominid skull recovered at the Olduvai Gorge in Tanzania is punctured by the tooth marks of a large crocodile.

The chronicles of the nineteenth-century explorers and hunters contain accounts of many fatal attacks. On New Year's Day 1896, the English big-game hunter Arthur H. Neumann had just finished bathing in a tributary of Lake Rudolf and was lacing up his boots when he heard a cry of alarm. Looking up he saw "a huge crocodile" seize his Swahili servant, Shebane, as he was bathing in shallow water. The crocodile held the man in his jaws "like a fish in a heron's beak," and before he could even move, there was a swirl, a splash, and the crocodile and victim disappeared, never to be seen again.

No accurate records have ever been kept of the exact number and location of crocodile attacks in Africa. Throughout the first half of the twentieth century, however, there was a rapid decline in the populations of alligators and crocodiles everywhere due to unregulated hunting of the species for meat and skins. Dr. Wilfred T. Neill, one of the world's leading authorities on these animals, wrote in 1971, "I suspect that the present book will be not only the first to deal broadly with crocodilian biology, but also the last: the last, that is, to be written by someone who had the chance to see almost all of the modern species . . . in their natural habitats."

But the passage of the Lacey Acts in 1970 and 1971 in the United States and the gradual adoption of protective measures elsewhere have shown that, contrary to the Renaissance bestiary, the crocodilians do have a "few friends in the world." As a result, populations of these highly evolved predators have exploded. In Malawi, for example, eight hundred crocodiles were formerly culled annually, but since the country's signing of the International Convention on Endangered Species in the late 1990s, there have been at least two people killed by crocodiles every day in the Lower Shire Valley there.

This may have been inevitable; to the predatory reflexes of a crocodile, there is no difference between an antelope approaching the edge of a river or lake to drink and a woman bending over to fill a drinking gourd or to wash clothes. The *British Medical Journal* reported that in the Korogwe District in Tanzania, when a village pump failed in 1994, there were eighteen deaths in one week as people resorted to collecting water at the river's edge.

In Kenya, in September 2001, the *East African Standard* reported an increase in aggressive behavior among the crocodiles of the Sio River, in the Busia region on the Kenya-Uganda border. After two people were killed within a few weeks, district official, Nathan Hiribae, asked the Kenya Wildlife Service, the country's conservation authority, to intervene and authorize the killing of some of the crocodiles. Increasingly, the besieged local population, who rely on rivers and lakes for water, washing, and their fishing livelihood, are pitted against conservation-minded government authorities, who see crocodiles as lucrative tourist attractions.

This strategy may backfire, however, when crocodiles eat the very tourists the governments hope to attract. In March 2002, an eighteen-year-old named Amy Nicholls and her fellow conservation volunteers set off for a picnic at Lake Challa on the Tanzania-Kenya border. Off the main tourist track and located in the extinct crater of a volcano, the beautiful turquoise-blue waters reflect Mount Kilimanjaro. It is recommended by a popular tourist guidebook as "a pleasant place to swim." But according to Elipba Mwakamba, a local administrative officer, people have been known to "disappear" in its deep waters.

Arriving at the lake without an experienced guide, Ms. Nicholls's group decided to take a twilight dip. Amy is reported to have told her friends that something was "tugging at her" before vanishing beneath the water. When Kenya police, wildlife rangers, and army divers found her body after two and a half days, it was missing an arm.

Later that same month, officials in Uganda finally decided to take action after crocodiles killed at least forty people—the majority of the victims being fishermen and women fetching water—along the shores of Lake Victoria, Africa's largest freshwater lake, and home to an estimated one hundred crocodiles. The Uganda Wildlife Authority killed the four it considered to be the troublemakers, but, according to the BBC, the agency "aims to help villagers coexist with wild animals by promoting tourism and the sale of hides and eggs."

This may prove to be a difficult task, however, as native beliefs and superstitions in Uganda contribute to the villagers' susceptibility to attack and their unwillingness to take action against crocodiles.

Many of the villagers believe that crocodiles attack men and women alternately and that, for example, "boys may bathe safely after an attack on another male." If a person is missing, and the villagers suspect a crocodile attack, they will seek advice from certain authorities, who then "consult with" the crocodiles to determine whether they are involved. If a body then turns up, the men apply special medicines and, believing themselves under the protection of witchcraft, wade into the water to retrieve it.

Yet the villagers are reluctant to harm crocodiles, because they fear retribution from the human owners they believe have tamed them for service. These tamed crocodiles are thought to work as assassins and even kidnappers, to procure women, whom they subdue and bring to their human handlers.

People coexist with crocodiles in many tropical waterways throughout the world. In April 1975, the Indian government established the Bhitarkanika Wildlife Sanctuary in Orissa State on the eastern coast. This one-hundred-square-mile park, criss-crossed with rivers and creeks, is the ideal habitat for the saltwater crocodile, *Crocodylus porosus,* the world's largest reptile. The sanctuary was home to sixteen male crocodiles between sixteen and twenty-seven feet long, and to some five hundred people per square mile. In an article published in 1983, the authors were happy to report that in the ten years from 1971 to 1981, there were only four fatal crocodile attacks on humans. The victims were "an old man" (aged fifty-three), who used to visit a river to collect grasses for basket-making; an eighteen- or nineteen-year-old-girl, who was washing her feet; a thirteen-year-old girl, who was fishing; and a thirty-eight-year-old man, swimming across a river with il-legally collected firewood. "In our experience," they wrote, "in-stances of man-eating have been greatly exaggerated." It seems that wildlife conservation is taken very seriously in India—even to the extent of willingness to suffer human casualties.

Sporadic fatal attacks by crocodiles on humans are not diffi-cult to find in the media. In September 1999, a seventy-year-old woman fishing along the Black River in Jamaica was pulled into the water and killed by a crocodile. In October 2000, the bottom half of a victim was found in a river in Eastern Malaysia. In June

2002, a man accused of killing a judge in Panama broke out of jail in Costa Rica, but was eaten by a crocodile while attempting to swim across the river Terraba. And in that year, a *Crocodylus porosus,* the dreaded estuarine or saltwater crocodile, killed a thirty-five-year-old British tourist as he was swimming in a river in Borneo.

This same estuarine crocodile was responsible for the worst animal attack on human beings ever recorded. British troops retaking Burma during World War II drove Japanese infantrymen into the mangrove swamps between Ramree Island and the Burmese mainland. The Japanese had expected to be evacuated by ship, but the British Navy blockaded the coast and, on the night of February 19, 1945, the Japanese soldiers were trapped in a wilderness of mud and water, unable to either advance or retreat.

An American biologist Bruce Wright, who was with the British troops, recorded what happened:

> That night was the most horrible that any member of the M.L. (marine launch) crews ever experienced. The scattered rifle shots in the pitch black swamp punctured by the screams of wounded men crushed in the jaws of huge reptiles and the blurred worrying sound of the spinning crocodiles made a cacophony of hell . . . Of about 1000 Japanese soldiers that entered the swamps of Ramree, only 20 were found alive.

Estuarine crocodiles, which the Australians call "big salties," are known to have killed seventeen people there. Fatalities among aboriginal people in remote areas may go unreported, however. The crocodiles are limited to the tropical waters of Northern Australia, where they have been a protected species since 1971. In a study of crocodile attacks in the Northern Territory from 1981 through 1991, the authors report that most attacks result from swimming or wading in shallow water, often in failing light or at night. Half of the victims were intoxicated. In all of the four fatal attacks, the crocodile killed by biting its victim in half, or by decapitation. The recoveries of survivors were frequently complicated by bite-wound infections, and the causative bacteria were similar to those found in Komodo dragon and alligator mouths. The victims frequently ignored warning signs, as in the following case.

At 11:30 P.M. on October 22, 2002, eight young German tourists decided to dive into Sandy Billabong, in Kakadu National Park in the Northern Territory. According to the *Daily Telegraph,* "It was hot, a near full moon was out and the water looked inviting." However, Sandy Billabong is the home of eight "big salties," and there were prominent warning signs (usually a swimmer inside a red circle with a cross through it and, above that, a croc's head with its mouth open).

Within a minute of entering the water, "24-year-old Isabel Von Jordan was in the jaws of a fifteen-foot crocodile and being spun underwater in a death roll." The crocodile was tracked by rangers and found over a mile from the attack site. In the inimitable style of law enforcement everywhere, Northern Territory police commander Max Pope told reporters, "This morning the crocodile was located still holding the deceased. It was harpooned by wildlife officers, which caused it to drop the deceased. The crocodile was secured and is now deceased."

The *Daily Telegraph* appended to the end of the article a list of the seventeen known Australian fatalities. They include:

Lee McLeod, 39, September 25, 1986, sleeping on bank of McArthur River, Northern Territory.

Ginger Meadows, 24, March 29, 1987, an American model who was partially eaten by a crocodile while swimming in the mouth of the Prince Regent River in northwestern Australia's Kimberly region.

Graham Freeman, 28, November 27, 1994, a crocodile handler at the Johnstone River Crocodile Farm in north Queensland, who was attacked during a tourist demonstration.

Nowhere in the world are the pros and cons of crocodile conservation more hotly debated than in Australia. Between the mid-1940s and 1971, crocodile hunting eliminated over fifty percent of the population, and big specimens became rare. But within a decade of protection that started in 1971, their numbers shot up to prehunting levels. In Queensland, where there are an estimated twenty thousand crocodiles, they enjoy full protection except in a "croc-free zone" around the city of Cairns. Even there, crocodiles are captured instead of being killed and are relocated hundreds of miles away. But crocodiles, like alligators, will often find their way home, even if it takes several years.

Fearing for their safety, people living in the small coastal settlement of Cooktown in Queensland are protesting the government's policy of strict protection, which includes two-year jail sentences and fines of over eighty thousand British pounds for anyone caught killing a wild crocodile. Inhabitants complain of a sixteen-foot croc at the fishing wharf, which is situated on the town's main shopping street, and of sighting crocodiles wandering across the town's golf course. They also have to contend with a local crocodile named Oscar, who is eighteen feet long and over ninety years old. John King, editor of the *Cooktown News,* is quoted as saying, "We've already lost several dogs over the last few months and it's only a matter of time before we lose a man or woman—and the crocs pose a real danger to children up here."

The Northern Territories, which has about seventy thousand crocodiles, does have a program for culling them: since the 1980s, landowners have been allowed to sell five hundred crocs a year to special farms, where they are processed for skin and meat. Landowners are also issued permits to harvest eggs from crocodile nests on their properties. The eggs or hatchlings are then sold to the farms. The program motivates landowners not to disturb crocodile habitats where nests are made, because they are earning money from the eggs and crocodiles they are allowed to harvest.

But even if this program were set up in Queensland, it would not satisfy die-hard hunters like "Crocodile Mike" Pittman. He favors a return to the old way of controlling crocodile populations. Quoted in a recent article, the forty-two-year-old said, "I've offered my services to any of the councils free of charge. I've got my own dinghies. I've got my own catching gear. But not one will take me on. All I want is the animals. I got Harrods interested in crocodile skin cured in bark but they won't take farmed crocodiles."

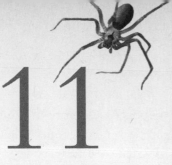

11

Rage

On Wednesday, March 8, 1995, a four-year-old girl was brought to a hospital in Lewis County, Washington. She had been drowsy and listless for two days and had been eating poorly. Her stomach and throat hurt. The examining physician noted the child's stuffy nose and red, runny eyes. He concluded that the girl had a routine cold. However, to be absolutely safe, the doctor wrote a prescription for antibiotics. The chart also noted that the girl was drooling and felt pain in the left side of her neck. In retrospect, these were clear signs of the terrible illness to come.

The following day the little girl was brought back to the emergency room. She had trouble standing and was hallucinating. She could not fall asleep and had been refusing to drink water. The admitting nurse noted that the tremulous child had a temperature of 104 and a racing pulse. The child's right pupil was larger than the left, and tests of her blood showed that it was dangerously concentrated, possibly because of her unwillingness to drink.

The ER physician was puzzled. Had the girl been drugged or poisoned? Ordering urine tests, the doctor admitted her to the hospital. A few hours later she had a seizure. A plastic tube was inserted into her airway to control her breathing. Her doctors loaded her onto a helicopter ambulance and took off for the regional medical center. While airborne, she went into cardiac arrest. By the time she arrived, she was in a coma.

The physicians met with family members and looked for clues in her recent medical history. Had a dog bitten the child in the last six months? Had she had any contact with wild animals, a coyote, fox, or raccoon?

No, there had been no animal bites—but there was one unusual event. In mid-February, a bat had been found in her bedroom. Since the child did not appear to have been bitten, the bat was simply taken out of the house, destroyed, and buried in the yard. Based on this history, doctors removed a tiny piece of skin from the back of the child's neck. No matter where a rabies patient is bitten, skin at the nape of the neck will frequently harbor the virus. On March 14, tests of the skin returned positive for the disease. That same day, local health department officials exhumed the body of the bat. "Despite trauma, decomposition, and partial consumption of the specimen by maggots, the brain was positive for rabies." On March 15 the girl died. At autopsy, her brain was positive, too.

Rabies, which is an almost uniformly fatal viral disease that attacks the brain, has been with us for all recorded history. The Babylonians described it in the twenty-third century BC. The Greeks called it *lyssa* ("frenzy"). Our term, rabies, comes from the Roman name *rabere,* Latin for "madness," but the Romans themselves borrowed the name from an ancient Sanskrit word *rabhas,* meaning "violence."

The rabies virus is transmitted in the saliva of a biting animal. But it isn't like malaria, which we contract from the saliva of mosquitoes in their natural search for food. As Berton Roueché writes in "The Incurable Wound," "There is nothing natural about the transfer of the rabies virus. It wrings collaboration from its carrier hosts by torturing them into a homicidal fury." We know now that rabies infection targets the limbic system, the part of the brain that controls rage.

The rabies agent is a small, bullet-shaped RNA virus. Almost any mammal can become its host. Researchers have infected mice, rats, rabbits, guinea pigs, dogs, foxes, monkeys, bats, and chickens. Baby hamsters are particularly susceptible to even minute doses, but mice are used most frequently to test vaccines, because mice and humans share the same one-to-three-month incubation period. Also, the disease in mice clinically resembles illness in dogs and people.

The rabies virus grows in the salivary glands of its host and usually enters its next victim through a bite. It then reproduces within the muscle cells of the new host and, weeks or months later, it gains access to the central nervous system by entering nerve endings near the bite site, and makes its way up the nerve's length to the brain. We know this from experiment; if the virus is injected into the mouse's footpad, amputating the large nerve in the animal's leg will block spread of infection.

Rabies is found on all continents except Antarctica and has probably existed in wild animals long before human beings appeared. In the developing world, where animals are rarely vaccinated, dog bites cause the majority of human cases. In the United States and Europe, most rabies infections are traced to wild animal exposures, in particular, bats, which are found in all forty-nine of the continental United States. Raccoons have also become an increasingly important rabies reservoir since the 1970s, after a hunt club brought raccoons, not suspected of being rabid, from Florida into the Virginia–West Virginia border. The result has been a smoldering rabies epizootic that has moved gradually northward as far as Ohio.

The World Health Organization (WHO) estimates that there are fifty thousand cases of rabies in the world each year, virtually all fatal. Rabies causes more deaths each year than yellow fever, polio, and meningococcal meningitis combined. Tragically, the victims of this agonizing disease are often school-aged children who come in contact with stray dogs.

The incubation period of rabies ranges from a few days to over a year, but about three-quarters of patients fall ill within three months after exposure. Rabies begins with a few days of vague, feverish symptoms, as with a cold or flu. About a third of patients then develop a telltale, classic symptom of the disease, but usually neither the patient nor the doctor realizes its terrible significance. This symptom is itching, pain, or tingling at the site of the original and now healed bite. These sensations are the first sign that the brain is aware of the deadly invader that has taken hold of the nerve endings, made its slow ascent up the long nerve tails, and begun to multiply in the central nervous system.

From this point on to the almost inevitably fatal end, all rabies victims take one of two paths. The majority of humans and most dogs develop agitated (furious) rabies. Paralytic (dumb) rabies claims the rest.

Furious rabies begins with anxiety and a mild sore throat that over the next few days progresses to hydrophobia. Hydrophobia is an excruciating contraction of the muscles of the throat, which is brought on by the act of swallowing water. After a few days, the sight of a water glass or even the sound of a faucet being turned on is sufficient to bring on the spasms, which are accompanied by intense terror. In some patients, hydrophobia progresses to aerophobia, in which a draft of air on the skin can induce the contractions. Spasms may spread to the muscles of the torso and mimic tetanus, heaving the patient into an arch supported by his head and heels. In other patients, the spasms lead to convulsions, during which the patient may be unable to breathe or may die of sudden cardiac arrest.

Patients then have periods of intense agitation with hallucinations. They may become aggressive or terrified. There are often lucid intervals in which they are oriented, resume their former personalities, and may even apologize for behavior over which they have no control.

However, the rabies virus then travels down the nerve cells of the brain and spinal cord, and attacks other parts of the nervous system. Soon it spreads to organs such as the heart. Patients may sweat profusely and cry, secrete copious amounts of thick, frothy saliva— the dreaded foaming at the mouth. Blood pressure and pulse may fluctuate wildly; body temperature may jump between burning fevers and abnormal coolness. The pupils of the eyes may dilate or contract, either separately or together. Male patients may have painful, persistent erections, and both male and female patients may have spontaneous orgasms. After one to two weeks, the patient slips mercifully into a coma and dies.

The child described at the opening of this chapter succumbed to furious rabies. The following patients illustrate further the features of the illness in human beings.

On April 21, 1992, an eleven-year-old boy was taken to a clinic in California because of pain in his left shoulder. The doctor thought that the boy had sustained an injury and treated him with Tylenol and codeine. The next day, the boy's parents were unable to give him his medication, because he refused to drink. The following morning, he could not bathe, because he was afraid of water. He became increasingly anxious and was taken to another clinic. That evening, when he began having hallucinations, he was brought to a hospital emergency room.

The emergency room doctors noted a combative boy with excessive salivation, who had trouble breathing. They placed him under heavy sedation, slipped a plastic tube into his airway, and attached him to a mechanical ventilator in the intensive care unit. The next day his temperature rose to 105.4°F. Despite a normal X-ray scan of his brain and a normal spinal tap, he continued to deteriorate and had two episodes of cardiac arrest from which he was successfully resuscitated. The doctors then transferred the child to a pediatric hospital.

On arrival, the boy had unstable cardiac function and evidence of inflammation and damage to the heart muscle. Over the next fourteen days, all brain activity ceased and he died.

Before his death, his doctors were able to isolate rabies virus antigens from a skin biopsy from the nape of his neck. They discovered that the child had a type of rabies found in dogs in Pakistan and India. The patient was born in India and had returned to visit between December 1991 and February 1992. One day, probably while he was playing with his friends, a stray dog bit him on the finger. He went to a local pharmacist, who gave him a bandage to apply to the wound site, but he never told his parents about the bite, which healed uneventfully.

The next patient with furious rabies was a twenty-six-year-old man from Mexico, who went to a private physician's office in Immokalee, Florida, on December 29, 1996. He complained of "anxiety, difficulty breathing while speaking," pain in his left lower abdomen, "left leg pain, lower back pain, and lethargy." He had bloodshot eyes, a common sign in early rabies. His temperature was below normal, but his pulse was rapid and he had a tender abdomen. The treating physician sent him by ambulance to a local emergency room, where he was treated for constipation and, when he said he felt better, released.

The next day he returned to the emergency room, because he had become anxious and short of breath when he tried to swallow. He now had a rectal temperature of 102°F. Over the next two to three hours, according to the account in the *Morbidity and Mortality Weekly Report,* he "became disoriented and agitated. During the lumbar puncture procedure, he jumped off the stretcher and became violent. After being restrained, he continued to scream and spit."

The man was intubated and placed on a mechanical ventilator in the intensive care unit. His doctors sent a biopsy of the skin on the back of his neck and saliva samples to CDC. Both samples were positive for rabies. On further study, it was found to be a strain associated with rabid dogs near the Mexico-Guatemala border. After the patient died, a friend reported that a puppy had bitten the victim in Chiapas, Mexico, two months before the onset of his illness. The patient killed the stray puppy at the time of the bite, and it was not available for testing.

In paralytic, or "dumb" rabies, patients tend to suffer less before they die, but delays in diagnosis make this form of the disease more hazardous to those around them, who may not take as stringent precautions to protect themselves from infectious secretions. Two of the most tragic cases in the history of transplant medicine occurred because the diagnosis of paralytic rabies was not considered in a patient dying of encephalitis.

A patient with paralytic rabies does not develop hydrophobia, aerophobia, or agitated behavior. The first symptom is usually weakness in the bitten extremity, sometimes with pain and trembling in the muscles of that limb. The weakness then creeps up the legs until the victim is paralyzed from the waist down and loses control of the bladder and bowels. After a few days the paralysis reaches the torso and arms, and the patient may lose the power to breathe unaided. In addition, there may be headache and a stiff neck, but the victim will usually not be confused until just before slipping into a coma. Death follows quickly. It is said that in South America most human rabies cases contracted from the bite of the vampire bat are of this type.

The following patient, also described in the *Morbidity and Mortality Weekly Report* of November 27, 1987, illustrates the clinical features of paralytic rabies. In March 1987, a rabid dog "severely bit a ten-year-old Thai boy on the left calf and forehead and on the right eyelid." The dog's tooth penetrated the outer membrane of his right eye. Although the child received rabies immune globulin and vaccine, he fell ill twenty-one days after the bite with "fever, headache, lethargy, vomiting, and progressive paralysis of all extremities." He died fifteen days later.

This patient's short, twenty-one-day incubation period and the failure of rabies preventive treatment reminded the editors of a similar case of vaccine failure in a twenty-year-old South African man who had been bitten on the finger by a rabid mongoose. He, too, became ill just three weeks after exposure despite preventive treatment. Severe bites by rabid animals to the face and digits, because of their rich nerve supply, are the most likely to lead to rabies and have the shortest incubation periods. The editors speculated that, in these two very high-risk bites, the fact that both patients received rabies injections in the buttocks led to vaccine failure. For optimal absorption, modern rabies vaccines should always be given in the upper arm.

Prompt diagnosis of rabies does not change the clinical outcome for the patient, who virtually always dies despite treatment. However, failure to diagnose paralytic rabies before death has had tragic consequences. In March 1979, physicians at the National Institutes of Health in Bethesda, Maryland, reported the following case of human-to-human transmission of rabies virus by corneal transplant.

The donor, a thirty-nine-year-old forester-rancher, was in excellent health until six days before his first hospital admission, when he developed lower-back pain and numbness over the lower right portion of his chest. The next day, his gait became unsteady, and his legs grew weak. The weakness spread upwards and soon reached his arms. He was admitted to a local hospital, and by the following day was too weak to swallow or breathe effectively. His doctors transferred him by air ambulance to St. Alphonsus Hospital in Boise, Idaho. On arrival he was intubated and placed on a mechanical ventilator.

The examining physicians found an alert but frightened man without a fever. He had weakness, not only of his extremities but of the muscles moving his eyes and face as well. His doctors thought he might have myasthenia gravis, a condition in which muscles are weak because nerve impulses to them are blocked, but tests for the disorder were negative. On the sixth hospital day, the man began having convulsions. Over the next three days he slipped into a coma. An electroencephalogram showed near shutdown of the brain's electrical activity. As the automatic functions of the central nervous system failed, his body temperature and blood pressure fell. On the sixteenth hospital day, the patient died. The cornea of his right eye was harvested for immediate transplantation, and the left one was frozen for later use.

The recipient of the cornea from the rabid rancher was a thirty-seven-year-old woman who had impaired vision due to an abnormally shaped cornea. Four and a half weeks after transplantation of his right cornea onto her right eye, she began to have a headache behind that eye and pain in the back of her neck and in her right shoulder. Her speech became slurred and she couldn't write properly. Her gait was unsteady. The next day she, too, was admitted to St. Alphonsus in Boise, where, after rapidly deteriorating, she lapsed into a coma and died fifty days after her transplantation surgery.

At autopsy, both patients had Negri bodies in stained microscopic sections of their brain cells. Negri bodies, which are specific for rabies, are clumps of virus particles within the nerve cells. After the autopsy, scientists at the National Institutes of Health then inoculated mice with specimens from the donor's frozen left cornea and the recipient's right eye. The mice developed rabies.

Since the publication of this case, patients dying of neurological syndromes of unknown cause have been excluded as organ donors. And for health care workers and others at risk after being exposed to rabies, we have rabies immune globulin and rabies vaccine. More than twenty thousand postexposure prophylaxis regimens are given each year in the United States alone.

The rabies vaccine has alleviated some of the terror of the disease and has undoubtedly saved countless lives. But it is important for us, the beneficiaries, to remember the courage that went into its creation.

Louis Pasteur halted an epidemic of silkworm-destroying parasites, saved the French wine industry by inventing pasteurization, and developed vaccines to prevent infections in chickens and pigs. Two common threads run through his work: a patriotic interest in the industries of France and a fascination with all things microscopic, particularly agents of disease.

By the time he turned to rabies, he was already in his sixties, and partially paralyzed on his left side from a stroke. To study rabies was a seemingly eccentric decision. Rabies is a tragic disease, but there were no more than two hundred cases in France each year. Furthermore, Pasteur was not a medical doctor nor had he ever experimented on human beings. But perhaps his childhood experience with rabies influenced his decision to pursue a cure.

When he was a boy, a mad wolf went on a rampage in the French Jura, attacking and biting both people and animals. Pasteur remembered seeing the wounds of one of the victims as it was being cauterized with a red-hot iron at the blacksmith's shop near his father's house. Those who had been bitten on the face or hands all died, including eight people in Pasteur's immediate neighborhood of Arbois.

Pasteur knew that the infectious agent of rabies was found in the saliva of its victims. He obtained a sample of saliva from a five-year-old child dying of the disease. Then he turned to the study of rabid dogs. An army veterinarian named Bourrel would send Pasteur a telegram when he heard of a new sighting of a mad dog. Greer Williams tells the following anecdote in his book *Virus Hunters*:

> One day, two of Bourrel's assistants threw a noose around a mad bulldog's neck, hauled him foaming from his cage, and then held him down on a table while Pasteur took a glass tube between his lips and through it sucked up a few drops of the deadly saliva from the animal's mouth. One slip could have meant a fatal bite on his face.

After a number of experiments in which he compared the bacteria growing in normal saliva to that in rabid saliva, Pasteur concluded that rabies was not a bacterial disease but was caused by some as yet unknown ultramicroscopic organism. Not deterred by this limitation in his knowledge of the ultimate cause of rabies, Pasteur worked to shorten the lengthy incubation period of the disease by injecting bits of a rabid dog's spinal cord directly into the brain of a rabbit. Then by harvesting the infected spinal cord from one rabbit and using it to infect another, he obtained a steady supply of the infectious agent in his laboratory.

Pasteur and his associate Emile Roux discovered that when an infected rabbit spinal cord is hung in a flask containing dry, sterile air, by the fourteenth day the virus is so weakened that it can no longer kill a rabbit. So, to build up immunity in a dog, Pasteur reversed this process. On the first day, the dog received an injection of fourteen-day-old rabid rabbit spinal cord. On the second day, he injected it with thirteen-day-old spinal cord. This continued until the fourteenth day, when the dog received an injection of one-day-old spinal cord. A healthy dog, thus treated, could be caged with a rabid one and emerge with multiple bites but no rabies. When vaccinated dogs were given chloroform anesthesia, and fully virulent rabies virus was injected directly into their brains, they proved likewise to be immune to the disease.

Based on these preliminary experiments, in May 1888, Pasteur began what he thought would be the first steps toward the development of a rabies vaccine for human beings. He requested that the Ministry of Public Affairs appoint a commission to verify his results, and he set up kennels to perform more extensive experiments on dogs.

Then, on July 4, 1888, in the Alsace region of northeastern France a mad dog attacked a nine-year-old boy named Joseph Meister as he walked to school. By the time a bricklayer drove the dog off with an iron bar, Joseph had received fourteen deep bites on his hands, arms, and thighs. Joseph's parents took him to Dr. Weber of Ville, who cauterized each wound painfully with carbolic acid. Despite this, the doctor thought the boy was at such high risk for contracting rabies that he advised the parents to take him to Paris to consult the eminent rabies researcher, Louis Pasteur.

On July 7, two and a half days after the attack, Joseph arrived in Paris. There was a brief but turbulent discussion in Pasteur's laboratory, in which Pasteur enlisted the advice of outside experts. Whether to vaccinate Joseph Meister with his live virus vaccine was a decision that Pasteur could not make by himself. Emile Roux was adamantly against using the vaccine, which was still in an early developmental stage, and resigned from the rabies research team. If the vaccine failed or killed the patient, its premature use would not only jeopardize future efforts to develop it but could potentially destroy the careers of everyone in the laboratory. In the end, Pasteur decided to administer the vaccine to Joseph Meister.

Dr. Jacques Grancher, one of Pasteur's physician advisors, agreed to administer the weakened virus preparation to the boy. The first of the fourteen inoculations were begun just three days after the attack. Every night following an inoculation, the normally calm Pasteur would lay awake in a state of anxiety. When he finally did fall asleep he was tormented by nightmares. He dreamed that Joseph was locked in the choking spasms of hydrophobia—the same agonies he had seen five years before in the child from whom he first obtained rabies-infected saliva.

Then, as the boy was being inoculated with progressively less attenuated rabbit-spinal-cord preparations, an accident occurred. As Dr. Grancher was taking the needle charged with the virus and moving toward the boy, he fumbled and plunged the syringe into his own thigh.

A second drama unfolded as Dr. Grancher told the laboratory staff that he had decided to submit to the vaccine series himself rather that risk contracting rabies. A second debate began, this one in secrecy. Pasteur's lab assistant Adrien Loir agreed to inject Dr. Grancher with the vaccine series. For reasons not entirely clear, Loir and his laboratory colleague, Viala, decided to share in the risk and undergo vaccination as well.

Grancher, Loir, Viala, and Joseph Meister survived fourteen injections of live, weakened rabies virus, and neither Joseph nor his doctor developed rabies. In Joseph's case, at least, it was clear that Pasteur's vaccine had saved his life. He grew up and became the gatekeeper of the Pasteur Institute. In 1940, at the age of sixty-four, he committed suicide rather than open the door to Pasteur's crypt to the invading Nazis.

A stream of bite victims now converged on Pasteur's laboratory from all over Europe. They included a fifteen-year-old shepherd who had been badly bitten saving a group of children from attack; nineteen wolf-bitten Russians, three of whom died despite vaccination; four children from New York, who all survived; and ten-year-old Louise Pelletier.

Louise had been bitten on the head by a rabid mountain dog thirty-seven days before she was brought in to Pasteur's lab. Although hers was a hopeless case, especially given the short incubation period of bite wounds to the head, Pasteur felt he could not refuse the pleas of her mother and father. Louise completed the fourteen injections, but eleven days after her last injection the unmistakable signs of hydrophobia began. Pasteur climbed the stairs to the family's rooms in the Rue Dauphine and sat with the child all day, holding her hand between the terrible spasms. As he was leaving, he said to her parents, "I did so wish I could have saved your little one."

There is still no cure for rabies. Once the disease begins, all patients, with very rare exceptions, die. Fortunately, we have rabies vaccines and immune globulins, which can prevent the disease in man and animals. And these products are the direct descendants of Pasteur's crude spinal cord vaccines.

Unfortunately, poor countries lack the infrastructure and money to vaccinate their populations of dogs and cats. And everywhere, including in the United States, many people do not fully grasp the risk of rabies following animal bites and exposures. On the flip side, vaccines are also often overused, because fear of rabies by paranoid patients and their overzealous doctors lead many people with low risk of exposure to rabid animals to undergo preventive injections.

In general, wild animal bites and some nonbite exposures merit consideration for rabies prophylaxis. Of especially high risk in the United States are bites by bats, wolves, foxes, skunks, coyotes, and raccoons. Since bat bites may be painless and almost invisible, anyone who has been possibly exposed to a bat while asleep (as when a bat is found in a bedroom) or who has even slight physical contact with a bat should seek medical consultation. In cases where the bat can be safely recovered and studied, vaccination may be delayed by a professional pending results of testing. Otherwise such persons should receive prophylactic treatment for rabies immediately.

On the low-risk side are bites by wild rodents (squirrels, rats, mice, chipmunks) and lagomorphs (rabbits, hares). These animals are almost never infected with rabies in the wild. One exception to this rule is the groundhog, which may become rabid following contact with infected raccoons.

However, the decision whether or not to recommend rabies prophylaxis following dog and cat bites may be difficult. It involves consideration of the vaccine status of the biting animal, the rabies risk in unvaccinated animals in the community, and the circumstances of the bite. Physicians caring for these patients often seek help in assessing rabies risk from infectious disease specialists or animal control agencies.

Rabies—being an ancient viral disease that most likely began in bats, a theory supported by many scientists—will always find a safe haven in the wild, as bats and their voracious appetites protect us from a world overrun by insects. Thus we must continue our uneasy coexistence with this terrible illness. But we can do so with a measure of calm, because we have the vaccine. Within two years of his saving Joseph Meister, Pasteur's health began to break down. He endured internal broils in his laboratory, lawsuits from the families of patients who died, and, worst of all, the burden of producing enough vaccine and administering it in time to the desperate patients who streamed into Paris. By 1887, weakened by heart disease, Pasteur suffered two more strokes. But he lived long enough to receive the love and homage of people all over the world, and their contributions helped establish the Pasteur Institute that endures to this day.

Toward the end of his life, Louis Pasteur received a letter from the father of Louise Pelletier, the child who had received the vaccine too late to be saved from the mountain dog's bite. M. Pelletier wrote, "Among great men whose lives I am acquainted with . . . I do not see any other capable of sacrificing, as in the case of our dear little girl, long years of work, of endangering a great fame, and of accepting willingly a painful failure, simply for humanity's sake."

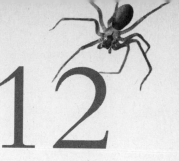

12

Bitten

Man's Best Friend

In 1994, dogs bit an estimated 4.7 million people in the United States and, in 1986, dog bites ranked twelfth among the leading causes of nonfatal injury in this country. Between 1979 and 1996, the Centers for Disease Control and Prevention recorded 279 dog-bite fatalities in the United States. California ranked first, with 30 fatalities, and Texas second, with 26. Of the ten pure breeds and seven crossbreeds, rottweilers accounted for 60 fatal attacks. The majority of fatalities are due to massive injury, and most occur in infants and children. However, fatal attacks on adults do occur, as in the much-televised San Francisco dog-mauling case in 2001.

Of the fatal cases compiled by CDC, about half of the bites involved an unrestrained dog on the owner's property. Attacking dog packs away from home account for as many as a third of fatalities. This observation suggests that, under certain conditions, even domesticated dogs may revert to feral behavior.

Yet massive dog-bite injuries are rare when compared to the wound infections that commonly follow even minor bites. Dogs have a gum structure similar to human beings, with crevices harboring a wide variety of microbes. Although dog-bite infections had been recognized since the early days of medicine, it was not until the 1970s that microbiologists began conducting systematic studies of the "gingival flora of the dog." In one study from the College of Veterinary Medicine at Michigan State University, published in 1976, two microbiologists used sterilized gauze pads and forceps to sample the bacteria living inside the gum lines of fifty healthy dogs. Between a third and a half of the dogs harbored the familiar species of streptococci and staphylococci that are frequent causes of dog-bite infections.

But other bacteria growing on the agar plates were so novel that they didn't even have proper names—bacteria like groups EF-2 and IIj. In addition, one very special species of bacteria grew in the mouths of twenty-two of the dogs studied, *Pasteurella multocida*—*Pasteurella* after Louis Pasteur, and *multocida* from the Latin meaning "killer of many." This organism, one of the most virulent known, can invade the tissues around a bite wound and involve an arm, leg, or face in red raging infection within twelve hours of a bite. *Pasteurella multocida* turns up in the mouths of many animals, from rats to raccoons, but it is especially common in dogs and cats, including the big cats.

In 1984, Dr. David J. Webber and coauthors from the Infectious Disease Unit at Massachusetts General Hospital described one of the most common dog-bite scenarios. A twenty-four-year-old man tried to separate two fighting dogs and, in the process, suffered multiple bite wounds to his left palm and the base of his left thumb. He first sought treatment in a community hospital emergency room where, under local anesthesia, his wounds were sutured and a severed nerve in his hand was repaired.

However, as is the case with many patients who develop *Pasteurella* infections from bite-wound injuries, he was allergic to penicillin. So, instead of the usual penicillin or ampicillin-based antibiotic regimens, he was given a prescription for erythromycin to prevent infection in his wound. Erythromycin is active against the common streptococci and staphylococci, but it is ineffective against *Pasteurella*. Within twenty-four hours he developed fever. Two days later he was admitted to Massachusetts General Hospital with redness and swelling extending to the middle of his forearm. When surgeons opened the wound in the operating room, they found pus all the way down to the deep tendons of the palm. Cultures of it grew miscellaneous dog-mouth bacteria and *Pasteurella multocida*. Since the publication of these and similar reports, most ER doctors now know that in patients with a history of allergy to penicillin, other antibiotics, like doxycycline, must be added to the dog-bite cocktail to keep *Pasteurella* from invading the wound.

While *Pasteurella multocida* aggressively penetrates the tissues around bite wounds, it only occasionally invades the bloodstream. Other bacteria may leave few traces of their presence at the bite site, but spread widely throughout the patient's body via the bloodstream. In 1977, Drs. Butler, Weaver, and Ramani published a paper in the *Annals of Internal Medicine* titled "Unidentified Gram-negative Rod Infection: a New Disease of Man." The authors reported seventeen seriously ill patients with fevers. Fourteen of these patients had an underlying illness, like cancer, and five had previously had their spleens removed for various reasons. Of the seventeen patients, ten had recently sustained dog bites and four others had histories of contact with dogs or other animals. The most seriously ill patients were the ones that lacked spleens. Two of them had so many millions of bacteria multiplying in their blood streams that, under the microscope, germs were visible in the patients' blood. The new organism was initially given the designation DF-2, but eventually, as more case reports accumulated, microbiologists decided on the picturesque name *Capnocytophaga canimorsus,* which means "carbon dioxide–eating, dog-bite" germ.

The following case of probable *Capnocytophaga* infection appeared in the *New England Journal of Medicine* in 1986. The patient, a thirty-eight-year-old woman, arrived in a community hospital emergency room in septic shock—a condition brought on by microbial invasion of the bloodstream. Instead of the normal blood pressure of 120/80, hers was 60/40. Large blotches of purple, unclotted blood shone through the skin of her face, neck, chest, and legs, and, as the doctors examined her, the purple spots spread over her arms. She began to bleed from the tear ducts of both eyes.

It seemed clear on clinical grounds that the patient had an overwhelming infection of some kind. Laboratory tests showed that something was destroying both her platelets and blood-clotting factors. But the identity of this invader was a mystery. The doctors turned to the patient's husband for clues.

The couple, he reported, had been camping in Martha's Vineyard, Massachusetts, two days previously, when a dog bit his wife on the lower leg. The next day she had a chill and complained of pain, swelling, and a purplish discoloration in the bite wound. On the day of admission she became weak, suffering diarrhea, vomiting, and tingling of her hands and feet. When she began bleeding into her skin, her husband brought her to the hospital.

"Was she in good health before?" they asked him.

"Yes," he said. She worked as a pediatric nurse's aide back home. However, there was one consideration: seven years earlier she'd had her spleen removed because of a blood disorder.

The doctors and nurses in the emergency room swarmed over their critically ill patient. They infused massive doses of antibiotics and gave transfusions of platelets to control bleeding. Because of the circulatory collapse resulting from shock, acid began accumulating in her bloodstream, making it necessary for her doctors to infuse ampoules of bicarbonate solution through her intravenous line to neutralize the effects. But even after she was pumped with nearly seven liters of intravenous fluid, her blood pressure remained critically low, and the purple spots of bleeding were spreading over her face. The doctors decided to transfer her by helicopter to Massachusetts General Hospital in Boston.

The receiving doctors noted that the woman was drowsy and had dried blood in her nostrils and on her lips. Fresh blood flowed from her right eye and from her vagina. They noticed two puncture marks on her right shin, but there was no pus or redness around the site. Despite the platelet transfusions she had earlier received, her platelet count was no higher than when she had arrived in the first emergency room. Studies of blood clotting showed that the patient was suffering from disseminated intravascular coagulation, or DIC. Some infectious agent had activated the entire clotting system, setting off a chain reaction that was consuming the soluble clotting factors and the platelets. Paradoxically, this process left her both vulnerable to uncontrolled bleeding and caused clots to form in the tiny arteries of her fingers. The digits, choked of their blood supply, were turning cold and blue-black.

On the second day at Massachusetts General, the victim was still in shock. Her blood oxygen level dropped, as her capillaries, poisoned by the infection, leaked fluid into her lungs. The blood cultures from the first hospital were negative, but at this point a sharp senior resident, Dr. Stewart Shuman, remembered a description he had read of DF-2 infection in a dog-bite victim who lacked a spleen. He knew that in this rare clinical situation there could be so many bacteria multiplying in the bloodstream that they might be visible under the microscope. Dr. Shuman obtained a drop of the woman's blood, spread it on a glass slide, and stained it with Gram's stain. As the specimen came into focus under high power, he could see the clinical drama being played out.

The blood film was speckled with polymorphonuclear leukocytes, white blood cells that engulf bacterial invaders, killing germs with enzymatic bombs and usually dying in the process. Inside these "kamikaze" white cells, Dr. Shuman saw pink-staining rod-shaped bacteria. He showed the slide to his superiors, who concurred. The shape of this germ, the fact that the patient lacked a spleen, and the catastrophic nature of her illness were almost certainly the work of the microbe we now call *Capnocytophaga*.

This woman spent over three weeks in the hospital and was dependent upon a ventilator machine to support her failed lungs for over a week. She lost most of her fingers at the first joint to gangrene. However, she survived, a lucky exception to the usual outcome of this kind of infection. After some time in a rehabilitation hospital, she went home to her family.

In the article on dog bite–related fatalities, published in 1997, the CDC listed the following measures for preventing dog bites:

1. Realistically evaluate environment and lifestyle and consult with a professional (e.g., veterinarian, animal behaviorist, or responsible breeder) to determine suitable breeds of dogs for consideration.
2. Dogs with histories of aggression are inappropriate in households with children.

3. Be sensitive to cues that a child is fearful or apprehensive about a dog and, if so, delay acquiring a dog.
4. Spend time with a dog before buying or adopting it. Use caution when bringing a dog or puppy into the home of an infant or toddler.
5. Spay/neuter virtually all dogs (this frequently reduces aggressive tendencies).
6. Never leave infants or young children alone with any dog.
7. Properly socialize and train any dog entering the household. Teach the dog submissive behaviors (e.g. rolling over to expose abdomen and relinquishing food without growling).
8. Immediately seek professional advice (e.g., from veterinarians, animal behaviorists, or responsible breeders) if the dog develops aggressive or undesirable behaviors.
9. Do not play aggressive games with your dog (e.g., wrestling).
10. Teach children basic safety around dogs and review regularly:
    a. Never approach an unfamiliar dog.
    b. Never run from a dog and scream.
    c. Remain motionless when approached by an unfamiliar dog (e.g., "be still like a tree")
    d. If knocked over by a dog, roll into a ball and lie still (e.g., "be still like a log").
    e. Never play with a dog unless supervised by an adult.
    f. Immediately report stray dogs or dogs displaying unusual behavior to an adult.
    g. Avoid direct eye contact with a dog.
    h. Do not disturb a dog that is sleeping, eating, or caring for puppies.

i. Do not pet a dog without allowing it to see and sniff you first.

j. If bitten, immediately report the bite to an adult.

The Cat Bite

Proailurus, the ancestor of all modern cats, appeared in the Old World thirty-four million years ago. At a time when *Mesohippus* was a Dalmatian-sized, three-toed creature hardly recognizable as the ancestor of the horse, *Proailurus* was already an unmistakable member of the clan *Felidae.* All of the modern cat families evolved during the late Miocene epoch, between five and ten million years ago. One branch led to the extinct saber-toothed line and the other spawned modern forms. *Felis catus,* the house cat, probably descended from an African wild cat only about seven thousand years ago. Cats were domesticated much later than were dogs. It was not until people developed agriculture and began to store grain, about 2500 B.C., that cats were domesticated, probably to control rodents eating harvested crops.

The cat was a sacred animal to the Egyptians as far back as the fourth millennium B.C. In the nineteenth century, so many millions of mummified cats were exhumed that they were shipped to Britain as ballast and ground into fertilizer. Archeologists even found mummified mice with some of the cats, presumably interred to provide them with food in the afterlife.

There are far fewer cat bites each year in the United States than dog bites—about four hundred thousand—but the infection rate following cat bites exceeds fifty percent. The jaws and teeth of dogs inflict a crushing bite, often with extensive immediate injury. But cats have a different type of biting apparatus, one adapted to stabbing and anchoring food by means of the canine teeth and cutting and shearing off pieces with the molars. The knifelike surfaces and needle-sharp points of cats' teeth make them incapable of chewing food. It must be sheared off and swallowed in chunks to be digested by powerful acids in the cat's stomach.

Cat bites, then, are deep, penetrating injuries. On the surface, the damage may look trivial, but the act of biting injects bacteria from the cat's mouth into the victims' deep tendons and even into the joints. There are also significant differences between the predominant bacteria in the mouths of cats and dogs.

From April 1994 through December 1995, a group of microbiologists and physicians called the Emergency Medicine Animal Bite Infection Study Group carried out a collaborative study of bite-wound infections. The investigators, who included Dr. Ellie Goldstein, performed meticulous wound cultures on fifty patients who were bitten by dogs and fifty-seven who were bitten by cats. Their results were published in the *New England Journal of Medicine* in 1999.

In general, these infected bites proved to be dirty wounds with a median of five different bacterial isolates. However, fully three-quarters of infected cat bites yielded *Pasteurella multocida,* confirming the clinical impression of infectious disease specialists that it is this microbe that makes cat bites so dangerous.

The following case report shows how the tiny, sharp teeth of a cat can inject *Pasteurella* into the victim's joint. The patient was a thirty-nine-year-old man, admitted to the Massachusetts General Hospital with swelling, tenderness, and drainage of pus from his right index finger nine days after being bitten by a cat. Although the patient did not have fever, his right index finger was markedly swollen. The cat's sharp teeth had penetrated the first knuckle joint. The doctors noted red streaking up the patient's forearm and some swollen lymph nodes in his armpit.

Cultures of the pus draining from the patient's finger wound yielded *Pasteurella* and a mixture of three other bacteria native to cat mouths. Fluid removed from the infected knuckle joint grew *Pasteurella multocida* in pure culture.

After three drainage procedures and multiple courses of antibiotics, the patient was cured but left with some joint stiffness as a result of his cat-bite infection. This patient's natural defenses, combined with the treatment he received, were able to confine his *Pasteurella* infection to his hand. However, this is not always the outcome. Sometimes, the organism breaches the immune defenses and spreads outside the confines of the wound.

An eighty-nine-year-old woman came to a hospital in Canada twelve days after being bitten on the right calf by her neighbor's cat. Within two days of the bite she developed signs of a serious local infection: redness, swelling, fever, a red streak ascending the lymphatic vessels of her leg, and swollen lymph nodes in her groin. Her family doctor gave her a prescription for erythromycin tablets, and her leg infection slowly subsided over the next eight days. However, eleven days after she was bitten, her caregivers found her lying on the bedroom floor with a purple bruise around her left eye. She said she had headache and was having trouble staying awake.

Physical examination in the emergency room disclosed sleepiness and fever. There was no sign of her original cat-bite infection. Even the swollen lymph nodes had subsided. However, when her doctors performed a spinal tap, her spinal fluid was creamy with pus cells, and *Pasteurella multocida* grew on culture. The microorganism had invaded the patient's bloodstream and penetrated the lining of her brain, causing meningitis. Fortunately, she responded to a course of treatment with intravenous penicillin.

The severity of any bite-wound infection is the result of the interplay of three factors: the virulence of the infecting germ, the adequacy of host defenses, and the extent of the original injury.

The last factor, severe initial injury, predominates when the attacker is not *Felis catus,* the house cat, but *Panthera leo,* the African lion.

The following case appeared in the *Journal of the American Medical Association* in 1985. The patient, "a young Masai warrior," came to the Kenyatta National Hospital in Nairobi two days after a lion bit him on the left shoulder. The young man had passed his test of manhood, slaying a lion while armed only with a spear, a long knife, and a shield. But during the battle the lion clawed the warrior's left thigh and bit his upraised left forearm and shoulder. The patient walked nine miles to his home, where he collapsed.

His family took him to a rural nursing station where his wounds were cleaned and bandaged. The next day, he had a high fever and pain in his left shoulder. He was given capsules of penicillin but he vomited most of them. The following day, his fever climbed to 105°F, and he became delirious. His shoulder was markedly swollen, and he could not move his arm without great pain. The health care workers at the rural station loaded him on an air ambulance and sent him to Nairobi.

The emergency room doctors found a confused, dehydrated young man with hot skin and a low blood pressure. There were deep, jagged tears over the left arm, but they did not appear infected. The lion's big canine tooth had gouged a hole the size of a dime in the back of his left shoulder. The wound was draining pus, and the entire shoulder was hot and swollen. On the youth's left thigh were multiple, linear lacerations, extending deep into the muscle and also oozing pus.

A Gram's stain of the drainage exiting the bite wound on the warrior's shoulder showed the short pink rods of *Pasteurella multocida,* which grew in pure culture. He was given a blood transfusion and intravenous antibiotics, including penicillin. Within two days the young man markedly improved, although his doctors had to perform skin grafts to repair his thigh wounds. The man spent about a month in the hospital and did not return to the clinic for his follow-up appointment. However, the outstation nurse reported that "the patient was received like a hero in his village."

The cat-bite story described above involves *Pasteurella multocida,* like the episode of the elderly woman. The following case is reminiscent of the October 2003 attack on illusionist Roy Horn, in which immediate neurological injury occurred following a tiger bite to the neck.

The patient, a young girl, had been helping with the care of animals at a children's zoo in British Columbia. She had been allowed to enter the cage of a Bengal tiger and to pet the animal, but when she turned to leave, the tiger suddenly seized her by the back of the neck. "After being held in the tiger's mouth for approximately 20 seconds, she was given a gentle shake and dropped to the ground."

In the hospital emergency room, doctors found an alert child who was paralyzed from the neck down. Over the next few hours the girl began to move her left leg and arm. She was then transferred to British Columbia Children's Hospital. On arrival there she was alert and had begun to move her leg a little, but her right arm and hand were still paralyzed. There was a three-inch gash on the upper right side of her neck and a half-inch puncture wound behind the right ear. However, as there were no signs of infection in these wounds, they were sutured.

Twenty-four hours after being bitten, the victim developed a fever of 103°F, began breathing rapidly, and had a seizure. An X-ray scan of her brain showed blood and fluid in the bony sinus behind her ear where the tiger's tooth had apparently penetrated. There was also a fracture visible in the arch of the first neck bone, with a fragment of bone loose near the spinal cord on the right side. Her doctors performed a spinal tap and found evidence of bleeding into the brain. In addition to blood, the spinal fluid showed a high white blood cell count and protein level, and a low level of sugar, all suggestive of infection. When the laboratory performed a Gram's stain of the fluid, the technicians saw the telltale pink rods of *Pasteurella*.

Because infected wounds cannot be surgically closed, the sutures in the child's neck were removed, and the wound was left open to drain. She was given intravenous antibiotics, including penicillin. Wound cultures grew *Pasteurella* and four other bacteria native to cat's mouths. The cerebrospinal fluid grew *Pasteurella* in pure culture.

In spite of the extent of the infection, the child survived, slowly recovering her mobility. However, she required several surgeries to repair her fractures and the torn lining of her brain. Ten months after her injury, she still had mild weakness of the right arm and leg, but was able to walk.

Immediate Treatment of Dog and Cat Bites

1. All cat bites and all high-risk dog bites should be evaluated by a physician within six hours and treated preventively with an oral antibiotic effective against *Pasteurella multocida,* staphylococcus, streptococci, and *Capnocytophaga*.
2. High-risk dogs bites include: bites to the hand or face, deep puncture wounds, wounds associated with extensive injury, or those occurring in patients lacking spleens or who have diminished immunity due to underlying disease or its treatment (some examples are HIV, cancer, rheumatoid arthritis, and organ transplants).
3. Except for disfiguring facial injuries, cat bites should not be sutured closed because of the high risk of infection.

4. Whether to suture a dog bite closed depends upon the time elapsed since the injury (under twelve hours for extremity or torso, under twenty-four hours for the face) and upon the judgment of the treating physician.

5. All patients who sustain dog or cat bites should receive tetanus toxoid if they have not received a booster in more than five years.

Human beings function, in part, as predators, and we seem to have an affinity with other predatory animals, probably because species that live by attacking and eating other creatures are often quick and intelligent. The agility and grace of cats and the social behaviors of dogs that have evolved for hunting have attracted human attention since antiquity. Those slow vegetarians, the turtle and the rabbit, though sometimes kept as pets, never elicit the same passionate devotion.

But every predator is equipped to kill, and no predatory animal can ever be completely tamed. Dogs and cats, both large and small, evolved in violence, and they must always be treated with vigilance and respect.

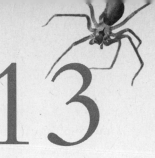

13

Menagerie

The Escape Artists

In 1988, physicians in Denver, Colorado, reported three cases of severe facial injuries to infants from attacks by pet ferrets. All three involved babies less than five months old, left briefly unattended in their cribs. In one of the cases a three-month-old girl was placed in her crib with her bottle. In just a few minutes, the family ferret managed to climb in and chew off forty percent of both her ears. Another patient in the series, a six-week-old boy, lost most of his left ear and, in another report, a baby girl lost her nose to a ferret attack.

The European ferret, *Mustela putorius,* is a predator in the weasel family. Ferrets are long, slender animals with short legs. Adult females are about a foot long (not including the tail), and males are about four inches longer. The ancient Egyptians kept ferrets as pets, and muzzled animals have been used to hunt small, burrowing game up to modern times. Attracted by the scent of milk, ferrets attack suckling animals in their dens. They were kept onboard sailing ships to control rodents and were the official mascots of the colonial navy of Massachusetts.

Mustela putorius was domesticated from the wild European polecat, and these animals should not be confused with the black-footed ferret, *Mustela nigripes,* which lives on the Great Plains and is an endangered species. Escaped European ferrets have established self-sustaining feral populations, and their attacks on commercial poultry have prompted some states and municipalities to prohibit the sale or ownership of these adaptable predators. Pet ferrets are illegal in California, Massachusetts, South Carolina, Georgia, New Hampshire, New York City, and Washington, D.C.

Ferrets have proved extremely valuable in medical research. Much of what we know about the natural history of influenza, for example, was learned in the laboratory by studying the infection in the European ferret, an animal exquisitely susceptible to this virus. Pet ferrets may contract influenza from their owners and, in turn, may transmit the flu to people.

Of greater concern, however, is the risk of contracting rabies from ferret bites. The skunk, a close relative of the ferret, is a notorious carrier of the disease, and ferrets readily contract the infection when they kill animals in the wild. According to the Centers for Disease Control and Prevention, nine cases of rabies were confirmed in ferrets in the United States between 1980 and 1987. One escaped ferret was found to be rabid when its owner recovered it ten days later. Since 1990, there has been a vaccine to prevent rabies in ferrets, and many states require animals over twelve weeks of age to be immunized. However, the efficacy of the vaccine in ferrets has not been rigorously demonstrated and, in fact, at least one vaccinated ferret has contracted rabies. In states where ferrets are prohibited, the many ferrets kept illegally are not usually vaccinated for rabies.

Unlike dogs and cats, which show symptoms of rabies within ten days of infection, ferrets and skunks may harbor the virus without symptoms for several weeks. A ten-day quarantine, as for dogs and cats, will not detect all rabid ferrets, and rabies vaccination of a bitten person may thus be dangerously delayed. Many authorities recommend that any ferret biting a human should be humanely killed and its brain examined for rabies.

Despite restrictions on their sale, there are an estimated five to seven million pet ferrets in this country. Ferrets are clean, intelligent, feisty, and friendly, and they are easily housebroken. For many years, ferret proponents have conducted a national campaign in print and online to repeal laws banning the animals as pets. In a letter to the *Journal of the American Medical Association* in 1989, Ferret Friends maintained that as long as they are not allowed to run freely about the house unsupervised, ferrets are safer pets than many other domestic animals. The letter cites a January 1989 attack in which a child in southern Arizona "had a sizable chunk taken out of her face while feeding a horse." Drs. Brian Lauer and John Paisley, authors of the report with which this chapter opened, wrote in answer to the letter that ferrets, unless caged at all times, are a constant danger to babies, and they add, "We are not aware of horses biting infants asleep in their cribs."

Ferrets may launch rapid attacks when supervision is allowed to lapse, even for a few minutes. In June 2000, a ten-day-old girl was attacked by two pet ferrets that may have been attracted by milk on the child's breath. The child's mother had let the ferrets out of their cage and had dozed off as she was watching television. A short time later, she awoke to her child's cries and found the baby's face covered with blood as a result of more than a hundred scratches, gashes, and bites. Had the family dog not jumped into the crib to save the infant, the attack could easily have proved fatal.

Confining the animals, however, has not always prevented attacks, as ferrets are escape artists. A 1998 report in the *Journal of Emergency Medicine* described two such attacks. In one, a ferret slipped out of its cage and attacked a four-month-old infant girl as she was riding in a safety seat in the back seat of her parents' car. In a few seconds the animal had inflicted three deep lacerations around the child's left eye. In the second case, a pet ferret attacked a sleeping five-year-old boy after it got loose. The parents had to pry the animal's jaws off the child's hand.

Since most ferret bites go unreported, statistical estimates of their frequency are inconclusive. Early in 1986, the California Department of Health Services solicited reports about ferret attacks from neighboring states, federal and local government agencies, and professional organizations. They were able to compile reports of 452 ferret attacks between 1978 and 1987. One hundred of these attacks occurred in California, where ferrets have been banned since 1935. Overall, there were sixty-three unprovoked attacks on infants and small children. In addition, a fatal attack on an infant was reported by the London Humane Society. One finding of note was that the majority of the biting ferrets belonged to a household other than the victim's. The four-month-old infant who lost 40 percent of her ears, for example, was attacked by a ferret at her baby-sitter's home.

Analysis of the available evidence suggests that the risk of a ferret bite from any individual animal is approximately the same as from a pet cat. But ferret attacks, while rare, are devastating, as these animals may "unleash frenzied, rapid-fire bite and slash attacks on all parts of the face . . . the result resembling ground beef," according to the California Department of Health Services.

Sleeping Barefoot

Worldwide, nearly four million rats are born every day, about ten for every person on earth. Rats carry more than seventy diseases, although only a few are transmitted directly by their bites. In the United States alone, rat-control programs cost nineteen billion dollars each year. Despite eradication efforts, rat populations are increasing, possibly as a result of global warming. A recent survey in the United Kingdom, for example, found rodent populations up 43 percent since the 1970s.

Unlike ferret attacks, rat bites are relatively common, especially among the urban poor. Rats bite ten in every one hundred thousand people each year in large cities, and most cases occur in children under age five. A survey in Philadelphia published in 1999 reported a total of 264 rat-bite cases over the twelve-year period from 1985 to 1996. The majority of bites occurred in sleeping children between midnight and eight a.m. and involved the face and hands. Bites were more common during the warmer months of the year, and victims were usually Hispanic or African-American.

In Philadelphia, the risk for rat bite was highest in old buildings constructed over sections of the city where sewer lines dated back to the turn of the last century. Cracks and breaks in the pipes allowed the Norway rat—the main American biter—to tunnel upward from their sewer homes and into human dwellings. The rats, which are dependent on humans for food, then established residence in the basements and first floors of the buildings.

Rat bites occur among poor people in newer urban dwellings as well. In 1985, physicians working in the emergency room at the Martin Luther King Hospital in Los Angeles reported a series of fifty rat-bite cases treated at their hospital between 1980 and 1983. Of those patients, 64 percent were Hispanic, and 36 percent were black. The majority of these bites occurred while the victims were asleep, though one person was bitten while trying to feed a wild rat. The patients ranged in age from five months to forty-two years, but 44 percent were under five years old. Most of the bites were to areas of the body exposed while the patients were sleeping. Although 30 percent of the bite wounds had positive cultures for bacteria, almost no serious infections occurred, probably because the patients usually sought treatment within hours of being bitten. When social workers made visits to the homes of some of the bite victims, they found that many of the patients were living in squalor. Investigation of these families revealed that other members had been previously bitten, in one case seven of a boy's siblings.

In most of the large series of rat bites, the injuries have been minor. However, there are isolated reports of serious biting injuries, and, as with ferret bites, infants are usually the victims.

In March 1985, a three-month-old boy was brought to a hospital in South Wales. The mother had placed the baby in his cot in the morning while she attended to her older son downstairs. She hurried upstairs when she heard the baby crying. When she reached him, she found multiple bites on the left side of his face. However, the most serious injury was to his left upper eyelid, half of which had been bitten off. At first the family suspected a wild ferret, which had been seen near their cottage. The ferret was subsequently captured and killed, and the body, along with photographs of the child's injuries was sent to a forensic dentist at the School of Dentistry in Cardiff. Based on the evidence, the dentist concluded that a rat, rather than a ferret, had probably attacked the baby. Plastic surgeons reconstructed the victim's eyelid, but he was left with facial disfigurement. However, in South Carolina, another baby was not so lucky.

In the fall of 1991, not long after Hurricane Hugo had flooded neighborhoods all around South Carolina, a father found his seven-week-old infant boy crying in a "pool of blood." The boy had cuts on the left side of his face and on his left hand. He was examined under anesthesia, where surgeons found and sutured four deep lacerations in the globe of the left eye. The bite wounds healed without infection, but the vision in the injured eye was effectively destroyed. The injuries were thought to be the result of a rat attack, probably by hungry rodents displaced by hurricane flooding.

Another group especially susceptible to rat bites are people with numb hands or feet—a consequence of certain diseases that damage nerves carrying sensory impulses. Barefoot diabetics, for example, have trod on carpet tacks and unknowingly proceeded to walk around with them lodged in their feet, unaware of their injury until serious infections occurred. Sleeping barefoot diabetics with nerve damage are uniquely susceptible to rat-bite injuries, as the following 1989 series of cases from the West Indies illustrate.

A diabetic on insulin therapy awoke one morning to see a rat eating his left great and second toe. He had suffered from diabetic nerve damage for about four years, with numb feet, absence of reflexes, and sexual impotency, and he could not feel the bites. Another patient, a diabetic woman, also woke up to find a rat biting her left big toe, which was gangrenous from diabetic blood-vessel damage and completely numb. This woman had to have her leg amputated below the knee.

Another important cause of nerve damage is leprosy, or Hansen's disease, which affects an estimated six million people worldwide. In leprosy, a bacterium related to the tubercle bacillus, lives inside the cells of the skin and, in some cases, destroys the sensory nerves of the hands and feet. In his book *Anatomy of an Illness,*

Norman Cousins describes the work of Drs. Paul and Margaret Brand, surgeons who cared for leprosy patients in the 1940s at the Medical College at Vellore, India.

In India, leprosy is a deforming and disabling disease, in which the hands become contracted like claws, and fingers and toes are gradually lost, joint by joint. When the Brands started their work, the prevailing idea was that the infection directly destroyed the patients' tissues, causing the flesh to atrophy and slough off. Despite this tissue damage, leprous patients were said to have prodigious strength in their hands.

But the Brands discovered that profound numbness was the explanation for both the tissue destruction and the apparent muscle power of leprosy patients. One day a leprous boy of twelve, watching Paul Brand try unsuccessfully to turn a key in a large rusty lock, stepped up and turned the key with ease. However, when he examined the boy's hand afterward, Dr. Brand found that the key had cut the flesh of his thumb and forefinger to the bone. Profoundly numb, the boy had been unaware of the damage that was occurring and kept exerting force long past the point where a person with normal sensation would have known to stop.

This was an important clue, but it still did not explain why the couple's patients kept turning up with parts of their fingers and toes missing. If they had fallen off, what happened to the pieces? In a flash of insight, Paul Brand realized it must be the nocturnal work of rats. He set up observation posts at night in the huts and wards, and it was just as he thought. Cousins writes:

> The rats climbed the beds of lepers, sniffed carefully, and, when they encountered no resistance, went to work on fingers and toes. The fingers hadn't been dropping off; they were being eaten.

The Brands were able to control the problem in their hospital by building barriers around the legs of the beds, but in parts of the world where leprosy and poverty coexist, rats continue to play their distinct role.

While rat-bite injuries only rarely threaten the life of the victim, the germs they carry in their mouths can cause a serious, and even fatal, infectious syndrome called rat-bite fever. Rat-bite fever actually describes two distinct diseases—Haverhill fever, first reported in the United States, and *sodoku* (Japanese for rat-bite fever), first recognized in Japan.

Descriptions of an infectious syndrome called rat-bite fever were recorded in the United States in the first half of the nineteenth century. In 1914, Dr. H. Schottmüller isolated a pink-staining bacterium growing in beadlike chains from the blood of a man who had become ill after a rat bite. However, the organism was forgotten until 1934, when eighty-six people in the town of Haverhill, Massachusetts, become sick after drinking milk contaminated with rat excretions. The outbreak was eventually traced to Dr. Schottmüller's bacterium, now called *Streptobacillus moniliformis* (from Latin *monile,* a necklace). Although occasional outbreaks of food- or waterborne illness caused by this organism still occur, *Streptobacillus moniliformis* infection most commonly follows bites by rats and other rodents, as in the following case described by physicians in Seattle in 1969.

A twenty-one-year-old laboratory technician was bitten at work by a rat, on the index finger of his left hand. Forty-eight hours later, he started having shaking chills, fever, vomiting, and pain in his muscles and joints. The pain was especially severe in his left shoulder and hip, and in both elbows. Shortly thereafter, he broke out with a rash on his palms, soles, legs, and torso. The man was admitted to the hospital, and after specimens of his blood were drawn for culture, he was given injections of penicillin. Six days later, when he was already feeling well, his blood cultures became positive for *Streptobacillus moniliformis*.

In the days before antibiotics, rat-bite fever often entered a chronic phase, with intermittent attacks of fever and persistent arthritis, lasting up to two years and leaving the patient with damaged joints. On rare occasions, *Streptobacillus moniliformis* infects a heart valve, and this condition is always fatal if not treated in time, as in the following tragic case reported in the *Annals of Emergency Medicine* in 1985.

The parents of a three-month-old boy in South Carolina brought him to a local physician's office after they noticed puncture wounds and scratches on the baby's arms. They had seen rats in the house and suspected that the child had been bitten. Since the wounds did not look infected, the doctor sent the boy home without treatment. However, the next day the child began having fever and diarrhea.

His parents then took him to the emergency room of the Richland Memorial Hospital in Columbia. On examination, the infant had a temperature of 104 and a rapid pulse, but otherwise looked well. He was alert, sucked actively on a bottle of Pedialyte, and clutched the doctor's stethoscope. There were two half-inch-long scratches on his left wrist and four puncture wounds on his right hand, none of which looked infected. Laboratory tests were reassuringly normal.

The emergency room physicians thought the child had a viral syndrome and sent him home with directions to the parents to give him Tylenol drops every four hours for fever. They were given an appointment to return in twelve hours.

The next morning the parents brought the boy back for his follow-up appointment. His temperature was down to 101°F, and he continued to look well. However, over the next day he became increasingly lethargic. Eighteen hours after he left the emergency room, and three and a half days after his rat bites, his parents found him dead in his crib. An autopsy showed infection of his heart valves, and cultures of his blood taken after death grew *Streptobacillus moniliformis.*

The second type of rat-bite fever was first described in Japan where, for over a hundred years, the Japanese have been familiar with a disease contracted from the bites of rodents called *sodoku, so* meaning rat and *doku* meaning poison. The causative organism, *Spirillum minus,* was discovered in the nineteenth century, and in 1908, a Japanese microbiologist named Ogata described spiral organisms in the wounds, lymph glands, and blood of *sodoku* patients. *Spirillum minus* belongs to a family of corkscrew-shaped bacteria called spirochetes. Other members of this family include the agents of syphilis and Lyme disease. *Spirillum minus* has never been grown on artificial media, and there are no blood antibody tests. Diagnosis depends entirely upon seeing characteristic spirochetes in blood or tissue from suspected cases.

Spirillary rat-bite fever is never food- or waterborne, but is almost always contracted as a result of a bite. The bite wound heals uneventfully, but one to four weeks later it becomes red-purple, swollen, and painful. A red streak of infection in the lymphatic channels then extends from the wound to the nearest draining lymph glands, which begin to swell. The patient runs a temperature, but the joints are spared in this form of rat-bite fever. Sometime during the first week of the illness, the patient's skin breaks out everywhere with a blotchy, red-purple to red-brown rash. The white blood-cell count climbs, and up to half of patients will have a falsely positive blood test for syphilis. Without treatment, victims have fevers on and off for a month or two. Left untreated, six to ten percent of patients will have a fatal spread of infection to the heart. But ten to fourteen days of penicillin treatment given early promptly cures most people.

In 1969, a thirty-five-year-old physician was bitten on the left index finger by a white laboratory rat. The wound healed promptly, but, twelve days later, he developed swelling, redness, and tenderness at the site of the healed bite. The next day, there was a red streak extending up his left forearm and he had shaking chills and fever. The patient, who was a hematologist, made a stained smear of his own blood and saw spiral-shaped bacteria. He took penicillin pills and felt better within twenty-four hours.

At least ten percent of people who work with laboratory animals face another occupational hazard—hypersensitivity to allergens present in urine and dander. Typically these workers suffer various combinations of wheezing, runny nose and eyes, facial swelling, and hives. On occasion, rat bite victims may develop acute anaphylactic reactions to substances in the rat's saliva, the same kind that occur after stings in patients highly allergic to bee or fire ant venom. The following case was reported in 1995.

A thirty-five-year-old research director at the University of Virginia School of Medicine sustained a rat bite while supervising an experiment in her laboratory. Within two minutes, her face became red and swollen, and she began to wheeze. Gasping for breath, she managed to walk the two hundred yards from her laboratory to the medical center. Five minutes after the rat bite, she staggered into the emergency room and collapsed. Within seconds, she turned blue, lost consciousness, and went into cardiac arrest.

Doctors and nurses in the ER performed cardiopulmonary resuscitation, inserting a plastic tube into her lungs and administering epinephrine (adrenaline) and hydrocortisone. After she recovered, she told her doctors that, beginning about a year before her attack, she had been having bouts of runny eyes and nose, and most recently wheezing when she worked with rats. She was discharged twenty-four hours after admission with an epinephrine-containing emergency kit and instructions to avoid all contact with rodents.

Not Horsing Around

In March 2002, a plastic surgeon at my hospital consulted me regarding antibiotic treatment for a horse bite. The patient, an eighteen-year-old woman, had been in the corral with a stallion when the horse clamped her entire right hand and wrist in its jaws. Although no bones were broken, the horse's teeth had lacerated the skin on the top and bottom of her hand. She first sought treatment in an outlying hospital, where the doctor ordered a tetanus shot, irrigated the wound, sutured it closed, and began empiric antibiotics by vein.

However, three days later, the young woman came to our hospital with redness, pain, and swelling in her hand and arm, and a relapse of fever and chills. There was so much swelling that the skin of the original suture line was stretched tight. I recommended adding another antibiotic to her regimen, and, by the next day, some of the redness on her forearm had receded. That day I examined the patient for the first time. Her hand was still tensely swollen, and she was unable to make a fist. Looking into her eyes as she tried to move her injured extremity, I was struck by the look of fear and vulnerability I saw there. She told me the stallion's attack had shaken her, and, though she was an experienced horsewoman, I wondered if she would ever be able to handle the animals again with the same confidence.

Later that day, the plastic surgeon took the woman to the operating room and removed all of the original sutures, irrigated the wound with sterile saline solution, and inserted a rubber drain. Her physical wounds healed slowly but uneventfully over the next two weeks.

Horse-bite injuries are fairly uncommon, relative to other

bites. In 1985, for example, American military personnel in central Germany reported that of 178 animal bites treated in that year, only 2 were due to horses. And in a review published in 1978, of 622 injuries caused by horses, only 24 were due to bites.

Donkeys

Although we usually think of donkeys as mild little animals, they can, on occasion, inflict nasty injuries. A twenty-year-old woman in Sweden had kept a donkey as a companion for her horse for some time. When she separated the donkey from the horse, it turned violent and clamped its jaws firmly on her thumb, refusing to let go. After the donkey was pried loose with a crowbar, the woman was taken to the emergency ward of the hospital in Gävle.

She had deep teeth marks on both sides of her thumb, but no fracture or joint injury. The physician ordered a tetanus vaccine and gave her narcotic tablets for pain, but no antibiotics.

Five days later, at the health center in Skutskär, she visited her primary care physician who noted pus draining from her thumb wounds. A culture of the wound was sent to the laboratory, and the patient was given antibiotic tablets. Interestingly, the cultures grew an organism, *Staphylococcus hyicus,* which is native to horses' mouths but which had never caused human infection before. The woman did well, though some residual nerve damage seemed to have occurred, as the tip of her thumb continued to be numb despite the wounds having healed.

Beast of Burden

Much more serious and even fatal injuries are inflicted by the camel, which is not only a beast of burden but also an essential source of wool, milk, meat, and hides. Camels, whether Arabian or the two-humped Bactrian, can stand over seven feet tall. Although normally docile when properly trained, the males are liable to have fits of rage during the rutting season. According to Dr. Ahmad Amer Al-Boukai of the King Khalid University Hospital in Riyadh, Saudi Arabia, handlers are typically bitten when they raise an arm to pull on the reins of the camels' heads to make them kneel. In his opinion, the bites "are usually a sudden vengeance for offences committed previously and which might have been forgotten by the handlers."

Dr. Al-Boukai and his colleagues described four extraordinary cases of severe osteolysis, or dissolved bone, in victims of camel bites, often many years previously. These case histories are testimonies to the stoicism and adaptability of the camel drivers.

The first patient was admitted to the hospital one year after a camel bit him on the left side of his chest. He had a cough, and doctors found a bulge at the site of the bite where four ribs had been destroyed by chronic infection following the injury. The surgeons reconstructed his chest wall with a synthetic mesh.

The other three patients had remote histories of camel bites to the arms. In each case, one of the arm bones had become infected and partially dissolved. Each man had adapted to some extent to his injury, including one camel driver who had lost most of the bone of his right upper arm to a bite thirty years previously. He had learned how to splint the boneless segment by forcefully contracting the muscles between shoulder and elbow, shortening the extremity so that the forearm and hand could be used. He was actually consulting the physician in Riyadh for an unrelated respiratory ailment.

However, some camel-bite injuries are too severe to be treated with folk remedies or merely endured. Doctors at the Usmanu Danfodiyo University Teaching Hospital in Sokoto, Nigeria, published a series of cases featuring four camel-bite wound infections, including that of a forty-year-old man who sought help twelve days after a camel bit his face down to the muscle. He tried to take care of the injury at home but sought treatment after developing symptoms of tetanus. Unfortunately, this condition proved fatal despite hospital care.

In another report from the same hospital, two surgeons describe how they saved the life of a sixteen-year-old boy. After a camel attacked him, his lower jaw was broken in many places, and three teeth were pulled out of their sockets. In the operating room the doctors reconstructed his shattered jaw using metal bridges and stainless-steel wires. After six weeks they removed the hardware and provided the boy with an acrylic partial denture. He returned home with good jaw function and without facial disfigurement.

Flying Spears

Mention fish bites, and the shark or much-maligned piranha come to mind. Sharks have been extensively covered elsewhere; as for piranhas, despite their fierce appearance, there is actually not a single documented case of a person being killed by one. But certain silver-colored members of the order Beloniformes that inhabit the warm Indo-Pacific Oceans have caused serious injury and death. Known by various names—garfish, needle-fish, long tom, and *aiguille* (French for needle)—these fish are surface predators, grow as long as four feet, and streak through the water in schools, at speeds of up to forty miles an hour. Their slender, spear-shaped beaks consist of two narrow jaws lined with rows of small, pointed teeth. They are capable of high-speed leaps of up to six feet out of the water, particularly when attracted by light.

In 1982, Dr. Peter G. Barss published a report in the *British Medical Journal* that described ten patients who were treated for garfish injuries at the Provincial Hospital in Alorau Milne Bay Province, Papua, New Guinea. All of the injuries occurred under similar circumstances: all of the victims were using lights to fish from canoes at night. There were three fatalities, among them the following case. A thirty-year-old man was spearing fish at night from a canoe, using a lantern, when a garfish leaped up from the water. He speared it. A second garfish followed, piercing the left side of his chest. He was taken to a nearby aid station, where the wound was quickly sutured closed. Then he began to deteriorate. Several hours passed before a boat could be found to take him to the hospital. He died in transit. At autopsy, the coroner found a quart of blood in the man's chest and more still in the abdomen. The fish's beak had pierced his chest, missing his lung, but perforating his stomach. The man had died from shock due to bleeding and leakage of his stomach contents.

Another patient in this series, a nine-year-old girl, required surgery when a garfish had perforated her stomach and liver. Two patients were blinded in one eye, one of whom was left paralyzed on one side of his body. Dr. Barss noted a further twenty-three patients injured by these fish—eight of which were additional fatalities. Other patients had come to the hospital to have the tip of the garfish beak removed after it became embedded in their bodies. He cautioned health care workers to remember that a garfish wound that appears trivial on the surface may be a sign of serious internal injury.

Seal Finger

In 1907, one J. H. Bidenknap, a Norwegian, reported the first official account of an affliction greatly feared by generations of seal hunters in the North Atlantic. Called seal finger in English, it was known as *spaek* finger—or "blubber finger"—by Norwegians. Following the bite of a seal or contact with its tissues, usually during skinning, a small pimple occurs at the site of the exposure. Over the next several weeks the afflicted individual begins to have throbbing pain at the bite site, aggravated by the slightest movement. The joint nearest the pimple and then the entire finger become swollen and stiff. Except for the agonizing pain, the sealer is generally well and without fever. But unable to sleep or to work, some of these men amputated their own fingers.

The cause of seal finger remained a complete mystery for many years. By trial and error, sealers and their doctors had found that the antibiotic tetracycline, if taken soon enough after the symptoms first appeared, could cure the illness. But all attempts to culture the causative organism from the sealer's wounds failed to yield a consistent result. Ironically, most recent reports of seal finger have involved people interested in the welfare of seals, as in the following 1981 case report from the *Journal of Hand Surgery*.

A twenty-three-year-old woman working as a volunteer at a marine mammal rehabilitation station near San Francisco was bitten by a baby elephant seal on the right index finger. Within twenty-four hours, her finger became painful and swollen. She was given erythromycin and an antibiotic in the penicillin family to take by mouth, but two weeks later, the joint nearest the knuckle was so swollen and tender that she had to be taken to the operating room for drainage under anesthesia.

Despite this treatment, the infection continued to progress. By eight and a half weeks after the bite, the woman had severe pain and stiffness affecting both joints of that digit, which she was now unable to bend. The site of the original bite was open and draining. Finally, her physicians decided to try tetracycline therapy. The pain and drainage diminished, but X-rays showed that the first finger joint had been destroyed. She underwent a second surgery, this time to fuse the joint, which relieved the pain. However, as a result of the baby elephant seal bite and her infection, the woman lost half of her pinch strength (the ability to grasp objects between the forefinger and thumb).

The first break in the seal finger puzzle came in 1979 and 1980, when an epidemic of pneumonia began killing seals along the New England seaboard. Cultures of the animal's lungs after death revealed a finicky, slow-growing bacterium called *Mycoplasma*. A species of *Mycoplasma* is a cause of pneumonia in people, as well. During a second epidemic of seal pneumonia in the Baltic in 1988 and 1989, two new species of *Mycoplasmas* were isolated from dead and dying animals.

Then in 1990, a young trainer at the New England Aquarium sustained a seal bite on her right forefinger. Six days after the bite, the trainer's finger had become swollen, painful, and red, and a clear discharge seeped from the wound. The clear fluid was cultured with careful attention to the strict growth requirements of the organism. One of the organisms from the Baltic epidemic, *Mycoplasma phocacerebrale* appeared on the culture plates. This bacterium was susceptible to tetracycline, but resistant to the antibiotics in the penicillin family usually given for skin infections. *Mycoplasma phocacerebrale* and other related organisms are likely to be the long-sought infectious agents of seal finger. Based on these preliminary reports, all patients bitten by marine mammals should be offered treatment with tetracycline as early as possible after the injury in an effort to prevent this devastating condition.

Birds

In 1987, in Walton, New York, a three-month-old boy was brought to the hospital with several deep, half-inch-long scalp lacerations. When his two physicians retracted the skin margins of the cuts to explore and clean the wounds, they found that the infant's skull had been fractured. According to the child's grandparents, the boy had been lying on a blanket in their rural backyard when "an unprovoked rooster attacked him with [its] beak and possibly claws."

Rooster attacks are not uncommon and, no doubt, most minor ones go unreported. The ancient sport of cock fighting exploits the ferocity of these birds, which attack, not only with their beaks, but also with their claws and a sharp spur on each foot. The following fatality resulting from a rooster attack in South Africa was reported in 1987.

A sixteen-month-old girl was attacked by a rooster, which pecked her on the left side of her head. She was admitted to the hospital several days later because of facial swelling and seizures, and was given intravenous penicillin. After the convulsions she remained in a stupor and so was transferred to University Hospital in Johannesburg for further treatment. On admission, an X-ray scan showed a large abscess on the left side of her brain. She was taken to the operating room where neurosurgeons drained the pus. She never gained consciousness and died six days after her transfer. Most likely, bacteria invaded the girl's brain, having entered through a small skull fracture from the rooster pecking.

Rooster injuries are not limited to children. Doctors in Turkey reported the case of a sixty-year-old woman who was pecked by a rooster on the right side of her face. Ten days after the incident she had trouble opening her mouth (lockjaw) and difficulty swallowing. She eventually required a tracheotomy and spent a month in a dark room, sedated and on a ventilator, before she recovered and was able to go home. Since roosters peck food off the ground, the bacteria of tetanus were probably introduced into the flesh when she was pecked.

Newspaper reports occasionally appear of minor attacks on joggers, pedestrians, and hikers by crows and magpies. Three physicians in Switzerland wrote a letter to the *New England Journal of Medicine* in 1984 describing their experience over a period of two years of treating twelve joggers attacked by European buzzards. The attacks almost all occurred during the breeding season between April and July. The birds attacked by diving from behind, causing scalp scratches and lacerations.

Some of the most serious attacks on people have come from birds that can't fly at all. On February 15, 2001, an employee of the San Francisco Zoo suffered deep cuts on his left leg when an eighty-pound New Zealand cassowary attacked him after he entered its cage. These homely birds grow up to six feet tall and weigh up to one hundred pounds. The males attack to defend their territory.

Ostriches, too, will attack in defense of territory. In 1997, a sixty-three-year-old woman in South Africa was kicked and stomped to death after taking a shortcut with her husband through an ostrich herd on an adjacent farm. The husband, who had also been seriously injured by the ostriches, was unable to come to his wife's aid.

On Christmas Eve 2001, in Dallas, Texas, a man named Kevin Butler was found stabbed to death in his apartment along with the body of his eighteen-inch crested cockatoo, named Bird, also stabbed. The prime suspect was Butler's coworker, Daniel Torres.

Bird provided the key piece of evidence that lead to Torres's eventual conviction. Apparently while Torres was attacking Butler, Bird flew at Torres and pecked his forehead. Torres then wiped his bleeding wound with his hand and touched a light switch, leaving his DNA at the crime scene. Police investigators also found his DNA on the handles of the two knives he used to attack Butler and Bird.

"This bird spoke; he spoke to us," prosecutor George West told jurors. "We know this bird will attack anybody who is attacking his owner. And who did he attack? Daniel Torres." Torres was convicted of capital murder and sentenced to life in prison.

And finally, doctors treating victims of animal attacks need to consider what the animal is normally eating when it's not attacking people. Consummate nocturnal predators with excellent night vision and silent flight, owls eat mice and other small animals, intestines and all. As a result, their claws and beaks are teeming with gut bacteria, including oxygen-hating anaerobes.

In a case reported in 1992, a fifty-eight-year-old man came to the general medicine clinic at the University of Iowa College of Medicine because of a laceration extending all the way from his right jaw to the left side of his head. He told the doctors that four days earlier he had been sitting by a campfire at midnight, when he was unexpectedly "attacked by a large bird" and knocked out of his lawn chair. He "saw feathers fly" and though he didn't get a look at his assailant, as an avid outdoorsman, he was confident it was an owl.

The cut didn't appear infected, and no antibiotics were prescribed. However, four days later he returned to the clinic, because the wound had become red and was draining a little fluid. His physicians took careful cultures, but because of concern about a drug allergy, the antibiotic cocktail they prescribed did not include an agent that is active against oxygen-hating anaerobes.

Three days later, the patient again returned to the clinic, because his head wound was now draining foul-smelling pus. The cultures taken previously were growing two species of the anaerobe *Bacteroides,* probably from rodent intestines. He was then given an antibiotic active against the organism, and his wounds healed. The patient seemed to take the adventure in stride and even came to the clinic wearing a baseball cap that read OWL FOOD.

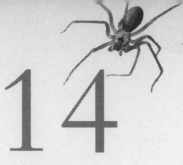

14

Monkey Business

I was sitting at my desk near the emergency room of the Sepulveda Veterans Hospital late one Friday afternoon in October 1987 when my telephone rang. The male voice on the other end was talking fast, stumbling over words, and at first not making much sense at all.

"She bit me, doc, and she's B-virus positive!"

"Who bit you?" I asked.

"Adelaide. She's a rhesus in the primate colony."

The young man I'll call Jim collected himself enough to tell me that he worked as a research assistant in the VA psychology laboratory on the hospital grounds. They were doing experiments with rhesus monkeys, each of which had been tested for infection with B-virus, a common infection in macaques.

Most herpesviruses are numbered. This one is named after the first researcher it was known to have killed, W.B.

"I want you to come over to Building 3 right away. I'll meet you in the emergency room," I said.

. . .

On October 22, 1932, William B. Brebner, a twenty-nine-year-old physician who was engaged in experimental work on poliomyelitis, was bitten on the ring and little fingers of his left hand by a healthy-appearing rhesus monkey. Brebner painted his wounds with iodine and alcohol and continued his work.

Three days later, he noticed that the bites were somewhat red and swollen. Most alarming, in this era before antibiotics, was the red line of infection streaking up his arm. Soon the lymph glands near his elbow and in his left armpit started to swell. Six days later, on October 28, Dr. Brebner was admitted to the Third Surgical Service of Bellevue Hospital in New York City. On admission he had a temperature of 101.4°F. With the exception of his sore arm, he appeared well. His doctors prescribed an injection of tetanus antitoxin and kept him under observation.

Over the next few days, Dr. Brebner seemed to improve. Several small blisters, similar to chicken pox spots, appeared near the site of his bites, each containing a small amount of cloudy fluid. However, by this time, the red streak had disappeared, and the swollen glands were smaller and only slightly tender. He experienced two days of abdominal cramps, but by November 2 they had stopped.

Between November 2 and 4, Dr. Brebner appeared well, and it seemed that he was out of danger. In reality, he was only passing through the eye of a viral hurricane. The incubating infection was moving inexorably toward his brain and spinal cord. On November 4, thirteen days after the bite, he was unable to pass urine. The muscles of the bladder wall were paralyzed. In addition, his skin from the waist down was painfully oversensitive. Even the lightest touch was unpleasant, in the same way a limb, which has fallen asleep, feels as it begins to wake up. His knee jerk reflexes disappeared.

Thinking that he may have contracted poliomyelitis, Dr. Brebner requested an injection of serum obtained from patients recovering from the disease. But the treatment had no effect. By the next day, he was unable to move his legs at all. The doctors performed a spinal tap (lumbar puncture). The cerebrospinal fluid was clear to the naked eye, but under the microscope they found an increased number of the white cells called lymphocytes that suggest a viral infection of the central nervous system.

Over the next four days, Dr. Brebner lay helplessly paralyzed as the infection moved up his spinal cord. First he felt the ghastly pins and needles in his torso, then in his arms. His fever climbed to 104.8. The pins and needles became aching pains. He began to hiccup, as the virus irritated the nerves to his diaphragm. The respiratory muscles weakened, his breathing became shallow, and his lips turned blue. Like the polio victims he had been trying to help, Dr. Brebner had to be placed in an iron lung respirator. Mercifully, a seizure and coma ended his awareness, and he died five hours after being put into the machine and nineteen days after the monkey bite.

Thomas A. Gonzalez, deputy chief medical examiner of New York City, performed the autopsy on Dr. Brebner. He found severe inflammation of the deep structures of the brain and of the spinal cord at the base of the neck. The cerebral cortex, however, was spared, explaining why the doctor had been able to think clearly almost to the end.

Despite an extensive search using special stains, no bacteria could be identified in any of the microscopic sections. Two researchers from Columbia University obtained some of the brain tissue from Dr. Brebner's autopsy and announced in 1933 that they had isolated a strain of human herpesvirus. The cause of

Dr. Brebner's death, they asserted, was herpes simplex encephalitis, a well-known infection.

But Albert Sabin, a young physician researcher, an intern at Bellevue Hospital where Dr. Brebner had died, thought otherwise. Before his year in the hospital, Sabin had already begun the laboratory research on polio that would culminate twenty-four years later in the oral vaccine. Now, instead of returning to his polio studies, Sabin, who had known Brebner at the City Health Department Laboratories, began his own studies of the infected brain tissue of the tragic young man.

Sabin and his colleague Arthur Wright inoculated rhesus monkeys with samples from Dr. Brebner's brain, spinal cord, spleen, and lymph node tissue. The rhesus monkeys suffered no ill effects from the infected tissue, even when it was inoculated directly into their brains. Mice, guinea pigs, and dogs were similarly immune.

However, when the two researchers performed the same experiments on rabbits, many of the animals became paralyzed and died within a few days. Sabin and Wright then obtained infected brain tissue from the rabbits that had succumbed to the first injections, and produced a lethal infection in new rabbits by injecting the material into their brains. The researchers carried out serial transmission experiments through a series of fifteen rabbits. When an extract of the infected rabbit brain was passed through a filter with pores just small enough to stop a bacterium, the extract retained its death-dealing power. The infectious agent was definitely a virus, and it did cause clumping in the cell nucleus, the so-called intranuclear inclusions that were typical of the herpes family.

But Sabin pointed out that this virus attacked the spinal cord early and in all its victims, while herpes simplex attacked the spinal cord late in infection, if at all. Sabin and Wright published their findings in the *Journal of Experimental Medicine* in 1934. They named the new agent B-virus after its victim. Sabin was just twenty-eight years old, and his assertion that he and Wright had discovered a new, and very lethal, agent was based on inference and instinct, without benefit of the sophisticated techniques available today. Sabin said later, "Maybe because I wanted it to be a new virus I said it was a new virus. I was naive. If I had known more, I would have said it was herpes simplex."

But the virus that killed Dr. Brebner, *Herpesvirus simiae* or B-virus, was, in fact, a new addition to the large family of viruses known as the herpesviruses. Unlike bacteria and higher forms of life, which contain the two genetic molecules, RNA and DNA, viruses are based on either one or the other. The majority of viruses including the agents that cause AIDS, polio, influenza, and SARS are RNA viruses. The DNA viruses, though in the minority, contain some important members—smallpox and hepatitis B, for example.

But the largest group of DNA viruses are the herpesviruses, which contain over one hundred members and infect a broad range of animals. Besides herpes simplex, the agent of cold sores and genital ulcers, the human herpesviruses include the chicken pox virus, the agent of infectious mononucleosis, and cytomegalovirus, or CMV. If a pregnant woman contracts CMV, it can destroy the baby's brain. In the last stages of AIDS, CMV of the retinas can leave the patient to die in the dark.

Many of the herpesviruses share this tendency with CMV to attack the nervous system at some stage of infection. Everyone who has had chicken pox carries the virus somewhere in the nervous system, usually in a nerve cluster in the spinal cord or in one of the cranial nerves in the brain. Under the stress of another illness or, most commonly, in old age, the virus awakens and moves down the nerve tracts to the skin, like a fireman sliding down a pole. The resultant rash, called herpes zoster, or shingles, follows a stripe on the skin corresponding to the area served by the particular nerve whose body and tail are playing host to the virus. And because the nerve host of the virus is usually one that carries sensory impulses, not only is the rash painful, but also the stripe of skin may ache or burn for years after the zoster heals. This poorly understood condition, a kind of painful neural echo or memory, is called postherpetic neuralgia.

All of the herpesviruses, like the varicella virus of chicken pox, share this characteristic of remaining dormant in the host after the symptoms of the acute infection have subsided. The virus of infectious mononucleosis, Epstein-Barr, and CMV go to sleep in the cells of the lymphoid system, while the varicella virus, herpes simplex, and B-virus establish dormant infection in the cells of the nervous system.

The term herpes is one of most ancient in medicine. It comes from the Greek *herpein,* to creep, and, in the Hippocratic writings dating from about 400 BC, was used to denote sores in the skin. In the seventh century AD, the Byzantine physician Paul of Aegina wrote:

> When yellow bile, unmixed with any other humour is fixed in a part, the affection is called herpes: but if it is thicker and rather acrid it ulcerates the whole skin as far as the subjacent flesh, . . . but if it is thin, less acrid and hot, it raises small blisters on the surface of the skin like millet-seeds . . .

The first clear description of genital herpes was made by the French physician Jean Astruc (1684–1766). Today Astruc is remembered as the founder of modern biblical criticism. In 1753, he published the still controversial theory that the creation narrative in Genesis consists of two intertwined accounts, in one of which the creator is called Yahweh, and in the other Elohim.

But Astruc, who was King Louis XV's physician, was equally important in the history of medicine. He described hydrocephalus (water on the brain), and coined the term reflex. In his book on venereal diseases, *De Morbis veneris* (1736), he not only gives clear descriptions of syphilis and genital herpes, but he describes some of the earliest attempts at safe sex by men who "have been employing for some time sacs made of fine, seamless membrane in the form of a sheath, . . . called in English 'condum.'"

Human infections with herpes simplex and B-virus infection in macaques are remarkably similar. The viruses infect the moist membranes of the mouth or genital areas as a result of contact with infected saliva or genital secretions during social or sexual interactions. If a fetus or newborn encounters a herpesvirus, the outcome is often fatal. But, most frequently, infection occurs in childhood or adolescence. There may be numerous painful sores in the mouth or genital area, but, just as often, the human or the monkey has no symptoms at all. However, like all members of the herpesvirus family, herpes simplex and B-virus establish dormant or latent infection in cells of the central nervous system. If the human or the animal is stressed in any way, the virus tends to awaken, and just as in the case of shingles, it moves down the nerve tails and arrives on the skin innervated by the nerve in which is has lain dormant. Whether or not a herpes ulcer appears, at those times the human or animal host sheds the virus and is contagious to others. At any given time, between one and two percent of latently infected humans or macaques are shedding herpesvirus.

Because of its residence within nervous tissue, herpesvirus outbreaks tend to be itchy or painful. In many cases, the human sufferer will get an advance warning that he or she is about to have an outbreak—tingling or pain in the skin or moist membrane a few days before the herpes blister appears. Sometimes the premonitory symptoms will be more severe. There may be pain radiating down the leg from the genital area, headache, or a stiff neck, all signs that the awakening virus is causing more than just a localized disturbance in the nervous system. Thus warned, the human sufferer can take precautions to avoid transmitting infection to others. But it is important to emphasize that in both man and macaque, herpesvirus may be shed from time to time without any symptoms at all.

On rare occasions the balance between viral parasite and host may be upset; the virus may run amok and destroy its host in a week. When this happens, instead of sliding down the nerve tails to the skin, the virus turns inward and destroys the brain. Herpes encephalitis, as this condition is called, may attack anyone who has ever had a cold sore or a genital herpes outbreak, or even carries the virus without symptoms. It seems to occur arbitrarily, without regard to age, season of the year, or sex. The victims usually die if not treated, and, even with treatment, the survivors rarely escape unscathed. One of my patients, for example, was never able to return to work after her encephalitis, because she could no longer say the names of objects and ideas, even though she could still picture them in her mind. The macaque hosts of B-virus may also, on rare occasion, be attacked by encephalitis from their own herpes.

But, in its normal host, the herpesvirus rarely behaves in this way. Instead, it is a near perfect viral parasite, living peaceably within the nervous system for life. However, the lethal course that B-virus took in Dr. Brebner is typical of a zoonotic infection. Some of the deadliest human infections are actually zoonoses, accidental intrusions by animal infectious agents into human hosts. We have seen what East African sleeping sickness can do when it infects a person instead of the wild game to which it is adapted. But there are viral zoonoses as well. Hanta virus, for example, is harmless to the deer mouse, but lethal to man. And many researchers believe that the AIDS epidemic is a zoonosis on a global scale. A virus well tolerated by a primate host, it was accidentally introduced into the human population producing lethal infection.

Between one half and three-quarters of human beings and about the same proportion of macaques are infected with herpesviruses. In their natural habitats, macaques come into limited contact with people. The genus *Macaca* consists of about twelve species of Old World monkeys found primarily in Asia. They range in size from eight to eighteen pounds and live in troops led by the larger males.

All macaques have doglike muzzles and large cheek pouches for storing food. Their arms and legs are about the same length, and tails may be short, long, or absent. Macaques are omnivorous and eat roots, herbs, fruits, insects, crops, and small animals. They are adaptable, highly intelligent, and can live almost thirty years.

Humans have been aware of the macaques for centuries. They are important in myths and folktales and, in India, the Hindus hold them sacred. It is three macaques who are the models for the Buddhist saying "see no evil, hear no evil, speak no evil." The Barbary ape is a species of tailless macaque and is the only wild monkey in Europe. Just as the ravens are thought to protect the Tower of London, it is said that the British will hold the Rock of Gibraltar only as long as the Barbary apes flourish there.

Macaca mulatta, the rhesus monkey, is native to temperate cedar oak forests, tropical woodlands, and swamp habitats of western Afghanistan, India, and northern Thailand. The name "rhesus" comes from the Greek, Rhesos—the legendary king of Thrace and Priam's ally at Troy. Jean-Baptiste Audebert, the French nature painter who named the monkey around 1797, gave no reason for his choice.

Rhesus monkeys live in groups of eighty to a hundred individuals. They are active, social, and loud, but, aside from some sparring for dominance among males, are rarely violent within the band or with other bands of their species. Rhesus macaques have adapted to a wide range of habitats, from lowlands to up to ten thousand feet. Where tolerated by people, as around temples in India, they have proliferated and become urban pests. In the Indian countryside, they do significant damage to crops and gardens.

But scientific research has drawn humans and macaques into a much closer relationship than that resulting from the accidental overlap of human and monkey habitats in the wild. Rhesus macaques and related species, like crab-eating macaques, are the preferred subjects in laboratories conducting medical, pharmacological, and psychological research. PubMed, the standard database for the world's medical literature since about 1965, lists over nine thousand citations under *Macaca mulatta* alone. Research using macaques is an industry involving thousands of scientists and millions of dollars of government and private grants. While it has proved invaluable in advancing human knowledge in the basic and applied sciences, monkey research has also provoked controversial questions about the ethics of animal research in general and about the use of nonhuman primates in particular.

The first research colonies of rhesus macaques were established in the United States in the 1920s. The campaign to develop a polio vaccine led to an upsurge in their use from the 1930s through the 1950s. Nonhuman primates were used as experimental astronauts in rocket launches starting in 1949. The first nonhuman primates to survive and return to earth alive were a rhesus monkey named Able and a squirrel monkey named Baker. In 1959, the Army Ballistic Missile Agency rocketed them on a suborbital mission in a Jupiter nose cone. Four days later, the rhesus monkey Able died from a reaction to the anesthetic he had been given to remove an infected electrode.

Since the mid-1980s there has been a steady increase in the

use of nonhuman primates, mostly macaques, to study retro-viruses, the viruses of AIDS. In 1990, more than forty seven thou-sand nonhuman primates were used in research, the majority of which were macaques. Although many of the rhesus macaques used in research are obtained from breeding colonies in the United States, another species, the crab-eating macaque, *Macaca fascicularis*, also known as the cynomolgus monkey, is being im-ported more frequently and in increasing numbers from Mauritius in the Indian Ocean. Between 1995 and 2002, almost eighty thou-sand crab-eating macaques were imported into the United States, the majority going to commercial firms supplying primates to re-search laboratories.

Anyone who has taken a college psychology course can prob-ably recall the photograph of a baby rhesus monkey clinging to a surrogate mother of wire mesh and fabric. In 1961, Dr. Harry Harlow reported that rhesus macaques that were separated from their mothers shortly after birth displayed severe anxiety, depres-sion, and social withdrawal as infants and continued to be impaired through adulthood. Animal advocates maintain that maternal dep-rivation experiments, which are still common citations in the psy-chology literature, are cruel to both infant and mother. Another current area of active research in macaques, with dozens of articles listed, concerns the effect of alcohol exposure during pregnancy upon maternal behavior and infant development.

Given the rarity and enormous expense of chimpanzees, the rhesus macaque and related species have for many years been the experimental animal of choice for the neurophysiologist. Macaque brain function in both awake and anesthetized monkeys has been mapped in microscopic detail using implanted elec-trodes. To place electrodes in the part of the brain of interest, re-searchers first anesthetize the monkeys and make an opening in the skull through which the conducting wire is passed into the nervous tissue. Scientific knowledge of brain function has been remarkably advanced by these studies, which, it can be argued, can be performed in no other way.

But animal rights groups, like the controversial Primate Freedom Project, maintain that much primate research is unnecessary, redundant, and cruel. Their examinations of laboratory records on individual animals, if accurate, raise more disturbing ethical questions than any amount of vociferous general protest. According to their Web site, one representative subject, a female rhesus in a primate research center in the Midwest, was injected with male hormones before birth so that she was born a hermaphrodite, having both male and female characteristics. During twenty-one years of captivity so far, she has had blood drawn 191 times and has been subjected to forty-five procedures requiring ketamine, a veterinary anesthetic.

The injuries that humans have inflicted on these long-lived and intelligent animals makes the human death toll due to B-virus seem almost trivial in comparison. Since Dr. Brebner's death in 1932, there have been only about forty-five human B-virus infections. But B-virus encephalitis, while rare, is usually lethal and is especially tragic because many cases were preventable.

Prevention of transmission of the virus to monkey handlers depends upon understanding its natural history. Macaques may erupt with cold sores around the mouth that look very much like the outbreaks humans develop from herpes simplex, but, like people, they can also shed the virus without symptoms. Researchers have been able to grow B-virus from macaque saliva, semen, mother's milk, and from their cells in tissue culture. While monkey bites account for many of the human infections, fatal cases have followed from a variety of exposures. People have contracted B-virus by getting macaque saliva into a preexisting wound and by getting stuck with a needle used to draw blood from a macaque.

Infection has followed contact with virus on the sharp edge of a broken tissue culture bottle or the metal of a monkey cage, by inhaling infected saliva, and even by cleaning a rhesus skull without gloves.

The patients' case histories are similar to Dr. Brebner's and share the same depressing clinical features. On June 13, 1989, a twenty-two-year-old man was admitted to a hospital in Kalamazoo, Michigan, after he stopped breathing. The patient had been a monkey handler for two years in a research facility housing rhesus and crab-eating macaques. During that time he had been bitten and scratched on his hands and arms numerous times, the most recent being a bite to his right upper chest in May. The bite healed uneventfully, but on June 9 he began to have pain in his right shoulder. By the next day the pain had worsened and spread to the front of his chest. On June 11, he consulted a chiropractor, but by now the entire limb was becoming numb and weak. He also complained of a mild headache.

Forty-eight hours later his illness took an aggressive downhill course. First he began having tingling in his shoulder. His nose started to run; he felt sick to his stomach, couldn't swallow and began to drool. Soon he was weak and dizzy and could not walk without help. Finally, he had a seizure and stopped breathing.

Paramedics resuscitated him and brought him to the emergency room. The examining doctor found tiny, shinglelike blisters on the right side of his chest. Both of his eyes were inflamed and runny with conjunctivitis, his gaze was unfocused, and he had a stiff neck. When the doctor put a tongue depressor down his throat, there was no gag reflex. The muscles of his right arm were weak, but he had a spastic stiffness, jumpy reflexes, and, from the waist down, he was limply paralyzed and without any knee jerks.

He was given the antiherpes drug, acyclovir, by vein, but, despite this, over the next few hours he slipped into a coma. His face and extremities swelled, his temperature dropped, and on the eighth day in the hospital, his doctors withdrew life support. At autopsy, like Brebner, he had the classic signs of B-virus infection of the base of the brain and the upper spinal cord.

Although the Kalamazoo man did not respond to acyclovir, probably because the drug was started during too late a stage in his illness, this antiviral drug, available since 1982, and a related drug called ganciclovir, have been the most important breakthroughs in the treatment of human B-virus infections. The first account of their use in this infection appeared in the *Morbidity and Mortality Weekly Report* of May 22, 1987, which described a cluster of four cases of B-virus infection that occurred in Pensacola, Florida.

On March 4, 1987, a thirty-one-year-old male researcher working at the Naval Aerospace Medical Research Laboratory was bitten on the left thumb by a three-year-old rhesus monkey. Like the Kalamazoo man, the monkey that bit the researcher had B-virus conjunctivitis and was probably highly infectious, but the man was apparently not wearing the leather gloves he usually wore when handling monkeys. Five days after receiving the bite, he developed numbness in his left arm, followed thirteen days later by fever, chills, and muscle pains. Over the next four days, he started experiencing numbness and tingling on the left side of his body, double vision, and nausea. Unfortunately, he was not hospitalized until March 28, twenty-four days after his bite. Though he received both intravenous acyclovir and ganciclovir, he was left in a persistent vegetative state and eventually died five months later.

On March 10, 1987, a thirty-seven-year-old male biological technician was bitten on the left forearm, presumably by the same monkey that bit the researcher. Coworkers did not know if he had been wearing protective gear at the time of the bite. Five days later, he broke out with herpes blisters near his wound. The biological technician consulted a dermatologist, who diagnosed a herpes infection and prescribed acyclovir cream. The general diagnosis was correct, but of course this was no ordinary herpes infection. The biological technician did not fill the prescription for acyclovir, but it probably would not have made any difference if he had, since the concentration of the drug applied topically would have been too low to stop the infection that was racing toward his brain. As the precious days went by without effective therapy, the biological technician's wife applied various creams to the blisters on her husband's arm. She had a skin condition herself, an allergy called contact dermatitis. After she had applied zinc oxide or hydrocortisone cream to her husband's blisters, she smeared some on a particularly itchy and inflamed area on her left ring finger.

Over the next several days the biological technician became lethargic and confused. He had a fever, numbness in his left arm, double vision and trouble swallowing. But it wasn't until March 30, twenty days after his bite and more than two weeks after he fell ill that he was admitted to the hospital. On that day he stopped breathing and had to be attached to a ventilator. His doctors gave him high-dose acyclovir and then ganciclovir by vein, but, it was already too late. A little less than a month later he was dead. A skin biopsy of one of the lesions on his arm grew herpes B.

The day after the biological technician was bitten, a fifty-three-year-old laboratory supervisor in the same facility caught a healthy monkey while wearing leather gloves. Later, while holding the rhesus for a procedure, he exchanged his leather gloves for surgical gloves. The laboratory supervisor didn't recall any bites, but he did remember being scratched by a wire on the monkey's cage. On March 27, he noticed itchy blisters on his right third finger. The next day the first bite victim in the cluster, the researcher, was admitted to the hospital, followed two days after by the hospitalization of the biological technician. B-virus was suspected in all three patients, the laboratory supervisor was sent to a dermatologist who, on March 31, took a punch biopsy from the skin of his finger, near one of the blisters. The doctor sent the specimen for viral culture, and the next day the laboratory supervisor went into the hospital for observation and treatment with intravenous acyclovir.

Although the fluid from his blisters promptly grew B-virus, under acyclovir treatment, they healed uneventfully. After three weeks in the hospital he was allowed to leave with the promise that he would take acyclovir tablets. However, he did not take the medication as prescribed, and, a week later, he was growing B-virus from his eyes and mouth. The laboratory supervisor was again brought into the hospital and given an additional three weeks of acyclovir by vein. He did well and was sent home with instructions to take acyclovir tablets indefinitely.

This outbreak illustrated how important it was for macaque handlers to take certain precautionary measures: to wear protective gear at all times against monkey bites, but also, as the researcher's case showed, against being scratched by a contaminated sharp edge or object in a cage. Equally important, this report demonstrated that acyclovir could alter the course of B-virus by confining the infection to the skin and hindering its lethal spread to the brain and spinal cord.

However, these three cases were not the end of the outbreak. The fourth patient was the most extraordinary of all, because, to date, she is the only patient to have contracted B-virus not from direct contact with a macaque but from another person.

On April 1, the wife of the biological technician consulted a dermatologist, because the dermatitis on her ring finger, rather than improving with the creams she had been using, was becoming unbearably itchy and raw. By then her husband was critically ill and was in the intensive care unit. The dermatologist performed a punch biopsy of the patch of eczema and gave the woman a prescription for acyclovir tablets. One week later, the biopsy was growing herpes B. The patient was admitted to the hospital and given intravenous acyclovir. Despite this, she began to shed B-virus from her eyes, although she did not have the oozing and weeping eyes of the sick monkey with conjunctivitis.

After eighteen days on high-dose therapy, the virus was losing ground and could no longer be isolated from the woman's eyes. After a month, the patch of infected contact dermatitis had healed. On May 17, the wife was sent home on oral acyclovir with directions to take the medication indefinitely.

Since 1973, the 1987 Pensacola cluster of human B-virus infections was the first report of infection with this agent. The outbreak prompted an investigation by the National Institutes of Health and the Centers for Disease Control and Prevention, which subsequently published new guidelines for the prevention and treatment of this tragic illness.

In reviewing the first two cases, CDC noted that the patients may have been injured because "they alarmed or excited an ill and essentially blind animal by reaching into its cage to capture it, causing it to attack." Housing the monkey in a squeeze-back cage could have prevented infection. Such cages allow the animal to be immobilized without the handler having to reach in and grab the animal. Also emphasized were the importance of sedating macaques for procedures and of using loop-ended poles to capture them. Proper protective gear, which the two men were most likely not wearing, is, of course, essential when handling macaques.

In 1995, a B-virus Working Group sponsored by Emory University and the CDC updated the 1987 guidelines. According to the panel, the most critical period for the prevention of B-virus infection is the first few minutes after exposure. The panel suggested making available a bite/wound kit where macaques were housed. The kit would contain supplies for disinfecting wounds, sterile saline solutions for irrigating eyes or other membranes following exposures, and the proper tubes and swabs for obtaining viral cultures. Finally, each kit would include a procedure manual with emergency telephone numbers of on-call physicians and reference laboratories.

The panel also recommended that, before beginning work with macaques, all employees collect a baseline serum which would be frozen and made available for comparison with serum obtained in the event of suspected B-virus infection. Because the exact nature of the patients' exposure was often unknown in human B-virus infections, the Emory/CDC team recommended that monkey handlers keep a bite-and-scratch log in the monkey house.

Detailed algorithms were also provided to help physicians caring for injured or exposed workers in assessing the risk for virus transmission and the need for acyclovir therapy. The authors of the guidelines conceded that one of the chief difficulties in preventing human B-virus infections is that, while monkey bites and scratches continue to be common, human B-virus infections remain a rarity. Complex and cumbersome protocols for managing exposures are difficult to enforce among monkey handlers who have received traumatic injuries in the past without ill effects.

It is ironic that it was at Emory University's own Yerkes Regional Primate Center, which had never had an occupational fatality in its entire sixty-eight-year history, that the next B-virus infection occurred. On December 10, 1997, a twenty-two-year-old woman named Elizabeth Griffin contracted B-virus following an exposure, which before had never led to infection.

Griffin was apparently following the handling protocol as she took the caged rhesus monkey for a physical examination on

October 29: she wore a lab coat, boots, a mask, and gloves. But as she looked into the cage to check on the monkey, an unidentified fluid, possibly feces, hit her right eye. Griffin wiped her eye with a paper towel and, about three-quarters of an hour later, she irrigated it for two or three minutes with tap water. Thinking the exposure to be minor, she did not file an incident report, and the monkey involved was not identified. In fact, since this kind of exposure was not considered a high risk for infection, eye protection was not required at Yerkes for working with caged macaques.

In an interview with *The Scientist,* Dr. Stephen Strauss, chief of the laboratory of clinical investigation at the National Institute of Allergy and Infectious Disease, remarked, "[Monkeys] will . . . urinate or spit on you, throw things, and hurl feces." Apparently, such exposures are commonplace in the monkey house.

However, ten days after the incident, Griffin came down with a headache and a red, swollen right eye. She told the emergency department physician at Emory University Hospital that she worked with nonhuman primates and was at risk for B-virus infection. The physician put a drop of fluorescein into her eye and examined the eye under the weak ultraviolet illumination of a Wood's lamp. Eye infection with the human herpesvirus produces a characteristic branching pattern under UV light that looks like a bolt of lightning. Griffin's cornea was negative for these "dendritic" lesions.

The physician then consulted the B-virus protocol on file in the emergency department and telephoned an infectious disease specialist. The consultant listened to the doctor's account of Griffin's accident and, based on the lack of prior transmission following this kind of exposure, thought the B-virus risk was low. Griffin was prescribed antibacterial eyedrops.

On November 11, she consulted an ophthalmologist, because her eye symptoms were getting worse. In addition to her monkey exposure, Griffin had had a recent cat's scratch. The ophthalmologist suspected cat-scratch fever, which can begin with eye symptoms similar to Griffin's. But a blood test for this disease was negative. On November 13, Griffin consulted a second ophthalmologist, because, in addition to redness, she was having pain behind her right eye, visual discomfort in bright light, nausea, and abdominal pain. After consultation with the infectious disease specialist, Griffin was admitted to the hospital.

During the first day there, Griffin spiked a fever. The tissues around her right eye were swollen, and she had conjunctivitis. Just in front of her right ear, there was a tender, swollen lymph node. Her doctors performed a lumbar puncture and sent samples of cerebrospinal fluid and swabs of her right eye for culture to the B-virus reference laboratory of Dr. Julia Hilliard at Georgia State University. In addition, they tracked down the previous cultures taken from Griffin's eye, as they were potentially dangerous to anyone handling them outside proper containment facilities.

Griffin was treated with a high dose of acyclovir, but the next day she broke out with herpes vesicles on the right side of her face. Her doctors changed her to the more toxic but theoretically more effective drug, ganciclovir. Over the next six days, the herpes lesions healed. Griffin had one day of sharp pain in the neck and upper back, which resolved. A magnetic resonance imaging (MRI) study of her brain was normal. On November 24, she felt well and was sent home on outpatient intravenous ganciclovir.

But the next day Griffin woke with right foot weakness and was unable to urinate. As in the case of Dr. Brebner sixty-five years before, B-virus was beginning to destroy her spinal cord. By the time she returned to the hospital, she was having abdominal pain and weakness in her left leg. The right leg was now limp, and she could no longer make a tight fist with either hand. This time her MRI showed abnormalities of her spinal cord from her neck to upper chest. Within thirteen hours she was paralyzed from the neck down and on a mechanical ventilator.

Over the next two weeks, Griffin's desperate doctors tried every possible remedy to save her. They filtered her blood through a plasmapheresis machine, gave cortisone compounds, and added another antiviral drug on an experimental basis, but all to no avail. Bacteria invaded her weakened lungs and then her bloodstream, she progressed to the adult respiratory distress syndrome, a condition of refractory lung leak similar to SARS, and, on December 10, she died. Blood tests confirmed B-virus infection.

Following this young woman's tragic death, CDC conducted a review of biohazard exposures among workers dealing with nonhuman primates. Despite previous recommendations for eye protection, such as a face shield, goggles, or personal eyeglasses, when working with uncaged macaques, eye splashes of primate body fluids were the commonest reported exposures. Even when workers wore face shields, eye exposures sometimes occurred when droplet splashed to the head ran into the eyes or came in from the sides of the shield. The new recommendations require that workers use goggles designed for splash protection in combination with a mask to protect the nose and mouth whenever working with macaques. It remains to be seen whether workers will comply with these directives over the long haul.

None of these recommendations, however, address the trade in pet macaques. Since October 10, 1975, federal law has prohibited the importation of nonhuman primates as pets and their breeding outside of licensed research centers and zoos. However, enforcement has been spotty. Although exact figures are not available, the U.S. Fish and Wildlife Service indicates that illegal traffic in nonhuman primates is a significant part of the estimated three billion dollars of wildlife illegally traded in the United States. A quick Internet search revealed that a buyer could, with the click of a mouse on an auction site, purchase a "beautiful 19 month old Rhesus Macaque . . . all the paper's [sic] from his vet showing his shots are all up to date. He has never been in a lab, he was born in a private breed does not do well with children." The price, fifteen hundred dollars (negotiable).

In a 1998 paper published in the *Emerging Infectious Diseases* journal, Stephanie Ostrowski and coworkers examined nonoccupational exposure incidents, mostly bites and scratches, involving twenty-four people and eight macaques. Four of the six macaques tested were B-virus positive. Children were three times as likely to be bitten as adults. In addition to the injuries listed, owners reported kissing the macaque on the lips, letting it eat off the owner's plate, exposing children at a home day-care center, and sharing chewing gum with their pet. As yet there have been no reported B-virus infections in owners of pet macaques or in their children. But, as Dr. Bernard Roizman, professor of virology at the University of Chicago, cautions in a recent issue of *The Scientist,* "Any person who has a macaque as a pet is sitting on a time bomb."

As an infectious disease specialist, I came face-to-face with the B-virus problem on that Friday afternoon in October 1987, when, at about four thirty, Jim, the monkey handler bitten by Adelaide, arrived in the emergency room. Although I had been working at that Veteran's Hospital for five years, I wasn't even aware that primates were being housed on the grounds, and there were no B-virus protocols on file in our emergency department.

I remembered reading about the Pensacola outbreak the previous March. So by the time the young man arrived, I had pulled the MMWR report from my reference files. The patient was a sandy-haired man in his twenties, wearing a VA-issue green maintenance worker's uniform and work boots. His brisk walk across the hospital grounds seemed to have calmed him down somewhat.

Glumly, he held out his right hand palm down. I saw two

peg-shaped holes in the fleshy area between the thumb and the first finger. Luckily, the bite was superficial.

"When was your last tetanus shot?" I asked.

He wasn't sure, so I ordered a booster.

"Here's what we're going to do, Jim. I'm going to give you two prescriptions. This first one's for an antibiotic to prevent bacteria from infecting this bite. Take one pill every eight hours. This prescription is for acyclovir. Take two of these pills five times a day. Space them out so you take them the first thing when you wake up and the last thing before you go to sleep, and don't forget any doses. Do you understand?" He nodded his assent. I took down his work and home phone number and told him I would be calling him next week with the recommendations of the B-virus experts.

The following Monday, I called CDC. The switchboard operator put me through to Dr. Gary Holmes of the Viral Exanthems Branch. Dr. Holmes told me to call Dr. Julia Hilliard, then at the Southwest Foundation for Biomedical Research in San Antonio, Texas.

Dr. Hilliard, who is now the head of the Viral Immunology Center at Georgia State University, is internationally recognized as the leading expert on B-virus. In the late 1980s, one procedure for bite exposures to known B-virus-positive macaques was to start acyclovir, as I had done, and then to obtain punch biopsies of the bite wounds for viral culture and examination under the electron microscope.

A few days later Jim reported to the dermatology clinic. The doctor took biopsies of his wounds under local anesthesia, and I arranged for these to be sent to Texas on dry ice. While waiting for the results of the tests, Jim was to continue to take acyclovir. I was directed to call Dr. Hilliard immediately if Jim developed any skin lesions, itching, pain, or numbness in his bite wounds.

About two weeks later I received good news from Texas. The flesh from Jim's wounds yielded negative cultures for B-virus, and examination of the tissue under electron microscopy was negative for virus particles. Jim could stop taking acyclovir, though he had to be examined weekly for another month.

Research in macaques has helped humans to conquer polio, study AIDS, and explore space. Thanks to these accessible animals, we are beginning to understand the structure and function of a brain that is close in evolutionary terms to our own. But monkeys don't just have brains; they have minds. When we confine these intelligent, long-lived creatures and subject them to frightening or painful procedures, we have made a deal with the devil.

Macaques fight back obdurately, obnoxiously, and resourcefully, and at any given time, a few of them are shedding a virus that may be lethal to their human handlers. We must work with these primates as compassionately as possible, but we must never let our guard down or forget our adversarial role.

I'll always remember his answer when I asked Jim why he hadn't worn gloves to handle Adelaide.

He said, "I thought she liked me."

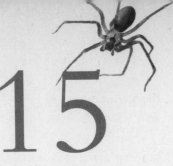

15

Human Bites

In September 1983, Dr. Ellie Goldstein and his colleagues in Los Angeles reported twenty-one serious hand infections due to *Eikenella corrodens,* a virulent bacterium in people's mouths. Ten of the infections were traced to human bites or to brawls in which the clenched fist of an assailant struck the teeth of an opponent, introducing germs into the knuckle joint. Case three in the paper describes an infection following a typical "clenched fist injury."

A thirty-one-year-old man came to a hospital emergency room in West Los Angeles five days after receiving a human bite injury to the knuckle of the ring finger of his right hand. At first the wound had not appeared serious, but gradually the area had become swollen, red, and painful, and by the time he came to the hospital, the patient was unable to move his finger. His doctors started two antibiotics by vein and took him to the operating room so that they could explore and drain his wound under general anesthesia. When the area was opened, they found that an infection had already destroyed all of the tendons on the top of the patient's ring finger. Pus from the wound grew *Eikenella corrodens* in pure culture.

Despite surgical drainage and antibiotics, the patient's infection spread into his palm, requiring a second incision for drainage. A few days later he began having high fevers, and on the tenth day, he was taken back to the operating room. The surgeon found, on opening the wound, that the knuckle joint had been consumed by infection. After thirty-six days in the hospital, the man's right ring finger and the adjoining bone were amputated.

Bite injuries represent one percent of all emergency room admissions in the United States, and of that percentage, human bites are the third most common, following dog and cat bites. After a human bite or tooth injury, the risk of infection is high. In the era before antibiotics, radical treatments of these wounds were recommended, such as surgical excision, electrocautery of the wound edge, and wiping the bite wound with fuming nitric acid. One paper published in the 1930s went so far as to recommend radiation therapy in the treatment of human bite–wound injuries.

Although the first systematic studies of human bite wounds and their infections go back only to 1910, the belief that human bites are particularly dangerous is an old one. The Orkneyinga Saga, written around 1200 AD, contains a chapter titled "A Poisoned Tooth," which describes the tenth-century death of Sigurd the Powerful, the first earl of Orkney. After he defeated Maelbrigte, an earl of Scots, and his men in battle, the following occurred:

> Sigurd had their heads strapped to the victors' saddles to make a show of his triumph, and with that they began riding home, flushed with their success. On the way, as

Sigurd went to spur his horse, he struck his calf against a tooth sticking out of Maelbrige's mouth and it gave him a scratch. The wound began to swell and ache, and it was this that led to the death of Sigurd the Powerful.

We have seen how bites by members of the cat family carry a high risk for invasive infection due to *Pasteurella*. Human bite and tooth wounds, particularly those on the hands, are also at high risk for infection, but for many years no one knew exactly why. As a rule, humans do not carry *Pasteurella* or even *Capnocytophaga*, the bacterium that makes dog bites so dangerous in patients lacking spleens. Human bite wounds seemed to be infected with the grab bag of bacteria that live either on the victim's skin or between the biter's teeth: staphylococci, streptococci of low virulence, and some oxygen-hating bacteria called anaerobes.

But hidden within this bacterial menagerie was a slow-growing, rod-shaped bacterium that grew reluctantly in the presence of oxygen and required an atmosphere enriched with carbon dioxide. It turned up in a microbiology lab in 1948, but the first clear description of the bacterium wasn't published until 1958. In that year, Dr. M. Eiken described twenty-one isolates of the germ taken from patients, most of whom had various abscesses and soft-tissue infections. Because of the bacterium's tendency to form pits in the surface of agar medium made with sheep's blood, he christened it *Bacteroides corrodens*.

However, the organism was difficult to recover in routine cultures, where it either failed to grow or was obscured by other bacteria that were less fastidious in their requirements. In 1971, F. L. Jackson and coworkers took another look at Eiken's germ and decided that it was a separate genus from *Bacteroides,* true anaerobes that are actually killed by the presence of oxygen. They renamed the bacterium *Eikenella corrodens*.

Unlike *Pasteurella,* which produces rapidly progressive, invasive disease that may occur within twelve hours of an animal bite, *Eikenella* infections are sneaky and insidious. It is the premier germ of the human fistfight in which the assailant punches his adversary in the mouth. Clenching the hand into a fist opens the knuckle joint and leaves it covered only by a thin layer of skin and tendons. All it takes to introduce *Eikenella* and other bacteria from the opponent's mouth is a small tooth cut. When the brawler relaxes his hand, the surface cut moves away from the underlying joint line, so neither the patient nor the doctor may suspect the seriousness of the injury.

If the assailant then seeks treatment, and the treating physician makes the mistake of suturing the little laceration closed, the diminished oxygen in the wound and the presence of the foreign material of the sutures sets the stage for serious infection. Although no cultures were taken in the following patient, this case reported in 1992 by Dr. Peter Thomas, an Australian physician, is a typical one.

Following a fistfight, a thirty-five-year-old metalworker in Queensland sought treatment from a local doctor for a tooth cut on his right third finger. A photograph of the patient's unclenched hand shows a half-inch-long laceration just beyond the knuckle. Not realizing that the opponent's tooth had breached the knuckle joint, the doctor simply cleaned up the wound and sutured it closed. No X-rays were taken or antibiotics prescribed.

Two days later the man sought treatment in the emergency department of the Princess Alexandra Hospital in Woolloongabba. By then the knuckle was red and swollen. He could not flex the finger, nor would he allow the doctor to move it passively, because of severe pain. Dr. Thomas reports that, during the operation, the knuckle joint was bulging with pus. After the joint was irrigated, the patient spent a week in the hospital on intravenous antibiotics.

He made a good recovery, but it was another three weeks before he could return to work.

Often people with clenched-fist injuries do not even seek medical attention until the infection is far advanced and irreversible damage to the delicate structures of the hand has already occurred. They may be fooled by the apparently trivial nature of the entrance wound, or, just as often, they delay treatment because of shame or fear of the legal consequences of the original brawl.

The most serious clenched-fist infections occur in parts of the world where people forgo modern medical aid in favor of traditional healers, or do not have ready access to medical care. In 1992, two orthopedic surgeons from the Dodoma Regional Hospital in Tanzania published a series of twenty-six human wounds and resulting finger infections treated at their facility. This hospital is one of four regional centers caring for a million people in the Tanzanian central plateau, where poor roads and lack of transport make timely referral of patients difficult, especially during the rainy season.

According to the authors, most human bites occur inside or around makeshift bars selling local maize liquor. Violent fights often break out among the intoxicated patrons. A few of the bites were inflicted "by angry wives in cases of love tangles." Many of these patients did not seek hospital care until weeks after the injury, by which time their fingers were monstrously swollen and X-rays showed bones dissolved by infection. In contrast to the animal bite wounds treated at the hospital (donkey, hyena, and snake), in which the finger can often be surgically salvaged, amputation was usually necessary in neglected fight bites.

While clenched-fist injuries are responsible for the most serious wound infections, they are only a part of the human bite problem. Occlusional bites, such as the one Mike Tyson inflicted on Evander Holyfield's ear in 1997, are an important cause of traumatic injury worldwide. Although, compared to the great apes, humans have smaller canine teeth and lack the skull development evolved to support massive jaws, the muscles that power the human jaw are among the strongest in the body. In addition, our sharp incisor teeth are capable of sheering off an opponent's finger, ear, or nose.

The clenched-fist style of fighting of Western society, perhaps conditioned by what people see in the movies and on television, is not universal. For example, the Marakwet tribespeople of the highlands of Kenya fight open-handed, which leaves the digits exposed. Doctors at the Kapsowar Hospital, a one-hundred-bed facility providing medical care in the region, in 1986 reported sixteen patients with human bite—wound injuries, mostly to the fingers rather than to the knuckle joint. Nine of these patients required amputation, but in four of their cases, the assailant had already bitten the finger off.

The large and delicate human ear is a vulnerable target in altercations. Dr. D. Datubo-Brown, a surgeon at the University of Port Harcourt Hospital in Nigeria, reported twenty-four patients treated for human bites to the face between 1983 and 1985. Ten of the patients lost part or all of the external ear—one twenty-eight-year-old woman lost her entire left ear in a fight with her female roommate, and another twenty-eight-year-old woman's right earlobe was bitten off by her husband's ex-wife.

Traumatic injuries to the face in general are not limited to Third World countries and Las Vegas boxing rings. In 1998, plastic surgeons in Rome, Italy, described a new surgical technique they used to restore the appearance of the mutilated left ear of a thirty-year-old man, a consequence of a brawl. In 1986, physicians at the Manhattan Eye and Ear Hospital described the surgical repair of five patients who had lost part or all of their upper eyelids due to fight bites.

But perhaps the most devastating bite-wound injuries are those involving the nose, not only because the nose is the most prominent and characteristic feature of the human face, but because the attack may be vengeful in nature.

According to both ancient Roman law and Indian custom, cutting off the nose was an acceptable punishment for certain crimes, such as theft and adultery. Plastic surgery began around 800 BC in India, with a technique that is still used today—"swinging" a flap of skin down from the forehead to reconstruct an injured nose. In some parts of the world, taking the law into one's own hands by vengeful nose-biting still occurs.

In 1995, Dr. Jacob Ollapallil and coworkers at the Port Moresby General Hospital in Boroko, near Papua, New Guinea, reported a series of ninety-five human bites treated in the Division of Surgery from 1986 to 1992. Twelve of the bites were to the nose—nine in women and three in men—and in most of the cases, the biter was an angry spouse. One twenty-eight-year-old man, who had lost a third of his nose to a bite by his wife, was treated with good results using the ancient Indian forehead flap technique.

Among the Kiribati (formerly Gilbert) islanders in Micronesia, biting off the tip of the nose as punishment for adultery is a traditional form of conjugal mutilation. In 1996, anthropologist Alexandra Brewis reported that there were still about ten to fifteen episodes of vengeful nose-biting each year. According to a report published in the *Lancet* in 1998, the purpose of biting off the nose of an adulterous wife is to *kabainranga* her (to "make despised"). The authors write: "One of the driving forces behind this behavior in Kiribati culture is a powerful sexual jealousy known as *koko*—'a murdering thing.'"

When a husband, after repeated warnings and beatings, bites off the tip of his wife's nose for immodesty or adultery he "not only destroys his wife's looks but also leaves her with a permanent and public sign of his *koko*." Fortunately, in recent years, regular visits by Australian plastic surgeons who reconstruct mutilated noses have alleviated some of the suffering resulting from these attacks.

Furthermore, as in New Guinea, vengeful nose-biting in Kiribati is not limited to men attacking women. The authors also tell the story of a forty-four-year-old Palauan schoolteacher who presented to a visiting physician for cosmetic restoration of his nose, which had been bitten off twenty-five years previously by his angry fiancée after she discovered his unfaithful liaisons.

According to the authors in the *Lancet* report, the nose may be regarded as a phallic symbol, because, like the penis, it is an unpaired organ that protrudes from the midline of the body. The ancient Romans believed that nasal and penile endowment were directly proportional. Perhaps when a woman bites off her husband's nose, she is symbolically castrating him, and when a husband bites off his wife's nose, he is castrating her lover. But whatever its psychological basis, vengeful nose-biting is an act of primitive, and even more than bestial, violence.

Also existing within the hazy border zone between sexuality and violence are the "love bites." Although at first sight these case reports appear to be straightforward records of assault, "love bites" are often accidental and unintentional injuries. A plastic surgeon colleague of mine, Dr. Avron Daniller, vividly recalls a woman some years ago, who was brought to the emergency room of his hospital bleeding profusely from one breast. Her lover had, in a paroxysm of passion during consensual sex, bitten her nipple off. Reports of such "coital love bites" caused by an involuntary jaw spasm initiated during the orgasmic climax are well described in the medical literature.

In heterosexual partners of about the same height, the most

common location for love bites is on the neck. Dr. M. Al Fallouji, surgeon at the Royal Victoria Hospital in Belfast, Ireland, reported seven bite-wound injuries incurred during sex. Four of the patients were men who had been bitten by women. One thirty-five-year-old man came to the doctor with a hard mass on his neck, which was initially thought to be a cyst. When the mass was opened in the operating room, the surgeon found a broken plastic tooth. After the patient regained consciousness he admitted that he had attended a Halloween party a year before where he had been bitten by a lady dressed as a vampire while they were both "drunk on lovemaking."

Although my plastic surgeon colleague couldn't give me details about the stature of the man who bit his patient's breast, Dr. Fallouji, in his article, recorded two cases in which women sustained bites to the breast during sex with short men. One of them, a twenty-three-year-old woman on her honeymoon had her left nipple completely bitten off "following a savage love biting by her drunk . . . husband." In cases like this one, it may be difficult to distinguish involuntary jaw clench from frank sexual assault and battery.

A special category of love bites is those to the penis. They are no doubt underreported in the medical literature, because victims are often too embarrassed to seek medical care. In cases that are documented, most penile bites occur among homosexuals, and serious infections have followed because patients have waited too long to seek medical care. Dr. Stuart Wolf Jr. and colleagues at the San Francisco General Hospital reported five gay men with penile bites. One bitten patient waited two weeks before going to the hospital, and by that time he had an abscess involving the entire penis. Another patient developed "flesh-eating strep" that had spread from a penile bite all the way to his lower abdomen. In this syndrome, more properly called necrotizing fasciitis, the same group-A streptococcus that causes sore throats invades and destroys the partitions or fascia that support the muscles. Surgeons removed a five-by-seven-inch piece of flesh and skin in order to save this man's life.

While the infections in the San Francisco report seemed to follow accidental injury during friendly sex, in a 1999 report from Texas, one sixty-six-year-old man was the victim of an assault brought on by extremely poor judgment. He apparently threatened to withhold payment from a prostitute while receiving fellatio. She bit him. Five days later, he came to the doctor with a nasty infected ulcer that grew *Eikenella corrodens*.

Most bite-wound infections are limited to the flesh near the bite site, but a few can lead to life-threatening bacterial infections, as in the patient whose penile bite turned into "flesh-eating strep." In a 1999 report in the *Lancet,* doctors in Munich, Germany, reported the case of a young man who came to the emergency room in shock, with low blood pressure, high fever, and a red, swollen right calf. After being given a massive dose of antibiotics by vein, he was rushed to the operating room where surgeons found necrotizing fasciitis due to group-A strep. The patient, who required a skin graft, told his doctors that two days previously he had been dancing on a beer table at Oktoberfest when an unknown woman had bitten him. He had apparently been the victim of a traditional biting known in the local Bavarian dialect as "Wad'lbeisser" or "calf biter."

On at least two occasions, tetanus has followed a human bite. In tetanus, a bacterium, *Clostridium tetani,* finds its way into a wound that is protected from oxygen. Rather than causing invasive infection, the germ releases a protein toxin that causes boardlike muscle spasms and uncontrolled discharges of the nerves that control blood pressure, pulse, and body temperature.

One patient, reported by surgeons in Pondicherry, India, in 1995 came to the hospital nine days after being bitten on the right ring finger by a drunken attacker. The forty-four-year-old man had been having lockjaw, trouble swallowing, fever, and finally spasms in all of his muscles. He was given tetanus antitoxin and antibiotics, but the badly infected fingertip had to be amputated. He eventually recovered after seventeen days in the hospital. A second patient, reported from Zimbabwe, was less fortunate.

Four days after being bitten in the left armpit by another woman during a domestic dispute, a forty-three-year-old woman was admitted to the Milo Central Hospital in Bulawayo, Zimbabwe. The bite wound looked only mildly inflamed, but the patient had a stiff neck and had been unable to open her mouth for twelve hours. While being examined, she started having agonizing spasms of opisthotonos in which the muscles of the back contract, lifting the patient off the bed in a belly-up arch. She had wild swings in blood pressure, from dangerous highs to shocking lows.

After her wound was surgically excised, and she received antitoxin and antibiotics, the woman, whose severe spasms interfered with breathing, was paralyzed with a nerve-blocking medication and attached to a ventilator. Despite treatment in intensive care, she died six days later.

Throughout this section, we have seen examples of how humans may acquire lethal zoonotic infections, such as B-virus, from animal bites. But bites by humans pose a special danger, because the biter may transmit a microorganism that readily infects another human host.

On May 15, 1980, a thirty-four-year-old man came to the

Skin Clinic of the Boston Dispensary because of ulcers on his penis. He told the examining physician that two months previously he had gone to a gay bar in another state while on a business trip, where, after several drinks, he invited a companionable man to his hotel room. However, during the act of fellatio, the man "bit him savagely." He ordered him out, wrapped his bleeding penis in a handkerchief, and sought emergency care. The victim was given antibiotic capsules and pain medication, and over the next two weeks the wound healed.

However, eleven weeks after the bite, the healed skin began to break down, and the patient developed a slowly growing painless ulcer. He sought treatment a week later—when the lymph glands in his groins began to swell. The treating physicians took a scraping from the ulcer base and examined it under the microscope using a technique of back lighting called dark-field examination. They saw telltale corkscrew bacteria, the spirochetes of syphilis. The original antibiotic the man had been given was not active against this infection. Fortunately, two penicillin injections cured him.

A variety of viral infections, however, mostly incurable, have also been transmitted to human-bite victims. In 1989, physicians from the University of Iowa reported the case of a licensed practical nurse, bitten on both wrists and on her right upper lip by a two-year-old pneumonia patient who had a fever blister on his lip. Two days later, the nurse came down with high fever, and swelling of her left wrist and the right side of her face, which lasted four days. Her blood showed a high level of antibodies to herpes simplex. Over the next year, the nurse suffered monthly episodes of fever, along with facial pain and swelling that disabled her for several days at a time. She was treated with acyclovir tablets and, fortunately, the recurrences eventually became shorter and less painful.

Human hepatitis viruses have also been transmitted by bites.

The following patient, reported in 1974, acquired hepatitis B in the days before the preventative vaccine.

On October 18, 1972, a fifty-two-year-old woman reported to a clinic in San Diego, California, with nausea, weakness, loss of appetite, dark urine, and jaundice. The patient, who worked at a school for retarded children, was found to have acute hepatitis B. She told the physicians that, five months earlier, a fourteen-year-old boy had begun choking while eating lunch. As the child turned blue, three teachers turned him upside down and pounded on his back, but were unable to relieve the obstruction. This teacher then stuck her fingers into the boy's mouth and pulled out a large amount of thick, bubbly material, relieving his distress. During the incident, she had been bitten on her right index finger. Testing that was conducted on the child, who was a known carrier of the virus, determined that the boy infected the woman with the same subtype of hepatitis B as he had.

Another person contracted hepatitis B while at work, this time in Ontario, Canada. On October 22, 1973, a middle-aged policeman was admitted to the hospital with nausea, vomiting, dark urine, jaundice, and itching. The officer, who had no other risk factors for hepatitis, recalled that on June 20 of the same year, a man resisting arrest had bitten him on the hand. The assailant was using illicit drugs by vein, and within a week, he came down with acute hepatitis B, from which he made a rapid and uncomplicated recovery. The officer, however, became so ill that he had to undergo exploratory abdominal surgery. A biopsy of his liver taken during his operation showed severe viral hepatitis. His recovery was slow and over many weeks, but, in the end, he was awarded financial compensation for his occupational injury.

The virus of hepatitis C is much less contagious than that of hepatitis B, which is fortunate, as there is yet no vaccine available to prevent hepatitis C. It is most commonly contracted through intravenous drug abuse, but may be occasionally transmitted through a human bite.

In a 1990 report in the *Lancet,* physicians from Australia described the case of a thirty-five-year-old bicycle courier who was bitten by a man in a barroom fight in Sydney. Several months after the fight, he sought medical care for jaundice, and his doctor's diagnosis was hepatitis C. The courier's only risk factor for infection was the bite he had received. Given that hepatitis C has been detected in the saliva of infected patients, his physicians reported him as a case of probable bite-transmitted infection, though they had no definite evidence.

The human immunodeficiency virus (HIV) is present in only trace amounts in saliva, and transmission by bites is very rare. In a letter published in *Clinical Infectious Diseases,* physicians at the University of São Paulo in Brazil report an interesting experiment of nature. On May 2, 1992, a fifty-nine-year-old man was bitten on the ring finger of his left hand by his own son, who was infected with both hepatitis C and HIV. Forty days after the bite, the patient came down with severe hepatitis C, but careful testing over many months showed that he remained negative for HIV.

However, there have been three reports of possible and one definite instance of HIV infection following a human bite. The following is one of the possible cases.

A twenty-year old Asian man living in South Carolina visited a nightclub for the first time in June 1995. He indulged in deep kissing with a call girl, during which he accidentally sustained a lip bite. He was uncertain whose teeth caused the bite, but he remembered the taste of blood. He became frightened and about a half-hour later went home and examined his mouth. He had a cut on the inside of his lower lip. The incident so unnerved him that he no longer pursued sexual contact with anyone. He became obsessed with the idea that he had contracted a venereal disease. Over the next several months, he requested multiple tests for HIV, which all came back negative. However, seven months after his initial exposure, his test converted to positive. His physicians interviewed the man numerous times, and he never wavered from his story. Seven months is an uncommonly long incubation period for HIV. The route of transmission in this patient still remains unproven. However, the following tragic case from Yugoslavia, involving a Good Samaritan, represents a definite instance of HIV transmitted through a human bite.

On May 12, 1995, a forty-seven-year-old man with advanced AIDS had a seizure at home. After he regained consciousness, he felt frightened and so went to his neighbor's house, where he then had a second seizure. During this convulsion, his fifty-three-year-old neighbor, unaware of his diagnosis, tried to prevent airway obstruction in the sick man by putting his fingers in his mouth. He received a slight bite on his left index finger and soon after noticed blood in the biter's saliva.

The man washed his hands about an hour after the incident, without using soap or disinfectants and an hour after that he consulted a physician who confirmed his injury. Ten hours later he began prophylactic treatment with zidovudine (AZT) capsules in high dose.

Despite the treatment, thirty-three days after his bite the neighbor started to have a sore throat, felt fatigued, and had a headache, all typical symptoms of acute HIV infection. He began to show antibodies to the virus on blood tests, and, fifty-four days after his bite, he had complete conversion to a positive HIV test on Western blot testing, which detects the whole family of antibodies to the virus. The biter, meanwhile, had died thirteen days after his seizure, which suggests that at the time of the accident he probably had a high concentration of viral particles in his blood. The neighbor had no other risk factors for HIV and no prior exposure to the AIDS patient, which makes this tragic accident an almost certain example of HIV transmission by human bite. Accidents are not the only scenario in which human bites have transmitted HIV. HIV-infected people have, on occasion, bitten others with malicious or criminal intent.

A prisoner in Minnesota tested positive for HIV, and, one month later, during a struggle over his smoking in a nonsmoking area, he bit two correction officers. He told the prison nurse that he "wanted to kill" the officers and hoped "that they [got] the disease" he had. The prisoner was indicted on and convicted of two counts of assault with a deadly and dangerous weapon—his teeth. In 1988 a federal appellate court for Minnesota upheld his conviction. Fortunately, the prison guards did not contract HIV from their bites.

Forensic dentistry deals, in part, with the criminal side of human bites. Before there was DNA evidence and even before fingerprints, bite marks were used to establish and validate identity. William the Conqueror was said to bite the wax seals of documents—validating them with his unique dentition. Debtors who came from Britain to the New World to work confirmed their agreements by biting the seal on the pact and becoming indentured servants.

Most people know that forensic dentists identify victims of fires and plane crashes by comparing recovered teeth with known dental records. But a lesser known branch of the discipline involves the identification of a criminal by analysis of the characteristic pattern left by his or her bite, usually in the flesh of a victim, but, in one case, in a cheese sandwich found at the crime scene.

The earliest recorded use of bite-mark evidence in the United States was in the case of Ohio versus Robinson in 1870. Ansil

Robinson was charged with the murder of his mistress, Mary Lunsford. The woman's body was found lying diagonally across a bed in her nightclothes, with her head hanging over the edge and her throat completely cut. "[H]er head was bruised, and she had a tremendous and ghastly cut on the left side of her mouth . . . a large cut in her abdomen and her arm showed five bites, the print of teeth being plainly visible."

According to the trial testimony of three dentists, Ansil Robinson lacked all but five teeth in his upper jaw, making his bite unique. Of the three suspects arrested in the case, only Robinson's bite mark matched the wounds left on Lunsford's body. Despite this evidence, Robinson was acquitted.

The admissibility of bite-wound evidence was not established until 1954, in Doyle versus State (of Texas). In this instance, a piece of cheese found at the crime scene had tooth marks. The defendant was asked to bite into another piece of cheese, and a firearm examiner, rather than a dentist, was asked to compare bite marks on the two pieces. The teeth matched. Doyle was convicted.

From these beginnings, the forensic analysis of human bite wounds has become a precise discipline in which special techniques are used to excise and preserve bitten skin in murder victims and to photograph bite wounds in survivors of assault. Suspects may be required to allow dental models to be made. Bite wound analysis was important in obtaining the 1979 conviction of famed serial killer Theodore "Ted" Bundy. Pediatricians and physicians working in emergency rooms are trained to recognize the characteristic pattern of bite marks. Suspected cases of child abuse have been detected and abusers have been convicted by means of bite wound analysis. In January 1990, pathologists from Albuquerque, New Mexico, reported the use of bite mark evidence in the solution of one of the most bizarre murder cases on record.

A nineteen-year-old woman wearing maternity clothes soiled

with blood and dirt brought a newborn infant girl to a hospital emergency room for examination. She told physicians that she had gone into sudden labor and delivered the baby after having been involved in a minor traffic accident. The infant was still partially covered with blood and the cottage cheese–like coating of newborns, called vernix. The infant's ragged umbilical cord stump was clamped and trimmed, and the woman and baby were admitted to the hospital for observation.

After several hours, the woman submitted to a physical examination, and it was immediately apparent that she had not recently given birth. Meanwhile, local police were searching for a young pregnant woman who had disappeared from a local obstetrical clinic earlier that morning. Summoned to the hospital, police detectives questioned the hospitalized woman, who admitted to "taking" the child.

The next day she led them to a remote canyon area, where the missing woman's body was found. She was lying on her back, her lower abdomen cut open and a length of umbilical cord protruding from beneath bloodstained maternity slacks.

The investigation revealed that the woman and a male accomplice had committed a horrible crime. While strangling the woman with a ligature, they had used a key to tear an incision on her abdomen and then seized the living infant from her dying body. Two types of bite marks were found at the crime scene. One set, on the front and sides of the victim's tongue were made by her own teeth. The second set was found at the torn and ragged edge of the umbilical cord. Dental casts made of the female suspect proved to be an exact match with the marks on the cord. Ultimately, the suspect admitted to having severed the umbilical cord by biting it in two. This evidence, combined with serological tests confirming the murder victim as the infant's mother, proved instrumental in bringing the woman and her accomplice to justice.

· · ·

As an infectious disease specialist, I have always thought of human bite wounds in terms of clenched-fist injuries. Beginning insidiously after what appears to be a trivial cut to a knuckle, the resulting infections are aggressive and often devastating assaults on that most delicate extension of the brain, the human hand.

Although our teeth and the germs on them cause these infections, technically, they are not really human bites, since it's the striking force of the assailant's own fist that creates the injury. However, it wasn't long before my research for this chapter took me into darker areas. In the quiet stacks of a university medical library, I glimpsed the border between the human and the bestial. And then, sitting on the floor with the *Journal of Forensic Pathology* on my lap, I came face to face with unspeakable crimes. I found a boundary no animal, no matter how ferocious, ever crosses: that place in the human mind where the merely violent and primitive becomes evil.

Conclusion

In writing *Bitten,* I was dazzled by the variety of survival strategies that animals have evolved. A tiny spider overwhelms prey many times its size, and swarms of little ants devour hatchlings in their nests. Powerful toxins make cone snails deadly predators, and insubstantial jellies, armed with stinging cells, draw heavy fish into their diaphanous mouths.

Larger than most animals, humans coerce a living from the world—thanks to brute force and a big brain. But to the tsetses, sandflies, and mosquitoes we are simply supersized blood meals.

When ecologists tell us that all life on earth is interconnected, we tend to think of the big picture, of the atmosphere enriched by oxygen from ocean phytoplankton or polluted by greenhouse gases. But sometimes the connections are more intimate and more direct: a bite from a spider we offend in our sleep or an opponent's tooth at the end of our own punching fist.

Glossary

Acetylcholine. A compound released from nerve endings that may depress heart contraction, dilate blood vessels, and cause intestinal spasms. Animal venoms may cause its massive release.

Aeromonas hydrophila. Rod-shaped bacteria that stain pink on Gram's stain and inhabit fresh and brackish water. They are an important cause of infections in traumatic injuries involving water exposure, including animal bites by aquatic species, such as alligators.

Amino acids. The basic structural units of proteins, which link together in chains.

Anaerobic bacteria, or **anaerobes.** Bacteria that fail to grow in air (eighteen-percent oxygen).

Anaphylactic reaction. A catastrophic, often lethal, allergic reaction that occurs within minutes after contact with a substance to which a person is previously allergic. The symptoms are hives, wheezing, and low blood pressure with shock.

Antivenin, or **antivenom.** A serum, usually produced in animals by injecting them with gradually increasing amounts of venom. It contains antibodies capable of neutralizing the venom's toxic effects.

Arachnida. The class of arthropods (joint-footed animals without backbones) that includes the araneida, or spiders, as well as scorpions, ticks, and mites.

Atrax robustus. The world's most lethal spider, the Sydney funnel web.

Autonomic nervous system. The nerves serving the heart, blood vessels, glands, and other organs that are not under conscious control. This system maintains such automatic functions as blood pressure, digestion, and perspiration.

B-virus, or **herpes B virus,** *Herpevirus simiae, Cercopithecine herpesvirus 1.* A DNA virus that causes mild skin and genital infection in macaques but serious and often fatal infection of the brain and spinal cord in humans.

Botulism. An intoxication due to a protein produced by the bacterium *Clostridium botulinum,* usually foodborne, that causes a descending paralysis, first of the face and eye muscles and then of the muscles controlling breathing.

Capnocytophaga canimorsus. A long, thin, rod-shaped bacterium that stains pink with the Gram's stain and lives in the mouths of members of the dog family. It may cause fatal infections in dog-bite victims who lack a spleen.

Carukia barnesi. A small jellyfish of the tropical waters off the northern Australian coast, whose stings cause the Irukandji syndrome.

Central nervous system. The brain, spinal cord, and their immediate connections such as the optic nerves and the olfactory organs.

Cerebrospinal fluid or **spinal fluid.** A clear fluid secreted inside the brain, in which the organ is suspended. In a lumbar puncture (spinal tap) this fluid is sampled with the aid of a long needle.

Cone snails. A large group of often strikingly beautiful but uniformly venomous predatory snails inhabiting warm coastal waters in Hawaii and the Southern Hemisphere.

Desensitization therapy. Sometimes called **allergy shots.** A series of injections of a substance to which a patient is allergic, such as fire ant venom, meant to induce antibodies that can block an anaphylactic reaction.

Disseminated intravascular coagulation. A state of uncontrolled clotting and bleeding, which may be initiated by bloodstream invasion by infectious agents.

Eflornithine, or the **"resurrection drug."** A promising new treatment for all stages of West African (Gambian) sleeping sickness.

Elapidae. A family of snakes—including cobras, mambas, coral snakes, sea snakes, and venomous snakes in Australia—in which the upper jawbone is shortened and not hinged, and in which there is a pair of short, fixed, hollow, poisoned fangs in front.

Encephalitis. An inflammatory condition of the brain.

Enzyme. A protein produced by cells, which acts as a catalyst to induce chemical changes in other substances without itself being consumed in the reaction.

Epinephrine. Also known as adrenaline. One of the hormones of the adrenal glands, it stimulates the heart, relieves wheezing, supports blood pressure, and is used to treat anaphylactic shock.

Epizootic. An outbreak of disease occurring among animals.

Fascia. The tough tissue that extends from skin to bone, enveloping the body and the muscle groups.

Gangrene. Tissue death caused by obstruction of its blood supply.

Gastropods. The class of mollusks that includes snails, slugs, and sea hares.

Gram's stain. A procedure developed by Dr. Hans Gram in which specimens are smeared on a glass slide and stained with a sequence of dyes so that the bacteria stand out from the background of cellular debris. Gram-positive bacteria stain blue, while Gram-negatives stain pink.

Guillain-Barré syndrome. An illness consisting of ascending weakness caused by the production in the patient of antibodies that impair nerve conduction to the muscles.

Hemoglobinuria. The presence of the oxygen-carrying compound hemoglobin and its breakdown products in the urine which may color it orange or red.

Hemolysis. Destruction of red blood cells releasing the oxygen-carrying compound hemoglobin.

Histamine. One of the compounds whose release induces the hives, wheezing, and dilatation of blood vessels that constitute an allergic reaction, sometimes progressing to fatal anaphylaxis.

Incubation period. The interval between the time an infection first enters the body and the time it manifests signs or symptoms of disease.

Ion channels. Protein portals in the cell through which sodium, potassium, and calcium move in and out.

Irukandji syndrome. Illness caused by the sting of the small jellyfish *Carukia barnesi* and consisting of restlessness, severe muscle spasms of the abdominal wall, vomiting, and, rarely, leakage of fluid into the lungs.

Kinetoplast. An intensely staining structure near the base of the flagellum in such organisms as *Trypanosoma* and *Leishmania*.

Latrodectus. Genus of spiders including *Latrodectus mactans*, the black widow, and similarly venomous species throughout the world.

Latrodectism. The syndrome of widow spider envenomation consisting of swollen glands near the bite, headache, vomiting, sweating, painful muscle spasms, tremors, fast pulse, and high blood pressure.

Leishman-Donovan body. The form the *Leishmania* protozoan takes inside the host cell. There is no flagellum (amastigote phase), but the parasite's nucleus and kinetoplast can be seen under the microscope.

Leishmaniasis. Parasitic diseases of the skin, moist membranes of the mouth and airway, the liver, spleen, and bone marrow transmitted by sandflies and caused by protozoa of the genus *Leishmania*.

Loxosceles reclusa. The brown recluse, or fiddle back spider, whose bite causes necrotic arachnidism.

Lymphatic system. A delicate system of channels that carries fluid from the tissues into the veins.

Mast cells. Cells filled with coarse granules that release histamine during allergic reactions.

Melarsoprol. A synthetic compound of arsenic, which, despite serious toxicity, must be used to treat patients with advanced East African (Rhodesian) sleeping sickness.

Meningitis. Inflammation of the membranes covering the brain and spinal cord.

Mustela putorius. The European ferret, sometimes kept as a pet.

Mycoplasmas. Bacteria causing diseases of the respiratory and genital tracts of humans and animals. They lack a fully developed cell wall, grow only on special, enriched media, and are the smallest free-living life-forms known.

Myasthenia gravis. A chronic weakness of the muscles, usually beginning with the face and throat.

Necrotic arachnidism. Tissue destruction and, rarely, red blood-cell breakdown (hemolysis) caused by certain spider venoms, notably that of the brown recluse and hobo spiders.

Necrotizing fasciitis. An invasive infection in which bacteria destroy the fibrous membranes covering muscle groups, leading to extensive tissue destruction.

Negri bodies. Clumps of rabies virus within stained nerve cells.

Nematocysts. Also called stinging cells. In the jellyfish family, coiled harpoonlike structures loaded with venom that impale animals coming into contact with their tentacles.

Pentamidine. A synthetic compound used to treat several parasitic diseases including sleeping sickness, leishmaniasis, and *Pneumocystis carinii* pneumonia in AIDS patients.

Pentostam. Sodium stibogluconate. A derivative of the antimony compound tartar emetic. Despite serious toxicity, it is the only reliable treatment for *Leishmania braziliensis.*

Phoneutria nigriventer. The wandering, or banana, spider, a dangerous species native to South America.

Phoneutrism. Syndrome caused by the bite of the wandering spider, *Phoneutria nigriventer,* which consists or drooling, sweating, priapism, shock, and paralysis of breathing.

Physalitoxin. The venom discharged by the stinging cells of the Portuguese man-o'-war that causes intense pain, abdominal cramps, vomiting, and muscle spasms in patients who are stung.

Platelet. A small blood particle that clumps in areas of injury to initiate clot formation and to stop bleeding.

Polymorphonuclear leukocytes, or **neutrophils.** Cells in the bloodstream, which form the first line of defense against tissue and bloodstream invasion by infection. They engulf and kill bacteria and other infectious agents, but are frequently destroyed in the process.

Priapism. Abnormal, prolonged penile erection that may follow animal envenomations.

Protozoa. A group of animals consisting of a single functioning cell or loose aggregate of several cells and including the parasites of malaria, sleeping sickness, and leishmaniasis.

Rat-bite fever. Either of two infectious diseases following rat bites. The streptobacillary form, due to *Streptobacillus moniliformis,* is most common in Europe and the United States, while the spirillary form caused by *Spirillum minus* occurs in Japan, where it is known as *sodoku*.

Rhesus macaques. Old World monkeys found primarily in Asia, which live in troops and are considered highly intelligent.

Robustoxin, or atrotoxin. A component of Sydney funnel web spider's venom that is toxic to humans. It causes massive discharge of autonomic nerves resulting in wide swings in pulse and blood pressure and shifts of fluid into the lungs.

Seal finger, or *spaek* finger. A chronic infection, usually of a finger and one or more of its joints, following seal bite or minor injury while handling seal flesh. It is probably caused by species of *Mycoplasmas*.

Serum sickness. An illness consisting of hives, fever, swollen glands, and joint pains, which appears one to two weeks after a patient is treated with an injection containing foreign serum, such as snake antivenin raised in horses.

Shock. A dangerous state of circulatory collapse with low blood pressure and inadequate flow of blood to the brain and other organs. It has many causes, including suffocation, bleeding, infection, toxins, and allergic reactions.

Sleeping sickness, or human African trypanosomiasis. A disease of the central nervous system caused by parasitic protozoa called trypanosomes and transmitted to humans and animals by the bite of the tsetse fly.

Solenospsis invicta. The imported red fire ant.

Suramin. A complex compound based on dyes, which is used to treat the early stages of sleeping sickness.

Sutherland pressure/immobilization technique. A procedure used in cases of spider bite and venomous snakebite, in which the wounded limb is wrapped in stretchy crepe and splinted until antivenin can be administered.

Sympathetic nervous system. A division of the autonomic

nervous system that regulates blood pressure, heart action, the airways of the lung, and metabolism by means of nerves that secrete chemicals in the epinephrine family.

Tetanus. A serious disease in which the bacterium *Clostridium tetani* grows in wounds not open to the air and produces a toxin that causes severe muscle spasms and unstable blood pressure and body temperature.

Tick paralysis. A syndrome of increasing weakness that ascends from the feet upward until the patient is unable to breathe. It is caused by toxins in the saliva of female hard-bodied ticks and occurs worldwide, although the most severe cases are reported in Australia.

Trypanosoma. A genus of protozoa that have a spindle- or eel-shaped body with a narrow membrane along the length ending in a lashing tail that, however, points forward. They are blood parasites causing sleeping sickness in Africa and also Chagas' disease in the New World.

Trypanosoma brucei gambiense. The protozoan that causes West African or Gambian sleeping sickness.

Trypanosoma brucei rhodesiense. The protozoan that causes the more acute East African or Rhodesian sleeping sickness.

Tsetse flies. A genus of bloodsucking insects that serve as intermediate hosts of the trypanosomes of sleeping sickness, supporting their multiplication and transmitting the infection when they feed on animal and human hosts.

Varanidae. The monitor family of lizards.

Variable surface glycoproteins. Proteins on the surface of trypanosomes to which sugars are attached. By changing their structure at intervals, the parasite evades the host's defending antibodies, allowing it to invade the central nervous system.

Viperidae. A family of venomous snakes that includes vipers, rattlesnakes, and water moccasins, in which the two upper jawbones ride on a hinged joint and are armed with a long, hollow tooth for venom injection.

Selected References

General

Caras, Roger. *Venomous Animals of the World*. Prentice-Hall, Inc., Englewood Cliffs, New Jersey, 1974.

Chandler, Asa C., Clark P. Read. *Introduction to Parasitology, with Special Reference to the Parasites of Man*. John Wiley and Sons, Inc., New York, 1967.

Cleland, Sir John B., R. V. Southcott. *Injuries to Man from Marine Invertebrates in the Australian Region*. A.J. Arthur, Commonwealth Government Printer, Canberra, 1965.

Encyclopedia Britannica, 15th Edition. Encyclopedia Britannica, Inc., Chicago, 1981.

Foster, W. D. *A History of Parasitology*. E. and S. Livingston LTD., Edinburgh, 1965.

Grice, Gordon. *The Red Hourglass, Lives of the Predators*. Delacorte Press, New York, 1998.

Mandell, Gerald L., John E. Bennett, Raphael Dolin, editors.

Principles and Practice of Infectious Diseases. Churchill Living-
stone, Philadelphia, 2000.

Matthews, Richard. *Nightmares of Nature.* HarperCollins Publish-
ers, London, 1995.

Mettler, Cecilia C. *History of Medicine.* The Blakiston Company,
Toronto, 1947.

Meier, Jürg, Julian White. *Handbook of Clinical Toxicology of Animal
Venoms and Poisons.* CRC Press, Boca Raton, 1995.

Sutherland, Struan K., James Tibballs. *Australian Animal Toxins.*
Oxford University Press, South Melbourne, 2001.

1: Invincible Invaders

Baer, Harold, T.-Y. Liu, Marsha C. Anderson, Murray Blum,
William H. Schmid, Frank J. James, "Protein Components of
Fire Ant Venom (*Solenopsis invicta*)." *Toxicon* 17 (1979):
397–405.

Clemmer, Dorothy I., Robert E. Serfling, "The Imported Fire Ant:
Dimensions of the Urban Problem." *Southern Medical Journal*
68, no. 9 (September 1975): 1133–1138.

deShazo, Richard, "The Continuing Saga of Imported Fire Ants:
Evolution Before Our Eyes." *Annals of Allergy, Asthma, and
Immunology* 77 (August 1996): 85–86.

deShazo, Richard, W. A. Banks, "Medical Consequences of Multiple Fire Ant Stings Occurring Indoors." *Journal of Allergy
and Clinical Immunology* 93, no. 5 (May 1994): 847–850.

deShazo, Richard, Brian T. Butcher, W. A. Banks, "Reactions to
the Stings of the Imported Fire Ant." *New England Journal of
Medicine* 323, no. 7 (April 16, 1990): 462–466.

deShazo, Richard, David F. Williams, Edward S. Moak, "Fire Ant
Attacks on Residents in Health Care Facilities: A Report of

Two Cases." *Annals of Internal Medicine* 131, no. 6 (September 21, 1999): 424–429.

deShazo, Richard, David F. Williams, "Multiple Fire Ant Stings Indoors." *Southern Medical Journal* 88, no. 7 (July 1995): 712–715.

Fox, Roger W., Richard F. Lockey, Samuel C. Bukantz, "Neurologic Sequelae Following the Imported Fire Ant Sting." *Journal of Allergy and Clinical Immunology* 70, no. 2 (August 1982): 120–124.

Hardwick, William, James A. Royall, Bruce A. Petitt, Samuel J. Tilden, "Near Fatal Fire Ant Envenomation of a Newborn." *Pediatrics* 90, no. 4 (October 1992): 622–624.

Hoy, Carol, "Single Gene Regulates Fire Ants' Behavior." *USA Today,* 15 November 2001.

Kemp, Stephen F., Richard deShazo, John E. Moffitt, David F. Williams, William A. Buhner, "Expanding Habitat of the Imported Fire Ant (*Solenopsis invicta*): A Public Health Concern." *Journal of Allergy and Clinical Immunology* 105, no. 4 (April, 2000): 683–691.

Leggett, Mike, "Fire Ants Killing Thousands of Trout on the Guadalupe." *Austin American Statesman,* 2 May 2002.

Lofgren C. S., W. A. Banks, B. M. Glancey, "Biology and Control of Imported Fire Ants." *Annual Review of Entomology* 20 (1975): 1–30.

Lofgren, Clifford S., Robert K. Vander Meer, editors *Fire Ants and Leaf-Cutting Ant: Biology and Management.* Westview Press, Boulder, 1986.

MacKay, William P., Said Majdi, James Irving, S. Bradleigh Vinson, Carroll Messer, "Attraction of Ants (Hymenoptera: *formicidae*) to Electric Fields." *Journal of the Kansas Entomological Society* 65, no. 1 (1992): 39–43.

Matus, Ron, "Imported Fly a Lethal Weapon in War on Fire Ants." *Gainesville Sun,* 20 November 2000.

Morrill, Wendell, "Red Imported Fire Ant Control with Mound Drenches." *Journal of Economic Entomology* 69, no. 4 (August 1976): 542–544.

Porter, Sanford D., Harold G. Fowler, William P. MacKay, "Fire Ant Mound Densities in the United States and Brazil (Hymenoptera: *formicidae*)." *Journal of Economic Entomology* 85, no. 4 (August 1992): 1154–1161.

Porter, Sanford D., Dolores A. Savignano, "Invasion of Polygyne Fire Ants Decimates Native Ants and Disrupts Arthropod Community." *Ecology* 71, no. 6 (December 1990): 2095–2106.

Rhoades, Robert B., Chester T. Stafford, Frank K. James, "Survey of Fatal Anaphylactic Reactions to Imported Fire Ant Stings." *Journal of Allergy and Clinical Immunology* 84, no. 2 (January 1989): 159–162.

Ross, Kenneth G., Edward L. Bargo, Laurent Keller, "Social Evolution in a New Environment: The Case of Introduced Fire Ants." *Proceedings of the National Academy of Sciences* 93, no. 7 (April 1996): 3021–3025.

Schwartz, Meyer P., "Fire Ants: The Death March." *Journal of Family Practice* 33, no. 4 (1991): 406–410.

Smith, J. D., Edgar B. Smith, "Multiple Fire Ant Stings, a Complication of Alcoholism." *Archives of Dermatology* 103, no. 4 (April 1971): 438–441.

Tankersley, Michael, Russell L. Walker, William K. Butler, Larry L. Hagen, Diane C. Napoli, Theodore M. Freeman, "Safety and Efficacy of an Imported Fire Ant Rush Immunotherapy Protocol With and Without Prophylactic Treatment." *Journal of Allergy and Clinical Immunology* 109, no. 3 (March 2002): 556–562.

Taylor, John, "Battle of the Ants." *ABC News Online,* 22 October 2001.

Triplett, R. Faser, "Sensitivity to the Imported Fire Ant: Successful

Treatment with Immunotherapy." *Southern Medical Journal* 66, no. 4 (April 1973): 477–480.

Vinson, S. Bradleigh, "Invasion of the Red Imported Fire Ant." *American Entomologist* (Spring 1997): 23–39.

Williams, David F. *Exotic Ants: Biology, Impact, and Control of Introduced Species.* Westview Press, Boulder, 1994.

Williams, William J., Ernest Beutler, Allan J. Erslev, R. Wayne Rundles, editors. *Hematology.* McGraw-Hill Book Company, New York, 1977.

2: Fangs in the Dark

Anderson, Philip C., "Spider Bites in the United States." *Dermatology Clinics* 15, no. 2 (April 1997): 307–312.

Atkins, James A., Curtis W. Wingo, William A. Sodeman, "Probable Cause of Necrotic Spider Bite in the Midwest." *Science* 126 (July 12, 1957): 73.

Broughton, Maj. George II., "Management of the Brown Recluse Spider Bite to the Glans Penis." *Military Medicine* 161, no. 10 (October 1996): 627–629.

CDC, "Necrotic Arachnidism—Pacific Northwest, 1988–1996." *Morbidity and Mortality Weekly Report* 45, no. 45 (May 31, 1996): 433–436.

Elston, Col. Dirk M., "What's Eating You? *Loxosceles reclusa* (Brown Recluse Spider)." *Cutus* 69, no. 2 (February 2002): 91–92.

Elston, Dirk M., Jeff S. Eggers, William E. Schmidt, Alan B. Storrow, Robert H. Doe, David McGlasson, Joseph R. Fischer, "Histological Findings After Brown Recluse Spider Envenomation." *American Journal of Dermatopathology* 22, no. 3 (2000): 242–246.

Fisher, Malcolm, John Raftos, Robert T. McGuinness, Ian T.

Dicks, John S. Wong, Keith R. Burgess, Struan K. Sutherland, "Funnel-web Spider (*Atrax robustus*) Antivenom 2. Early Clinical Experience." *Medical Journal of Australia* 2 (November 14, 1981): 525–526.

Fisher, Randall G., Patrick Kelly, Marvin S. Krober, Michael R. Weir, Robert Jones, "Necrotic Arachnidism." *Western Journal of Medicine* 160, no. 6 (June 1994): 570–572.

Gertsch, Willis J. *American Spiders*. D. Van Nostrand Co., Inc. New York, 1949.

Goto, Collin S., Thomas J. Abramo, Charles M. Ginsburg, "Upper Airway Obstruction Caused by Brown Recluse Spider Envenomation of the Neck." *American Journal of Emergency Medicine* 14, no. 7 (November 1996): 660–662.

Handel, Cheryl C., Luis A. Izquierdo, Luis B. Curet, "Black Widow Spider (*Latrodectus mactans*) Bite During Pregnancy." *Western Journal of Medicine* 160, no. 3 (March 1994): 261–262.

Hartman, Leonard J., Struan K. Sutherland, "Funnel-web Spider (*Atrax robustus*) Antivenom in the Treatment of Human Envenomation." *Medical Journal of Australia* 141, no. 12–13 (December 8/22, 1984): 796–799.

Levi, Herbert W., Lorna R. Levi. *Spiders and Their Kin*. Golden Books Publishing Co., Racine, Wisconsin, 1990.

Lucas, Sylvia, "Spiders in Brazil." *Toxicon* 26, no. 9 (1988): 759–772.

O'Malley, Gerald F., Richard C. Dart, Edwin F. Kuffner, "Successful Treatment of Lactrodectism with Antivenin after 90 Hours." *New England Journal of Medicine* 340, no. 8 (February 25, 1999): 657.

Majeski, James A., George G. Durst, "Necrotic Arachnidism." *Southern Medical Journal* 69, no. 7 (July 1976): 887–891.

Masters, Edwin J., "Images in Clinical Medicine, Loxoscelism." *New England Journal of Medicine* 339, no. 6 (August 6, 1998): 379.

Meadows, Paul E., Findlay E. Russell, "Milking of Arthropods." *Toxicon* 8 (1970): 311–312.

Newlands, G., P. Atkinson, "Review of Southern African Spiders of Medical Importance, with Notes on the Signs and Symptoms of Envenomation." *South African Medical Journal* 73, no. 4 (February 20, 1988): 235–239.

Phillips, Scott, Michael Kohn, Dale Baker, Rob Vander Leest, Hernan Gomez, Patrick McKinny, John McGoldrick, Jeffrey Brent, "Therapy of Brown Spider Envenomation: A Controlled Trial of Hyperbaric Oxygen, Dapson, and Cyproheptadine." *Annals of Emergency Medicine* 25, no. 3 (March 1995): 363–368.

Pincus, Steven J., Kenneth D. Winkel, Gabrielle H. Hawdon, Struan K. Sutherland, "Acute and Recurrent Skin Ulceration After Spider Bite." *Medical Journal of Australia* 171 (July 19, 1999): 99–102.

Reeves, Julie A., E. Jackson Allison Jr., Peggy E. Goodman, "Black Widow Spider Bite in a Child." *American Journal of Emergency Medicine* 14, no. 5 (September 1996): 469–473.

Srochosky, Barbara, "Necrotic Arachnidism." *Western Journal of Medicine* 131, no. 2 (August 1979): 143–148.

Sutherland, Struan. *A Venomous Life*. Hyland House, South Melbourne, 1998.

Sutherland, Struan K., "Antivenom to the Venom of the Male Sydney Funnel-web Spider *Atrax robustus*." *Medical Journal of Australia* 2 (October 18, 1980): 437–441.

Sutherland, Struan K., "The Sydney Funnel-web Spider (*Atrax robustus*) 3. A Review of Some Clinical Records of Human Envenomation." *Medical Journal of Australia* 2 (September 16, 1972): 643–647.

Sutherland, Struan K., "The Management of Bites by the Sydney Funnel-web Spider, *Atrax robustus*." *Medical Journal of Australia* 1 (February 11, 1978): 148–150.

Sutherland, Struan K., A. W. Duncan, J. Tibballs, "Local Inactivation of Funnel-web Spider (*Atrax robustus*) Venom by First-aid

Measure." *Medical Journal of Australia* 2 (October 18, 1980): 435–437.

Taylor, Eugene H., William F. Denny, "Hemolysis, Renal Failure and Death, Presumed Secondary to Bite of Brown Recluse Spider." *Southern Medical Journal* 9 (October 1966): 1209–1211.

Timms, Patrick K., Robert B. Gibbons, "Latrodectism—Effects of the Black Widow Spider Bite." *Western Journal of Medicine* 144, no. 3 (March 1986): 315–317.

Vest, Darwin K., "Necrotic Arachnidism in the Northwest United States and Its Probable Relationship to *Tegenaria Agrestis* (Walckenaer) Spiders." *Toxicon* 25, no. 2 (1987): 175–184.

3: Stingers from the Sea

Auerbach, Paul S., "Marine Envenomations." *New England Journal of Medicine* 325, no. 7 (August 15, 1991): 486–493.

Barnes, J. H., "Cause and Effect in Irukandji Stings." *Medical Journal of Australia* 1 (June 13, 1964): 897–904.

Burnett, Joseph W., Peter J. Fenner, Franco Kokelj, John A. Williamson, "Serious *Physalia* (Portuguese man o'war) Stings: Implications for Scuba Divers." *Journal of Wilderness Medicine* 5 (1994): 71–76.

Currie, Bart J., Yvonne K. Wood, "Identification of *Chironex Fleckeri* Envenomation by Nematocysts Recovery from Skin." *Medical Journal of Australia* 162, no. 9 (May 1, 1995): 478–480.

Fenner, Peter J., "Dangers in the Ocean: The Traveler and Marine Envenomations. I. Jellyfish." *Journal of Travel Medicine* 5, no. 3 (September 1998): 135–141.

Fenner, Peter J., John A. Williamson, "Worldwide Deaths and Severe Envenomation from Jellyfish Stings." *Medical Journal of Australia* 165 (1996): 658–666.

Fenner, Peter J., John A. Williamson, John A. Blenkin, "Successful Use of *Chironex fleckeri* Antivenom by Members of the Queensland Ambulance Transport Brigade." *Medical Journal of Australia* 151 (December 4/18, 1989): 708–710.

Fenner, Peter J., John Williamson, Vic I. Callahan, Ian Audley, "Further Understanding of, and a New Treatment for, 'Irukandji' (*Carukia barnesi*) Stings." *Medical Journal of Australia* 145 (December 1/15, 1986): 569–574.

Flecker, H., "Fatal Stings to North Queensland Bathers." *Medical Journal of Australia* 1 (January 12, 1952): 35–38.

Flecker, H., "Injuries by Unknown Agents to Bathers in North Queensland." *Medical Journal of Australia* 1 (January 27, 1945): 98.

Flecker, H., "Irukandji Sting to North Queensland Bathers Without Production of Weals (sic) but with Severe General Symptoms." *Medical Journal of Australia* 2 (July 19, 1952): 89–91.

Hartwick, Robert, Vic Callanan, John Williamson, "Disarming the Box Jellyfish. Nematocyst Inhibition in *Chironex Fleckeri*." *Medical Journal of Australia* 1 (January 12, 1980): 15–20.

Little, Mark, Richard F. Mulcahy, "A Year's Experience of Irukandji Envenomation in Far North Queensland." *Medical Journal of Australia* 169 (December 1998): 638–641.

Little M., R. F. Mulcahy, D. J. Wenck, "Life-Threatening Cardiac Failure in a Healthy Young Female with Irukandji Syndrome." *Anaesthesia and Intensive Care* 29, no. 2 (April 2001): 178–180.

Martin, John C., Ian Audley, "Cardiac Failure Following Irukandji Envenomation." *Medical Journal of Australia* 153 (August 6, 1990): 164–166.

Southcott, R. V., "Tropical Jellyfish and Other Marine Stingers." *Military Medicine* 124, no. 8 (August 1959): 569–579.

Southcott, R. V., C. W. Kingston, "Lethal Jellyfish Stings: A Study in 'Sea Wasps.' " *Medical Journal of Australia* 1 (March 28, 1959): 443–444.

Stein, Mark R., John V. Marraccini, Neal E. Rothschild, Joseph W. Burnett, "Fatal Portuguese Man-o'-war (*Physalia physalis*) Envenomation." *Annals of Emergency Medicine* 18, no. 3 (March 1989): 312–315.

Williamson, John A., Vic I. Callanan, Robert Hartwick, "Serious Envenomation by the Northern Australian Box Jellyfish (*Chironex fleckeri*)." *Medical Journal of Australia* 1 (January 12, 1980): 13–16.

4: Beautiful, Deadly Cones

Barinaga, Marcia, "Science Digests the Secrets of Voracious Killer Snails." *Science* 249 (July 20, 1990): 250–251.

Barnes, Robert D. *Invertebrate Zoology*. W. B. Saunders Company, Philadelphia, 1968.

Clench, William J., Yoshio Kondo, "The Poison Cone Shell." *American Journal of Tropical Medicine and Hygiene* 23 (1943): 105–121.

Concar, D., "Doctor Snail." *New Scientist* 19 (October 1996): 26–28.

Fegan, David, David Andresen, "*Conus Geographicus* Envenomation." *Lancet* 349 (June 7, 1997): 1672.

Flecker, H., "Cone Shell Mollusc Poisoning, with Report of a Fatal Case." *Medical Journal of Australia* 1 (April 4, 1936): 464–466.

Gibbs, W. W., "A New Way to Spell Relief: V-e-n-o-m. A Toxin from Killer Sea Snails Promises a Better Painkiller." *Scientific American* 274, no. 2 (February 1996): 20–21.

Hermitte, L. C. D., "Venomous Marine Molluscs of the Genus *Conus*." *Transactions of the Royal Society of Tropical Medicine and Hygiene* 39, no. 6 (June 1946): 485–512.

Kohn, Alan J., "Cone Shell Stings." *Hawaii Medical Journal* 17, no. 6 (July–August 1958): 528–532.

Kohn, Alan J., "The Ecology of *Conus* in Hawaii." *Ecological Monographs* 29, no. 1 (January 1959): 47–90.

Olivera, Baldomero M., "*Conus* Venom Peptides, Receptor and Ion Channel Targets, and Drug Design: 50 Million Years of Neuropharmacology." *Molecular Biology of the Cell* 8 (1997): 2101–2109.

Olivera, Baldomero M., Michael McIntosh, Craig Clark, David Middlemas, William R. Gray, Lourdes Cruz, "A Sleep-inducing Peptide from *Conus Geographicus* Venom." *Toxicon* 23, no. 2 (1985): 277–282.

Olivera, Baldomero M., Jean Rivier, Craig Clark, Cecilia A. Ramilo, Gloria P. Corpuz, Fe C. Abogadie, E. Edward Mena, Scott R. Woodward, David R. Hillyard, Lourdes J. Cruz, "Diversity of *Conus* Neuropeptides." *Science* 249 (July 20, 1990): 257–263.

Olivera, Baldomero M., Jean Rivier, Jamie K. Scott, David R. Hillyard, Lourdes J. Cruz, "Conotoxins." *Journal of Biological Chemistry* 266, no. 33 (November 25, 1991): 22067–22070.

O'Neil, Graeme, "Painkiller from the Sea." *Herald Sun* (Australia), (21 April, 1996): 5.

Scott, David A., Christine E. Wright, James A. Angus, "Actions of Intrathecal Omega-Conotoxins CVID, GVIA, MVIIA, and Morphine in Acute and Neuropathic Pain in the Rat." *European Journal of Pharmacology* 451 (2002): 279–286.

Sutherland, Struan K., James Tibballs. *Australian Animal Toxins.* Oxford University Press, South Melbourne, 2001.

Terlau, Heinrich, Ki-Joon Shon, Michelle Grilley, Martin Stocker, Walter Stühmer, Baldomero M. Olivera, "Strategy for Rapid Immobilization of Prey by a Fish-hunting Marine Snail." *Nature* 381 (May 9, 1996): 148–151.

5: The Limbless Ones

Amarasekera, N., A. Jayawardena, A. Ariyaratnam, U. C. L. Hewage, Anslem de Silva, "Bite of a Sea Snake (*Hydrophis spiralis*): A Case Report from Sri Lanka." *Journal of Tropical Medicine and Hygiene* 97, no. 4 (1994): 195–198.

Angel, Michael F., Feng Zhang, Matthew Jones, James Henderson, Stanley W. Chapman, "Necrotizing Fasciitis of the Upper Extremity Resulting from a Water Moccasin Bite." *Southern Medical Journal* 95, no. 9 (September 2002): 1090–1094.

Butner, Alfred N., "Rattlesnake Bites in Northern California." *Western Journal of Medicine* 139, no. 2 (August 1983): 179–183.

Davidson, Terence M., Susan Schafer, James Killfoil, "Cobras." *Journal of Wilderness Medicine* 6 (1995): 203–219.

Denis, D., T. Lamireau, B. Llanas, R. Bedry, M. Fayon, "Rhabodomyolysis in European Viper Bite." *Acta Paediatrica* 87 (1998): 1013–1015.

Department of the Navy, Bureau of Medicine and Surgery. *Poisonous Snakes of the World. A Manual for Use by U.S. Amphibious Forces.* NAVMED P-5099, United States Government Printing Office, Washington D.C., 1962.

Gold, Barry S., Richard Dart, Robert A. Barish, "Bites of Venomous Snakes." *New England Journal of Medicine* 347, no. 5 (August 1, 2002): 347–356.

Gold, Barry S., Willis A. Wingert. "Snake Venom Poisoning in the United States: A Review of Therapeutic Practice." *Southern Medical Journal* 87, no. 6 (1994): 579–589.

Goldstein, Ellie J. C., Diana M. Citron, Henry Gonzalez, Findley E. Russell, Sydney M. Finegold, "Bacteriology of Rattlesnake

Venom and Implications for Therapy." *Journal of Infectious Diseases* 140, no. 5 (November 1979): 818–821.

Grice, Gordon. *The Red Hourglass. Lives of the Predators.* Delacorte Press, New York, 1998.

Hodgson, Peter S., Terence M. Davidson, "Biology and Treatment of the Mamba Snakebite." *Wilderness and Environmental Medicine* 2 (1996): 133–145.

Isbister, Geoffrey K., Andrew H. Dawson, Ian M. Whyte, "Two Cases of Bites by the Black-bellied Swamp Snake (*Hemiaspis signata*)." *Toxicon* 40 (2002): 317–319.

Jorge, M. T., S. de A. Nishioka, R. B. de Oliveira, L. A. Ribeiro, P. V. P. Silveira, "*Aeromonas hydrophila* Soft-tissue Infection as a Complication of Snake Bite: Report of Three Cases." *Annals of Tropical Medicine and Parasitology* 92, no. 2 (1998): 213–217.

Jorge, Miguel Tanús, Lindioneza Adriano Ribeiro, Maria Lucia R. Da Silva, Elisa J. Uro Kusano, João Silva de Mendonça, "Microbiological Studies of Abscesses Complicating *Bothrops* Snakebite in Humans: A Prospective Study." *Toxicon* 32, no. 6 (1994): 743–748.

Jorge Miguel Tanus, Ida S. Sanos-Martins, Sandra C. Tomy, Sandra C. B. Castro, Ronney A. Ferrar, Lindioneza Adriano Ribeiro, David A. Warrell, "Snakebite by the Bushmaster (*Lachesis muta*) in Brazil: Case Report and Review of the Literature." *Toxicon* 35, no. 4 (1997): 545–554.

Lewis, James V., Charles A. Portera Jr., "Rattlesnake Bite of the Face: Case Report and Review of the Literature." *American Surgeon* 60, no. 9 (September 1994): 681–682.

Mara W. R. *Venomous Snakes of the World.* T.F.H. Publications, Inc., Neptune City, New Jersey, 1993.

Mellor Norman H., John C. Arvin, "A Bushmaster Bite During a Birding Expedition in Lowland Southeastern Peru." *Wilderness and Environmental Medicine* 3 (1996): 236–240.

Milani Jr., R., M. T. Jorge, F. P. Ferraz de Campos, F. P. Martins, A. Bousso, J. L. C. Cardoso, L. A. Ribeiro, H. W. Fan, F. O. S. França, I. S. Sanos-Martins, D. Cardoso, et al, "Snake Bites by the Jararacuçu (*Bothrops jararacussu*): Clinicopathological Studies of 29 Proven Cases in São Paulo State, Brazil." *Quarterly Journal of Medicine* 90 (1997): 323–334.

Minton, Sherman A., Madge Rutherford Minton. *Venomous Reptiles*. Charles Scribner's Sons, New York, 1969.

Morandi, Neil, Janet Williams, "Snakebite Injuries: Contributing Factors and Intentionality of Exposure." *Wilderness and Environmental Medicine* 8 (1997): 152–155.

Phillips, Charles M., "Sea Snake Envenomation." *Dermatologic Therapy* 15 (2002): 58–61.

Pochanugool, Charn, Henry Wilde, Kasien Bhanganada, Lawan Chanhome, "Venomous Snakebite in Thailand II: Clinical Experience." *Military Medicine* 163 (May 1998): 318–323.

Tanen, David, Anne-Michelle Ruha, Kimberlie A. Graeme, Steven C. Curry, Mark A. Fischione, "Rattlesnake Envenomations: Unusual Case Presentations." *Archives of Internal Medicine* 161, no. 3 (February 12, 2001): 474–479.

Russell, Findlay E., "Snake Venom Poisoning in the United States." *Annual Review of Medicine* 31 (1980): 247–259.

Tu, Anthony T., Gordian Fulde, "Sea Snake Bites." *Clinics in Dermatology* 5, no. 7 (July–September 1987): 118–126.

Watt, George, R., David G. Theakston, "Sea Snake Bites in a Freshwater Lake." *American Journal of Tropical Medicine and Hygiene* 34, no. 4 (July 1985): 770–113.

Wingert, Willis A., "Rattlesnake Bites in Southern California and Rational for Recommended Treatment." *Western Journal of Medicine* 148 (January 1988): 37–44.

6: Silent Stowaways

Anonymous, "Tick Paralysis on the Atherton Tablelands." athertontablelands.com, accessed 2/21/2003.

Bassoe, Peter, "Paralysis of Ascending Type in an Adult Due to Bite by a Woodtick." *Archives of Neurology and Psychology* 11 (May 1924): 564–567.

Beyer, Arthur B., Mark Grossman, "Tick Paralysis in a Red Wolf." *Journal of Wildlife Diseases* 33, no. 4 (October 1997): 900–902.

Botzler, R. G., J. Albrecht, T. Schaefer, "Tick Paralysis in a Western Harvest Mouse (*Reithrodontomys megalotis*)." *Journal of Wildlife Diseases* 16, no. 2 (April 1980): 223–224.

Costa, Joseph A., "Tick Paralysis on the Atlantic Seaboard." *American Journal of Diseases of Children* 83 (1952): 336–347.

Dworkin, Mark S., Phyllis C. Shoemaker, Donald E. Anderson, "Tick Paralysis: 33 Human Cases in Washington State, 1946–1996." *Clinical Infectious Diseases* 29 (December 1999): 1435–1439.

Felz, Michael W., Lance A. Durden, "Identifying Ticks: A Pictorial Guide." *Patient Care for the Nurse Practitioner* (March 1999): 40–51.

Felz, Michael W., Carrie Davis Smith, Thomas R. Swift, "A Six-Year-Old Girl with Tick Paralysis." *New England Journal of Medicine* 342, no. 2 (January 13, 2000): 90–94.

Ferguson, E. W., "Deaths from Tick Paralysis in Human Beings." *Medical Journal of Australia* 2 (October 4, 1924): 346–348.

Grattan-Smith, P. J., J. G. Morris, H. M. Johnston, C. Yiannikas, R. Malik, R. Russell, R. A. Ouvrier, "Clinical and Neurophysiological Features of Tick Paralysis." *Brain* 120 (November 1997): 1975–1987.

Greenstein, P., "Tick Paralysis." *Medical Clinics of North America* 86, no. 2 (March 2002): 441–446.

Hadwen, Seymour, "On 'Tick Paralysis' in Sheep and Man Following Bites of *Dermacenter Venustus,* with Notes on the Biology of the Tick." *Parasitology* 6 (October 1913): 283–297.

Jessup, David A., "Tick Paralysis in a Grey Fox." *Journal of Wildlife Diseases.* 15 (April 1979): 271–272.

Kaire, G. H., "Isolation of Tick Paralysis Toxin from *Ixodes Holocyclys.*" *Toxicon* 4, no. 2 (August 1966): 91–97.

Needham, Glen R., "Evaluation of Five Popular Methods for Tick Removal." *Pediatrics* 75, no. 6 (June 1985): 997–1002.

Pearn, John, "The Clinical Features of Tick Bite." *Medical Journal of Australia* 2, no. 10 (September 3, 1977): 313–318.

Spach, David H., W. Conrad Liles, Grant L. Campbell, Robert E. Quick, Donald E. Anderson, Thomas R. Fritsche, "Tickborne Diseases in the United States." *New England Journal of Medicine* 329, no. 13 (September 23, 1993): 936–947.

Todd, John L. "Tick Bite in British Columbia." *Canadian Medical Journal* 2 (July–Dec 1912): 1118–1119.

7: Nightmare

Anonymous, "Obituary: Joseph Everett Dutton." *British Medical Journal* (May 6, 1905): 1020–1021.

Bruce, Sir David, "The Croonian Lectures on Trypanosomes Causing Disease in Man and Domestic Animals in Central Africa. Lecture I." *Lancet* (June 26, 1915): 1323–1330.

Bruce, Sir David, "The Croonian Lectures on Trypanosomes Causing Disease in Man and Domestic Animals in Central Africa. Lecture III." *Lancet* (July 10, 1915): 55–63.

Case Records of the Massachusetts General Hospital (case

20–2002). *New England Journal of Medicine* 346, no. 26 (June 27, 2002): 2069–2076.

Conrad, Joseph. *Heart of Darkness.* Penguin Books, London, 1995.

Cook, G. C., "Sir David Bruce's Elucidation of the Aetiology of *Nagana*—Exactly One Hundred Years Ago." *Transactions of the Royal Society of Tropical Medicine and Hygiene* 88 (1994): 257–258.

Cloudsley-Thompson, J. L. *Insects and History.* Weidenfeld and Nicolson, London, 1976.

Desowitz, Robert, "The Fly That Would Be King." In *New Guinea Tapeworms and Jewish Grandmothers.* W. W. Norton and Company, New York, 1987.

Donelson, John E., Mervyn J. Turner, "How the Trypanosome Changes Its Coat." *Scientific American* 252, no. 2 (February 1985): 44–51.

Dutton, J. Everett, "Note on a Trypanosoma Occurring in the Blood of Man." *British Medical Journal* 2 (September 20, 1902): 881–884.

Fèvre, E. M., P. G. Coleman, M. Odiit, J. W. Magona, S. C. Welburn, M. E. J. Woolhouse, "The Origins of a New *Trypanosoma brucei rhodesiense* Sleeping Sickness Outbreak in Eastern Uganda." *Lancet* 358 (August 25, 2001): 625–628.

Gear, J. H. S., "African Sleeping Sickness—African Trypanosomiasis. The Story of Its Conquest." *Adler Museum Bulletin* 12, no. 1 (March 1986): 3–10.

Kappmeier, Karin, E. M. Nevill, R. J. Bagnall, "Review of Tsetse Flies and Trypanosomiais in South Africa." *Onderstepoort Journal of Veterinary Research* 65, no. 3 (September 1998): 195–203.

Kolata, Gina, "Scrutinizing Sleeping Sickness." *Science* 226 (November 23, 1984): 956–958.

MacArthur, Lieut.-General Sir William, "An Account of Some of Sir David Bruce's Researches, Based on His Own Manuscript

Notes." *Transactions of the Royal Society of Tropical Medicine and Hygiene* 49 (1955): 404–412.

Manson, Patrick, C. W. Daniels, "A Case of Trypanosomiasis." *British Medical Journal* 1 (May 30, 1903): 1249–2254.

Panosian, Claire B., Lee Cohen, David Bruckner, George Berlin, W. David Hardy, "Fever, Leukopenia, and a Cutaneous Le-sion in a Man Who Had Recently Traveled in Africa." *Reviews of Infectious Diseases* 13 (November–December 1991): 1131–1138.

Pecoul, Bernard, Pierre Chirac, Patrice Trouiller, Jacques Pinel, "Access to Essential Drugs in Poor Countries: A Lost Battle?" *Journal of the American Medical Association* 281, no. 4 (January 27, 1999): 361–367.

Petru, Ann M., Parvin H. Azimi, Susan K. Cummins, Albert Sjoerdsma, "African Sleeping Sickness in the United States. Successful Treatment with Eflornithine." *American Journal of Diseases of Children* 142 (February 1988): 224–228.

Ransford, O. N. "Sir Aldo Castellani—An International Man." *History of Medicine* 224 (August 1980): 861–863.

Sahlas, Demetrios J., J. Dick Maclean, John Janevski, Allan S. Detsky, "Out of Africa." *New England Journal of Medicine* 347, no. 10 (September 5, 2002): 749–753.

Sinha, Anushua, Christopher Grace, W. Kemper Alston, Fred Westenfeld, and Maguire, James H. "African Trypanosomiasis in Two Travelers from the United States." *Clinical Infectious Diseases* 29 (October 1999): 840–844.

Smith, David H., Jacques Pepin, August H. R. Stich, "Human African Trypanosomiasis: An Emerging Public Health Crisis." *British Medical Bulletin* 54, no. 2 (1998): 341–355.

Smith, G. Joan. "The Liverpool School of Tropical Medicine Expedition to Senegambia, 1902, as revealed in the Letters of Dr. J. L. Todd." *Annals of Tropical Medicine and Parasitology* 71, no. 4 (December 1977): 391–399.

Spencer, Harrison C., James J. Gibson Jr., Richard E. Brodsky, Myron G. Schultz, "Imported African Trypanosomiasis in the United States." *Annals of Internal Medicine* 82, no. 5 (May 1975): 633–638.

Stich, August, Paulo M. Abel, Sanjeev Krishna, "Human African Trypanosomiasis." *British Medical Journal* 325 (July 27, 2002): 203–206.

Taelman, Henri, Paul J. Schlecter, Luc Marcelis, Jean Sonnet, Gaston Kazyumba, Jean Dasnoy, Klaus D. Haegele, Albert Sjoerdsma, Marc Wery, "Difluoromethylornithine, an Effective New Treatment of Gambian Trypanosomiasis. Results in Five Patients." *American Journal of Medicine* 82 (March 23, 1987): 607–614.

Van Nieuwenhove, Simon, "Gambiense Sleeping Sickness: Re-emerging and Soon Untreatable?" *Bulletin of the World Health Organization* 78, no. 11 (2000): 1283.

Wendo, Charles, "Uganda Revises Cattle Treatment to Protect Humans from Sleeping Sickness." *Lancet* 359 (January 19, 2002): 239.

Wickware, Potter, "Resurrecting the Resurrection Drug." *Nature Medicine* 8, no. 9 (September 2002): 908–909.

Zimmer, Carl, "A Sleeping Storm." *Discover Magazine,* August 1998.

8: Sponge Face and Black Fever

Anonymous, "Information Material for Physicians from the Centers For Disease Control and Prevention About Pentostam (Sodium Stibogluconate)." Centers for Disease Control, August 19, 1995, 1–17.

Anonymous, "The Leishmaniases and Leishmania/HIV Co-infections." World Health Organization, www.who.int accessed 3/22/03.

CDC, "Cutaneous Leishmaniasis in U. S. Military Personnel—Southwest/Central Asia, 2002–2003." *Morbidity and Mortality Weekly Report* 52, no. 42 (October 24, 2003).

Berger, Robert S., Rafael A. Perez-Figaredo, Richard L. Spielvogel, "Leishmaniasis: The Touch Preparation as a Rapid Means of Diagnosis." *Journal of the American Academy of Dermatology* 5, p. 2 (May 1987): 1096–1105.

Campbell-Lendrum, Diarmid, Jean-Pierre Dujardin, Eddy Martinez, M. Dora Feliciangeli, J. Enrique Perez, Laura Ney Marcelino Passerat de Silans, Philippe Desjeux, "Domestic and Peridomestic Transmission of American Cutaneous Leishmaniasis: Changing Epidemiological Patterns Presenting New Control Opportunities." *Memórias do Instituto Oswaldo Cruz* 96, no. 2 (February 2001): 159–162.

Desowitz, Robert S., "In Search of Kala Azar." In *The Malaria Capers*. W. W. Norton and Company, New York, 1991.

Donovan C., "On the Possibility of the Occurrence of Trypanosomiasis in India." *British Medical Journal* 2 (July 11, 1903): 79.

Hatcher, Robert A., ed., Paul C. Barton, assoc. ed. *Useful Drugs, A Selected List of Essential Drugs with Brief Discussions of Actions, Uses and Dosage*. American Medical Association, Chicago, 1942.

Herwaldt, Barabara L., Susan Stokes, Dennis D. Juranek, "American Cutaneous Leishmaniasis in U.S. Travelers." *Annals of Internal Medicine* 118, no. 10 (May 15, 1993): 780–784.

Herwaldt, Barbara L., "Leishmaniasis." *Lancet* 354 (October 2, 1999): 1191–1199.

Herwaldt, Barbara L., Jonathan D. Berman, "Recommendations for Treating Leishmaniasis with Sodium Stiboglubonate (Pentostam) and Review of Pertinent Clinical Studies."

American Journal of Tropical Medicine and Hygiene 46, no. 3 (1992): 296–255.

Hoare, Cecil A., "Early Discoveries Regarding the Parasite of Oriental Sore, with An English Translation of the Memoir of P. F. Borovsky: 'On Sart Sore.' 1898." *Transactions of the Royal Society of Tropical Medicine and Hygiene* 32, n. 1 (June 1938): 67–92.

Hyams, Kenneth C., James Riddle, David H. Trump, John T. Graham, "Epidemic Infectious Diseases and Biological Warfare During the Gulf War: A Decade of Analysis and Final Concerns." *American Journal of Tropical Medicine and Hygiene* 56, no. 5 (November 2001): 664–670.

Jaffe, Ludwig, "Nasal Leishmaniasis in Panama." *Archives of Otolaryngology* 72 (1957): 601–611.

Jones, T. C., W. D. Johnson Jr., A. C. Barretto, E. Lago, R. Badero, B. Cerf, S. G. Reed, E. M. Netto, M. S. Tada, F. Franca, K. Wiese, L. Golightly, E. Fikrig, J. M. L. Costa, C. C. Cuba, P. D. Marsden, "Epidemiology of American Cutaneous Leishmaniasis Due to *Leishmania braziliensis*." *Journal of Infectious Diseases* 156, no. 1 (July 1987): 73–83.

Katz, Kevin C., Sharon Walmsley, Anne G. McLeod, Jay S. Keystone, Allan S. Detsky, "Where Are You From? (Clinical Problem Solving)." *New England Journal of Medicine* 346, no. 10 (March 7, 2002): 764–767.

Leishman, Major W. B., "On the Possibility of the Occurrence of Trypanosomiasis in India." *British Medical Journal* 1 (May 30, 1903): 1252–1254.

Magill, Alan J., Max Grögl, Robert A. Gasser, Wellington Sun, Charles N. Oster, "Visceral Infection Caused by *Leishmania Tropica* in Veterans of Operation Desert Storm." *New England Journal of Medicine* 328, no. 19 (May 13, 1993): 1383–1387.

Manson, Patrick. *Lectures on Tropical Diseases Being the Lane Lectures for 1905 Delivered at Cooper Medical College, San Francisco U.S.A.*

August 1905. Archibald Constable and Company, London 1905.

Marsden, Philip Davis, "Mucosal Leishmaniasis (Espundia Escomel, 1911)." *Transactions of the Royal Society of Tropical Medicine and Hygiene* 80 (1986): 859–876.

Marsden, P. D., R. N. R. Sampaio, R. Rocha, M. Radke, "Mucocutaneous Leishmaniasis—An Unsolved Clinical Problem." *Tropical Doctor* 7 (January 1977): 7–11.

Roberts, Lynden J., Emanuela Handman, Simon J. Foote, "Leishmania." *British Medical Journal* 321 (September 30, 2000): 801–804.

Rogers, Leonard, "Preliminary Note on the Development of Trypanosoma in Cultures of the Cunningham-Leishman-Donovan Bodies of Cachexial Fever and Kala-Azar." *Lancet* 2 (July 23, 1904): 215–216.

Ross, Major R., "Note on the Bodies Recently Described by Leishman and Donovan." *British Medical Journal* 2 (November 14, 1903): 1261–1262.

Seaman, Jill, Alec J. Mercer, H. Egbert Sondorp, Barbara L. Herwaldt, "Epidemic Visceral Leishmaniasis in Southern Sudan: Treatment of Severely Debilitated Patients Under Wartime Conditions and with Limited Resources." *Annals of Internal Medicine* 124, no. 7 (April 1, 1996): 664–672.

Snow, James S., E. M. Satulsky, B. H. Kean, "American Cutaneous Leishmaniais, Report of Twelve Cases from the Canal Zone." *Archives of Dermatology and Syphilogy* 57 (1948): 90–101.

Takafuji, Ernest T., Larry D. Hendricks, Joseph L. Daubek, K. Mills McNeil, Henry M. Scagliola. Carter L. Diggs, "Cutaneous Leishmaniasis Associated with Jungle Training." *American Journal of Tropical Medicine and Hygiene* 29, no. 4 (1980): 516–520.

Walton, Bryce C., Luis Valverde Chinel, Oscar Eguia Y Eguia,

"Onset of Espundia After Many Years of Occult Infection with *Leishmania braziliensis.*" *American Journal of Tropical Medicine and Hygiene* 22, no. 6 (1973): 696–698.

9: New York, Summer 1999

Altman, Lawrence K., "After a Phone Tip, Medical Detectives Track Down a Killer." *New York Times on the Web,* 9 September 1999.

Asnis, Deborah S., Rick Coneta, Alex A. Teixeira, Glenn Waldmann, Barbara A. Sampson, "The West Nile Virus Outbreak of 1999 in New York: The Flushing Hospital Experience." *Clinical Infectious Diseases* 30 (March, 2000): 413–418.

Case Records of the Massachusetts General Hospital (Case 17-2003). *New England Journal of Medicine* 348, no. 22 (May 29, 2003): 2239–2247.

CDC, "Acute Flaccid Paralysis Syndrome Associated with West Nile Virus Infection—Mississippi and Louisiana, July–August 2002." *Morbidity and Mortality Weekly Report* 51, no. 37 (September 20, 2002): 825–828.

CDC, "Guidelines for Surveillance, Prevention, and Control of West Nile Virus Infection—United States." *Morbidity and Mortality Weekly Report* 49, no. 2 (January 21, 2000): 25–28.

CDC, "Outbreak of West Nile–Like Viral Encephalitis—New York, 1999." *Morbidity and Mortality Weekly Report* 48, no. 38 (October 1, 1999): 845–849.

CDC, "Possible West Nile Virus Transmission to an Infant Through Breast-Feeding—Michigan, 2002." *Morbidity and Mortality Weekly Report* 51, no. 39 (October 4, 2002): 877–878.

CDC, "Update: Investigations of West Nile Virus Infections in Recipients of Organ Transplantation and Blood Transfusion."

Morbidity and Mortality Weekly Report 51, no. 37 (September 20, 2002): 833–836.

CDC, "West Nile Virus Activity—United States, October 30–November 5, 2003." *Morbidity and Mortality Weekly Report* 52, no. 44 (November 7, 2003): 1080.

CDC, "WNV Infections in Recipients of Blood Transfusions." *Morbidity and Mortality Weekly Report* 51, no. 41 (October 18, 2002): 930–931.

Chen, David W. "Lives That Were Changed Forever by the Aftereffects of a Mosquito Bite." *New York Times,* 19 August 2000, A13.

Glass, Jonathan D., Owen Samuels, Mark M. Rich, "Poliomyelitis Due to West Nile Virus." *New England Journal of Medicine* 347, no. 16 (October 17, 2002): 1280–1281.

Goodnough, Abby, "Encephalitis Strikes 3 People, 1 Fatally, In Queens, City Says." *New York Times on the Web,* 4 September 1999.

Jacobs, Andrew, "Exotic Virus Is Identified in 3 Deaths." *New York Times on the Web,* 26 September 1999.

Leis, Arturo A., Dobrivoje S. Stokic, Jo Lynn Polk, Victor Dostrow, Michael Winkelmann, "A Poliomyelitis-like Syndrome from West Nile Virus Infection." *New England Journal of Medicine* 347, no. 16 (October 17, 2002): 1279–1280.

Lueck, Thomas J., "Elderly Queens Resident Is 2d to Die of Encephalitis." *New York Times on the Web,* 5 September 1999.

Nash, Denis, Farzad Mostashari, Annie Fine, James Miller, Daniel O'Leary, Kristy Murray, Ada Huang, Amy Rosenberg, Abby Greenberg, Margaret Sherman, Susan Wong, Marcelle Layton, for the 1999 West Nile Outbreak Response Working Group, "The Outbreak of West Nile Virus Infection in the New York City Area in 1999." *New England Journal of Medicine* 344, no. 24 (June 14, 2001): 1807–1814, 1858–1859.

Manuelidis, Ellas E., "Neuropathology of Experimental West Nile Virus Infection in Monkeys." *Journal of Neuropathology and Experimental Neurology* 15 (1956): 448–460.

Marfin, Anthony A., Duane J. Gubler. "West Nile Encephalitis: An Emerging Disease in the United States." *Clinical Infectious Diseases* 33 (November 15, 2001): 1713–1719.

Petersen, Lyle, Anthony Marfin, "West Nile Virus: A Primer for the Clinician." *Annals of Internal Medicine* 137, no. 3 (August 6, 2002): 173–179.

Revkin, Andrew C., "West Nile Moving Faster and Wider." *New York Times on the Web,* 8 August 2003.

Sink, Mindy, "West Nile Virus Is Still a Threat as Fall Nears." *New York Times on the Web,* 16 September 2003.

Steinhauer, Jennifer, "African Virus May Be Culprit In Mosquito-Borne Illnesses." *New York Times on the Web,* 25 September 1999.

Steinhauer, Jennifer. "Outbreak of Virus in New York Much Broader Than Suspected." *New York Times,* 28 September 1999.

Tsai, T. F., C. Cernescu, G. L. Campbell, N. I. Nedelcu, for the Investigative Team, "West Nile Encephalitis Epidemic in Southeastern Romania." *Lancet* 352 (September 5, 1998): 767–771.

Nash, Denis, Farzad Mostashari, Annie Fine, James Miller, Daniel O'Leary, Kristy Murray, Ada Huang, Amy Rosenberg, Abby Greenberg, Margaret Sherman, Susan Wong, Marcell Layton, for the 1999 West Nile Outbreak Response Working Group, "The Outbreak of West Nile Virus Infection in the New York City Area in 1999." *New England Journal of Medicine* 344, no. 24 (June 14, 2001): 1807–1814, and editorial, 1858–1859.

Pealer, Lisa N., Anthony A. Marfin, Lyle R. Peterson, Robert S.

Lanciotti, Peter L. Page, Susan L. Stramer, Mary Grace Sto-
bierski, Kimberly Signs, Bruce Newman, Hema Kapoor, Jesse
L. Goodman, Mary E. Chamberland, "Transmission of West
Nile Virus Through Blood Transfusion in the United States
in 2002." *New England Journal of Medicine* 349, no. 13 (Sep-
tember 25, 2003): 1236–1245.
Wadler, Joyce, "Public Lives, Passionate Life in a Lab With Dead
Animals." *New York Times on the Web,* 1 October 1999.

10: "The Jaws That Bite"

Anonymous, "Alligators Are on the Move Right Now." *Florida
Fish and Wildlife Conservation Commission,* floridaconserva-
tion.org, 25 April, 2002.
———, "Alligator Bites Leg Off of 81-Year-Old Florida Man by
Canal in Third Fatal Attack This Year." Associated Press, 13
September 2001.
———, "American Alligator (*Alligator mississippiensis*)." www.
audubon.org.
———, *"Des Crocodiles du Fleuve Sio Font des Victimes."* PANA, 19
September 2001.
———, "Protected Crocodiles Eat Malawians." BBC News, 5 Janu-
ary 2000.
———, "Suspect Escapes Jail, Is Eaten by Crocodile." Reuters, 21
June 2002.
———, "Uganda Culls Man-eating Crocs." BBC News, 25 March
2002.
———, "Ugandan Officials Slaughter Man-eating Crocodiles."
Planet Ark/Reuters, 26 March 2002.
———, "Victim of Croc Attack." *Daily Express* (East Malaysia), 26
October 2000.

———, "Woman, 70, Killed By Crocodile in Jamaica." Reuters, 11 September 1999.

Auffenberg, Walter. *The Behavioral Ecology of the Komodo Monitor.* University Presses of Florida, Gainesville, 1981.

Cagel, Jess, "Transcript: Sharon Stone vs. The Komodo Dragon." TIME.com, 23 June 2001.

Casey, Marcus, "Should This Predator Be Protected?" *The Daily Telegraph* (Sydney), 26 October 2002.

Chipperfield, Mark, "Invasion of the Killer Crocs." *Salt Lake Tribune,* 5 November 2000.

Ciofi, Claudia, "The Komodo Dragon." *Scientific American* (March 6, 1999).

Conover, Michael R., Tami J. Dubow, "Alligator Attacks on Humans in the United States." *Herpetological Review* 28, no. 3 (1997): 120–124.

Doering, E. J., C. T. Fitts, W. M. Rambo, Gilbert B. Bradham, "Alligator Bite." *Journal of the American Medical Association* 218, no. 2 (October 11, 1971): 255–256.

Flandry, Fred, Major Edward J. Lisecki, MC, USA, Gerald J. Domingue, Ronald L. Guggisberg, C. A. W. *Crocodiles, Their Natural History, Folklore, and Conservation.* Stackpole Books, Harrisburg, 1972.

Herodotus. *The Histories,* Aubrey de Sélincourt (translator). Penguin Books, Harmondsworth, Great Britain, 1971.

Hines, T. C., K. D. Keenlyne, "Two Incidents of Alligator Attacks on Humans in Florida." *Copeia* 4 (1977): 735–738.

Kar, S. K., H. R. Bustard, "Saltwater Crocodile Attacks on Man." *Biological Conservation* 25 (1983): 377–382.

King, Dennis, Brian Green. *Monitors, The Biology of Varanid Lizards.* Krieger Publishing Company, Malibar, Florida, 1993.

Matheson, Ishbel, "Adventure that Ended in Tragedy." BBC News, 11 March 2002.

Mekisic, Allan P., Jonathan R. Wardill, "Crocodile Attacks in the Northern Territory of Australia." *Medical Journal of Australia* 157 (December 7/21, 1992): 751–754.

Nichols, Donald L. Greer, Ray J. Haddad, "Initial Antibiotic Therapy for Alligator Bites." *Southern Medical Journal* 82, no. 2 (February 1989): 262–266.

Pence, Angelica, "Editor Stable After Attack by Komodo Dragon. Surgeons Reattach Foot Tendons of Chronicle's Bronstein in L.A." *San Francisco Chronicle,* 11 June 2001.

Perry, Michael, "Crocodile Kills German Tourist in Australia." Yahoo! News (October 23, 2003).

Pianka, Eric R., "Evolution of Varanid Lizards." Department of Zoology, University of Texas, uts.cc.utexas.edu

Neill, Wilfred T. *The Last of the Ruling Reptiles, Alligators, Crocodiles, and Their Kin.* Columbia University Press, 1971.

Scott, Richard, Heather Scott, "Crocodile Bites and Tradition Beliefs in Korogwe District Tanzania." *British Medical Journal* 309, (December 24–31, 1994): 1691–1692.

Stewart, George L., Joel M. Montgomery, Don Gillespie, Putra Sastrawan, Terry M. Fredeking, "Aerobic Salivary Bacteria in Wild and Captive Komodo Dragons." *Journal of Wildlife Diseases* 38, no. 3 (July 2002): 545–551.

Vanwersch, Koen, "Crocodile Bite Injury in Southern Malawi." *Tropical Doctor* 28 (October 1998): 221–222.

Woodward, Allan R., Barry L. Cook, "Nuisance-Alligator (*Alligator mississippiensis*) Control in Florida, U.S.A." In *Crocodiles. Proceedings of the 15th Working Meeting of the Crocodile Specialist Group,* IUCN–The World Conservation Union, Gland, Switzerland, 2000.

11: Rage

Arellano-Sota, Carlos, "Biology, Ecology, and Control of the Vampire Bat." *Reviews of Infectious Diseases* 10, supplement 4 (November–December 1988): S615–S619.

CDC, "Extension of the Raccoon Rabies Epizootic—United States, 1992." *Morbidity and Mortality Weekly Report* 41, no. 36 (September 11, 1992): 661–664.

——, "Human Rabies Despite Treatment with Rabies Immune Globulin and Human Diploid Cell Rabies Vaccine— Thailand." *Morbidity and Mortality Weekly Report* 36, no. 46 (November 27, 1987): 759–765.

——, "Human Rabies—California, 1992." *Morbidity and Mortality Weekly Report* 41, no. 26 (July 3, 1992): 461–463.

——, "Human Rabies—Florida, 1996." *Morbidity and Mortality Weekly Report* 45, no. 33 (August 23, 1996): 719–727.

——, "Human Rabies—New Hampshire, 1996." *Morbidity and Mortality Weekly Report* 46, no. 12 (March 28, 1997): 267–270.

——, "Human Rabies—Washington, 1995." *Morbidity and Mortality Weekly Report* 44, no. 34 (September 1, 1995): 625–627.

——, "Update: Raccoon Rabies Epizootic—United States and Canada, 1999." *Morbidity and Mortality Weekly Report* 49, no. 2 (January 21, 2000): 31–35.

Dubos, René. *Louis Pasteur, Free Lance of Science.* Charles Scribner's Sons, New York, 1976.

Fishbein, Daniel B., Laura E. Robinson, "Rabies." *New England Journal of Medicine* 329, no. 22 (November 25, 1993): 1632–1638.

Houff, S. A., R. C. Burton, R. W. Wilson, T. E. Henson, W. T.

London, G. M. Baer, et al, "Human-to-Human Transmission of Rabies Virus by Corneal Transplant." *New England Journal of Medicine* 300, no. 11 (March 15, 1979): 603–604.

Messenger, Sharon L., Jean S. Smith, Charles E. Rupprecht, "Emerging Epidemiology of Bat-Associated Cryptic Cases of Rabies in Humans in the United States." *Clinical Infectious Diseases* 35 (September 15, 2002): 738–747.

Noah, Donald L., Cherie L. Drenzek, Jean S. Smith, John W. Krebs, Lillian Orciari, John Shaddock, et al, "Epidemiology of Human Rabies in the United States, 1980 to 1996." *Annals of Internal Medicine* 128, no. 11 (June 1, 1998): 922–930.

Plotkin, Stanley A., "Rabies." *Clinical Infectious Diseases* 30 (January 2000): 4–12.

Roueché, Berton. *The Incurable Wound and Further Narratives of Medical Detection*. Berkley Publishing Corporation, New York, 1966.

Williams, Greer. *Virus Hunters*. Alfred A. Knopf, New York, 1960.

12: Bitten

Anonymous, "Roy Horn Responding to Voices." USAToday .com, October 4, 2003.

CDC, "Dog-Bite-Related Fatalities—United States, 1995–1996." *Morbidity and Mortality Weekly Reports* 46, no. 21 (May 30, 1997): 463–467.

Burdge, David R., David Scheifele, David P. Speert, "Serious *Pasteurella multocida* Infections from Lion and Tiger Bites." *Journal of the American Medical Association* 253, no. 22 (June 14, 1985): 3296–3297.

Capellan, J., I. W. Fong, "Tularemia from a Cat Bite: Case Report and Review of Feline-Associated Tularemia." *Clinical Infectious Diseases* 16 (April): 472–475.

Case Records of the Massachusetts General Hospital (Case 17-1999). *New England Journal of Medicine* 340, no. 23 (June 10, 1999): 1819–1826.

Findling, James W., Guenther P. Pohlmann, Harold Rose, "Fulminant Gram-Negative Bacillemia (DF-2) Following a Dog Bite in an Asplenic Woman." *American Journal of Medicine* 68 (January 1980): 154–156.

Goldstein, Ellie J. C., "Bite Wounds and Infection." *Clinical Infectious Diseases* 14 (March 1992): 633–638.

Habif, Thomas P., James L. Campbell, Mark J. Quitadamo, Kathryn A. Zug. *Skin Disease. Diagnosis and Treatment.* Mosby, St. Louis, 2001.

Henderson, John A. M., Harry C. Rowsell, "Fatal *Pasteurella multocida* Pneumonia in an IgA-Deficient Cat Fancier." *Western Journal of Medicine* 150 (February 1989): 208–210.

Kullberg, Bart-Jan, Rudi G. J. Westendorp, Jan W. Van't Wout, and A. Edo Meinders, "*Purpura Fulminans* and Symmetrical Peripheral Gangrene Caused by *Capnocytophaga canimorsis* (Formerly DF-2) Septicemia—A Complication of Dog Bite." *Medicine* 70, no. 5 (1991): 287–292.

Kumar, A., H. R. Devlin, H. Vellend, "*Pasteurella multocida* Meningitis in an Adult: Case Report and Review." *Reviews of Infectious Diseases* 12, no. 3 (May–June 1990): 440–448.

Morgan, Marina S., "Tiger Bites." *Journal of the Royal Society of Medicine* 92, no. 10 (October 1999): 545.

Newman, Cathy, "Cats: Nature's Masterwork." *National Geographic* 191, no. 6 (June 1997): 54–76.

Saphir, D. A., G. R. Carter, "Gingival Flora of the Dog with Special Reference to Bacteria Associated with Bites." *Journal of Clinical Microbiology* 3, no. 3 (March 1976): 344–349.

Talan, David A., Diane M. Citron, B. S. Fredrick, M. Abrahamian, Gregory J. Moran, Ellie J. C. Goldstein, for the Emergency

Medicine Animal Bite Infection Study Group, "Bacteriologic Analysis of Infected Dog and Cat Bites." *New England Journal of Medicine* 340, no. 2 (January 14, 1999): 85–92, and editorial 138–140.

Walton, Robert L., W. Earle Matory Jr., "Wound Care." In *Current Emergency Diagnosis and Treatment,* Charles E. Saunders, Mary T. Ho, editors. Appleton and Lange, Norwalk, 1992.

Weber, David J., John S. Wolfson, Morton N. Schwartz, David C. Hooper, "*Pasteurella multocida* Infections." *Medicine* 63, no. 2 (1984): 133–154.

13: Menagerie

Al-Boukai, Ahmad Amer, Nour El-Din Hawass, Pravichandra J. Patel, Taiyewo M. Kolawole, "Camel Bites: Report of Severe Osteolysis as Late Bone Complications." *Postgraduate Medical Journal* 65, no. 770 (December 1989): 900–904.

Anonymous, "Bird Attack Said Key to Conviction." *Los Angeles Times,* 20 February 2003.

——, "Ostrich Kicks 63-Year-Old Woman to Death in South Africa." Associated Press, 29 December 1997.

——, "Rat Disease Set to Increase." BBC News, 10 February 2003. news.bbc.co.uk, accessed 2/19/2003.

——, "Rats Threaten to Engulf Streets." BBC News, 1 August 2002. news.bbc.co.uk, accessed 2/19/2003.

Applegate, James A., Marcia F. Walhout, "Childhood Risks from the Ferret." *Journal of Emergency Medicine* 16, no. 3 (1998): 425–427.

Baker, Ann Sullivan, Kathryn L. Ruoff, Sarabelle Madoff. "Isolation of *Mycoplasma* Species from a Patient with Seal Finger." *Clinical Infectious Diseases* 27, no. 5 (November 1998): 1168–1170.

Badejo, O. A., O. O. Komolafe, D. L. Obinwogwu, "Bacteriology and Clinical Course of Camel-Bite Wound Infections." *European Journal of Clinical Microbiology and Infectious Diseases* 18, no. 12 (December 1999): 918–919.

Barss, Peter G., "Injuries Caused by Garfish in Papua New Guinea." *British Medical Journal* 284, no. 6309 (January 9, 1982): 77–79.

Berkowitz, Frank E., David W. C. Jacobs, "Fatal Case of Brain Abscess Caused by Rooster Pecking." *Pediatric Infectious Disease* 6, no. 10 (October 1987): 941–942.

California Department of Health Services, "Need for Data on Ferrets that Bite, Eat Human Flesh, or Develop Rabies." *California Morbidity* 7 (February 21, 1986): 1.

Childs, Ginny, "Attack Ferrets?" *Journal of the American Medical Association* 261, no. 11 (March 17, 1989): 1583–1583.

Cole, James S., Ralph W. Stoll, Roger J. Bulger, "Rat-bite Fever." *Annals of Internal Medicine* 71, no. 5 (November 1969): 979–981.

CDC, "Rat-bite Fever—New Mexico, 1996." *Morbidity and Mortality Weekly Report* 47, no. 5 (February 13, 1998): 89–91.

Cooles, P., H. Paul, "Rat Bites and Diabetic Foot in the West Indies." *British Medical Journal* 298, no. 6677 (April 1, 1989): 868.

Cousins, Norman. *Anatomy of an Illness as Perceived by the Patient.* W. W. Norton and Company, New York, 1979.

Davis, Bradley, Richard P. Wenzel, "Striges Scalp: *Bacteroides* Infection After an Owl Attack." *Journal of Infectious Diseases* 165, no. 5 (May 1992): 975–976.

Hagelskjær, Inger Sørensen, Else Randers, "*Streptobacillus moniliformis* Infection: 2 Cases and a Literature Review." *Scandinavian Journal of Infectious Diseases* 30, no. 3 (1998): 309–311.

Hesford, Jessica D., Thomas A. E. Platts-mills, Richard F. Edlich, "Anaphylaxis After Laboratory Rat Bite: An Occupational

Hazard." *Journal of Emergency Medicine* 13, no. 6 (November–December 1995): 765–768.

Hirschhorn, Randall B., Robert R. Hodge, "Identification of Risk Factors in Rat Bite Incidents Involving Humans." *Pediatrics* 104, no. 3 (September 1999): e35.

Hoffman, Janaleigh, Gregory R. Hack, Bliss Clark, "The Man Did Fine, but What About the Wahoo." *Journal of the American Medical Association* 267, no. 15 (April 15, 1992): 2039.

Itin, P., A. Haenel, H. Stalder, "From the Heavens, Revenge on Joggers." *New England Journal of Medicine* 311, no. 26 (December 27, 1984): 1703.

Jones, Meg, "Pet Ferrets Attack 10-day-old Girl." *Milwaukee Journal Sentinel,* 28 June 2002.

Kara, Cuneyt O., C. Banu Cetin, Nevzat Yalcin, "Cephalic Tetanus as a Result of Rooster Pecking: An Unusual Case." *Scandinavian Journal of Infectious Disease* 34, no. 1 (2002): 64–66.

Kizer, Kenneth W., Denny G. Constantine, "Pet Ferrets—A Hazard to Public Health and Wildlife." *Western Journal of Medicine* 150, no. 4 (April 1989): 466.

Lauer, Brian A., John W. Paisley, "In Reply to Letter by G. Childs." *Journal of the American Medical Association* 261, no. 11 (March 17, 1989): 1584.

Marks, Kathy, "Mating Magpies Mob Suburban Australians." *Independent* (United Kingdom), 11 October 2000.

Markham, Richard B., B. Frank Polk, "Seal Finger." *Reviews of Infectious Diseases* 1, no. 3 (May–June 1979): 567–569.

Marshall, Kent R., "Ferrets as Pets." *Journal of the American Veterinary Association* 193, no. 2 (July 15, 1988): 160–161.

Mass, Daniel P., William L. Newmeyer, Eugene S. Kilgore, "Seal Finger." *Journal of Hand Surgery* 6, no. 6 (November 1981): 610–612.

McHugh, Terrence P., Robert L. Bartlett, James I. Raymond,

"Rat Bite Fever: Report of a Fatal Case." *Annals of Emergency Medicine* 14 (November 11, 1985): 1116–1118.

Morrison, Grant, "Zoonotic Infections from Pets." *Postgraduate Medicine* 110, no. 1 (July 2001): 24–48.

Myers, C. Blake, Linda M. Christmann, "Rat Bite—An Unusual Cause of Direct Trauma to the Globe." *Journal of Pediatric Ophthalmology* 28, no. 6 (November–December 1991): 356–358.

Ogunbodede, E. O., J. T. Arotiba, "Camel Bite Injuries of the Orofacial Region: Report of a Case." *Journal of Oral and Maxillofacial Surgery* 55, no. 10 (October 1997): 1174–1176.

Ordog, Gary J., S. Balasubramanium, Jonathan Wasserberger, "Rat Bites: Fifty Cases." *Annals of Emergency Medicine* 14 (February 2, 1985): 126–130.

Österlund, Anders, and Elisabeth Nordlund, "Wound Infection Caused by *Staphylococcus Hyicus* Subspecies *Hyicus* After a Donkey Bite." *Scandinavian Journal of Infectious Diseases* 29, no. 1 (1997): 95.

Paisley, John W., Brian A. Lauer, "Severe Facial Injuries to Infants Due to Unprovoked Attacks by Pet Ferrets." *Journal of the American Medical Association* 259, no. 13 (April 1, 1988): 2005–2006.

Preiser, Gary, Thomas E. Lavell, "Rooster Attacks on Children." *Pediatrics* 79, no. 3 (March 1987): 426–427.

Roughgarden, Jean W., "Antimicrobial Therapy of Ratbite Fever" *Archives of Internal Medicine* 116 (July 1965): 39–54.

Squatriglia, Chuck. "Giant Bird Attacks Worker at S.F. Zoo." *San Francisco Chronicle,* 16 February 2001.

Wykes, W. N., "Rat Bite Injury to the Eyelids in a 3-month-old Child." *British Journal of Ophthalmology* 73, no. 3 (March 1989): 202–204.

14: Monkey Business

Anonymous, "Before Human Spaceflight. The Able-Baker Mission." National Aeronautics and Space Museum, nasm.si.edu, accessed 2/22/03.

Anonymous, "From the Files of Wisconsin Regional Primate Research Center." The Primate Freedom Project, primate-freedom.com, accessed 4/26/03.

Anonymous, "Medical Services Herpes B Exposure Control, Standard Procedures." WRAMC Pamphlet No. 40-6, April 9, 1999. Department of the Army Headquarters, Walter Reed Army Medical Center, Washington DC 20307-5001.

Anonymous, "Primate Trade-imports to the United States 1995–2002." Aesop Project (Allied Effort to Save Other Primates), aesop-project.org, accessed 4/26/03.

CDC, "B Virus Infections in Humans—Michigan." *Morbidity and Mortality Weekly Report* 38, no. 26 (July 7, 1989): 453–454.

———, "B-Virus Infection in Humans—Pensacola, Florida." *Morbidity and Mortality Weekly Report* 36, no.19 (May 22, 1987): 289–296.

———, "Fatal *Cercopithecine herpesvirus* 1 (B Virus) Infection Following a Mucocutaneous Exposure and Interim Recommendations for Worker Protection." *Morbidity and Mortality Weekly Report* 47, no. 49 (December 18, 1998): 1073–1083.

Cohen, Jeffrey, David S. Davenport, John A. Stewart, Scott Deitchman, Julia K. Hilliard, Louisa E. Chapman, "Recommendations for Prevention of and Therapy for Exposure to B Virus (*Cercopithicine Herpesvirus* 1)." *Clinical Infectious Diseases* 35, no. 10 (November 15, 2002): 1191–1203.

Davenport, David S., David R. Johnson, Gary P. Holmes, Dennis

A. Jewett, Stephen C. Ross, and Julia K. Hilliard, "Diagnosis and Management of Human B Virus (*Herpesvirus simiae*) Infections in Michigan." *Clinical Infectious Diseases* 19, (July, 1994): 33–41.

Ergenzinger, E. R., M. M. Glasier, J. O. Hahm, T. P. Pons, "Cortically Induced Thalamic Plasticity in the Primate Somatosensory System." *Nature Neuroscience* 1, no. 3 (July 1998): 226–229.

Eron, Carol. *The Virus That Ate Cannibals*. Macmillan Publishing Co., Inc., New York, 1981.

Holmes, Gary P., Louis E. Chapman, John A. Stewart, Stephen E. Straus, Julia K. Hilliard, David S. Davenport, and the B Virus Working Group, "Guidelines for the Prevention and Treatment of B-Virus Infections in Exposed Persons." *Clinical Infectious Diseases* 20 (February 1995): 421–439.

Holmes, Gary P., Julia K. Hilliard, Karl C. Klontz, Angus H. Rupert, Christine M. Schindler, Eva Parris, Gary Griffin, George S. Ward, Norman D. Bernstein, Terrel W. Bean, Michael R. Ball Sr., James A. Brady, Michael H. Wilder, Jonathan E. Kaplan, "B Virus (*Herpesvirus simiae*) Infection in Humans: Epidemiologic Investigation of a Cluster." *Annals of Internal Medicine* 112, no. 11 (June 1, 1990): 833–839.

Hummeler, Klaus, Wallace L. Davidson, Werner Henle, Alfred C. LaBoccetta, Hilda G. Ruch. "Encephalomyelitis Due to Infection with *Herpesvirus Simiae* (Herpes B Virus). A Report of Two Fatal, Laboratory-Associated Cases." *New England Journal of Medicine* 261, no. 2 (July 9, 1959): 64–68.

Lutwick, Larry I., Robert O. Deaner, "Herpes B." *EMedicine* (March 18, 2002) at emedicine.com/med/topic3367.htm, accessed 4/19/03.

Ostrowski, Stephanie R., Mira J. Leslie, Terri Parrott, Susan Abelt, Patrick E. Piercy, "B-virus from Pet Macaque Monkeys: An

Emerging Threat in the United States." *Emerging Infectious Diseases* 4, no. 1 (January–March 1998): 117–121.

Palevitz, Barry A., Ricki Lewis, "Death Raises Safety Issues for Primate Handlers." *Scientist* 12, no. 5 (March 2, 1998): 1–5.

Palmer, Amos E., "B Virus, *Herpesvirus simiae:* Historical Perspective." *Journal of Medical Primatology* 16 (1987): 99–130.

Sabin, Albert B., Arthur M. Wright, "Acute Ascending Myelitis Following a Monkey Bite, with the Isolation of a Virus Capable of Reproducing the Disease." *Journal of Experimental Medicine* 59 (1934): 115–136.

Weigler, Benjamin, "Biology of B Virus in Macaque and Human Hosts: A Review." *Clinical Infectious Diseases* 14 (February 1992): 555–567.

15: Human Bites

Agrawal K., T. Ramachandrudu, A. Hamide, T. K. Dutta, "Tetanus Caused by Human Bite of the Finger." *Annals of Plastic Surgery* 34, no. 2 (February 1995): 201–202.

Al Fallouji, M., "Traumatic Love Bites." *British Journal of Surgery* 77, no. 1 (January 1990): 100–101.

Anonymous, "Prisoner with AIDS Convicted of Assault with Dangerous Weapon." *New Jersey Medicine* 85, no. 9 (September 1985): 705.

Basadre, Jesse O., Samuel W. Parry, "Indications for Surgical Débridement in 125 Human Bites to the Hand." *Archives of Surgery* 126, no. 1 (January 1991): 65–67.

Brooks, George F., J. Morgan O'Donoghue, J. Peter Rissing, Kenneth Soapes, James W. Smith. "*Eikenella Corrodens,* A Recently Recognized Pathogen." *Medicine (Baltimore)* 53, no. 5 (1974): 325–342.

Clark, Ellen G. I., Ross E. Zumwalt, Moses S. Schanfield, "The Identification of Maternity in an Unusual Pregnancy-Related Homicide." *Journal of Forensic Sciences* 35, no. 1 (January 1990): 80–88.

Datubo-Brown, D. D. "Human Bites of the Face with Tissue Losses." *Annals of Plastic Surgery* 21, no. 4 (October 1988): 322–328.

Dusheiko, G. M., M. Smith, P. J. Scheuer, "Hepatitis C Virus Transmitted by Human Bite." *Lancet* 336, no. 8713 (August 25, 1990): 503–504.

Earley M. J., A. F. Bardsley, "Human Bites: A Review." *British Journal of Plastic Surgery* 37, no. 4 (October 1984): 458–462.

Ellerstein, Norman S. "The Cutaneous Manifestations of Child Abuse and Neglect." *American Journal of Diseases of Children* 133, no. 9 (September 1979): 906–909.

Eyre, S. J., B. Carson, B. T. Johnson, "Human Bites in Rural Kenya." *Tropical Doctor* 16, no. 2 (April 1986): 61–63.

Farmer, C. Baring, Ronald J. Mann. "Human Bite Infections of the Hand." *Southern Medical Journal* (May 1966): 515–518.

Farrar, W. E., "A Poisoned Tooth." *Annals of Internal Medicine* 116, no. 5 (March 1, 1992): 429.

Ferri, Massimiliano. "Treatment of Partial Losses of the Helix." *Plastic and Reconstructive Surgery* 104, no. 1 (July 1999): 297.

Figueiredo, J. F., A. S. Borges, R. Martinez, Ade L. Martinelli, M. G. Villanova, D. T. Covas, A. D. Passas, "Transmission of Hepatitis C Virus but Not Human Immunodeficiency Virus Type 1 By a Human Bite." *Clinical Infectious Diseases* 19, no. 3 (September 1994): 564–547.

Fiumara, N. J., J. H. Exner, "Primary Syphilis Following a Human Bite." *Sexually Transmitted Diseases* 8, no. 1 (January–March 1981): 21–22.

Fuortes L., E. Melson, "Primary and Recurrent *Herpes Simplex*

Infection in a Pediatric Nurse Resulting from a Human Bite." *Infection Control and Hospital Epidemiology* 10, no. 3 (March 1989): 120.

Goldstein, Ellie J. C., Michel F. Barones, Timothy Miller, "*Eikenella corrodens* in Hand Infections." *The Journal of Hand Surgery* 8, no. 5, part 1 (September 1983): 563–567.

Goldstein, Ellie J. C., "Bite Wounds and Infection." *Clinical Infectious Diseases* 14 (March 1992): 633–638.

Hamilton, J. D., B. Larke, A. Qizilbash, "Transmission of Hepatitis B by a Human Bite: An Occupational Hazard." *Canadian Medical Association Journal* 115, no. 5 (September 4, 1976): 439–440.

Khajotia, Rumi R., "Transmission of Human Immunodeficiency Virus Through Saliva After a Lip Bite." *Archives of Internal Medicine* 157, no. 16 (September 8, 1997): 1901.

Loro, A., F. Franceschi, "Finger Amputations in Tanzania." *East African Medical Journal* 69, no. 12 (December 1992): 697–699.

Loro, A., F. Franceschi, "Human Bites and Finger Infecitons: A Survey at Dodoma Regional Hospital, Tanzania." *Tropical Doctor* 22, no. 1 (January 1992): 24–26.

MacQuarrie, Michael B., Bagher Forghani, Donal A. Wolochow, "Hepatitis B Transmitted by a Human Bite." *Journal of the American Medical Association* 230, no. 5 (November 4, 1974): 723–724.

Muguti, G. I., M. S. Dixon, "Tetanus Following Human Bite." *British Journal of Plastic Surgery* 45, no. 8 (November–December 1992): 614–615.

Muguti, G. I., M. Zvomuya-Ncube, E. T. Bvuma, "Experience with Human Bites in Zimbabwe." *Central African Journal of Medicine* 37, no. 9 (September 1991): 294–298.

Okimura J. T., S. A. Norton, "Jealousy and Mutilation: Nose-Biting as Retribution for Adultery." *Lancet* 352, no. 9145 (December 19–26, 1998): 2010–2011.

Ollapallil, Jacob J., John Beaso, David A. K. Watters, "Human Bite Injuries to the Nose." *Tropical Doctor* 25, no. 2 (April 1995): 85–87.

Pierce, Larry, Daniel J. Strickland, E. Steven Smith, "The Case of *Ohio v. Robinson*, an 1870 Bite Mark Case." *American Journal of Forensic Medicine and Pathology* 11, no. 2 (June 1990): 171–177.

Rosen Ted, Nicole Conrad, "Genital Ulcer Caused by Human Bite to the Penis." *Sexually Transmitted Diseases* 26, no. 9 (October 1999): 527–530.

Rothwell, Bruce R., "Bite Marks in Forensic Dentistry: A Review of Legal, Scientific Issues." *Journal of the American Dental Association* 126, no. 2 (February 1995): 223–232.

Senn, David R., John D. McDowell, Marden E. Alder, "Dentistry's Role in the Recognition and Reporting of Domestic Violence, Abuse, and Neglect." *Dental Clinics of North America* 45, no. 2 (April 2001): 343–363.

Spinelli, Henry M., John E. Sherman, Richard D. Lisman, Byron Smith, "Human Bites of the Eyelid." *Plastic and Reconstructive Surgery* 78, no. 5 (November 1986): 610–614.

Stoloff, Anthony L., Maree L. Gillies, "Infections with *Eikenella corrodens* in a General Hospital: A Report of 33 Cases." *Reviews of Infectious Diseases* 8, no. 1 (January–February 1986): 50–53.

Sweet, D., I. A. Pretty, "A Look at Forensic Dentistry—Part 2: Teeth as Weapons of Violence—Identification of Bitemark Perpetrators." *British Dental Journal* 190, no. 8 (April 28, 2001): 415–418.

Thomas, P., "A Case of Human Bite." *Australian Family Physician* 21, no. 9 (September 1992): 1359.

Vidmar, L., M. Poljak, K. Seme, I. Klavs, "Transmission of HIV-1 by Human Bite." *Lancet* 347, no. 9017 (June 22, 1996): 1762.

Wienert, P., J. Heiss, H. Rinecker, A. Sing, "A Human Bite." *Lancet* 354, no. 9178 (August 14, 1999): 572.

Wolf, J. Stuart, Reynoldo Gomez, Jack W. McAninch, "Human Bites to the Penis." *The Journal of Urology* 147 (May 1992): 1265–1267.

Wright, Franklin D., J. Curtis Dailey, "Human Bite Marks in Forensic Dentistry." *Dental Clinics of North America* 45, no. 2 (April 2001): 365–397.

Index

Accident and Emergency Department
of the Royal Darwin Hospital
(Australia), 54
acyclovir (antiherpes drug), 256–57
Adie, Helen, 136
Aeromonas hydrophila infection, 74–76
Africa; widow spiders in, 27
African lions and *Pasteurella multocida*,
215
AIDS/HIV
and human bites, 281–83
and leishmaniasis, 138–39
as a zoonotic infection, 251–52
Al Fallouji, M., 276
Al-Boukai, Ahmad Amer, 235
Aleppo boil, 131, 135
See also leishmaniasis
Allied Chemical Corporation, 12
alligator attacks, 178–79, 180–81
bite-wound infections, 179–80
fatalities from, 180
Alligator mississipiensis (American
alligator), 177–79
culling, 181
diet, 177
Florida, "nuisance alligators" in, 181
habitat, 177
hibernation, 178
procreation and egg incubation, 178
swimming ability, 178
translocation, 181
alligator, 176–77, 178–81
American alligator (*Alligator
mississipiensis*), 177–79

culling, 181
crocodile, distinguished from, 177,
182
diet, 177
habitat, 177
hibernation, 178
procreation and egg incubation,
178
swimming ability, 178
translocation, 181
See also crocodiles
American alligator (*Alligator
mississipiensis*), 177–79
culling, 181
diet, 177
Florida, "nuisance alligators" in, 181
habitat, 177
hibernation, 178
procreation and egg incubation, 178
swimming ability, 178
translocation, 181
American crocodile (*Crocodylus acutus*),
183
Lacey Acts and, 184
anaphylaxis (anaphylactic reaction)
fire ant sting and, 3–4, 14–15
immunotherapy and, 15–16
treatment for, 15
Anatomy of an Illness (Cousins), 227–29
ancient Egyptians
and cats, 215
and crocodiles, 182
and ferrets, 221
and snakes, 79, 86

Angola, sleeping sickness epidemic in, 122
Annals of Emergency Medicine, 230
Annals of Internal Medicine, 209
antihistamine and fire ant stings, 3
antihistamine, fire ant sting and, 3
Antimony, 146–48
araña capulina (cherry spider), 27
Araneida. *See* spider bites; spiders
Armstrong, William, 114
Asnis, Deborah S., 154–56, 164
Astruc, Jean, 249–50
Atkins, John, 102–3
Atrax robustus (funnel web spider), 33–38
  antivenin for, 37–38
  fatalities from, 34, 37, 95
Auffenberg, Walter, 172–73, 175
Australia
  crocodile attacks in, 187–90
  fire ant invasion of, 16–17
  funnel web spiders in, 33–38, 95
  jellyfishes, fatalities from, 43–45, 54–55
  and monitor lizards, 171
  and necrotic arachnidism research, 26–27
  snake bites in, 82–83
  tick epidemics in, 91–92
  tick paralysis in, 94–98
  widow spiders in, 27–28
Australian Commonwealth Serum Laboratory, 31, 46, 50, 82, 96
Australian *Daily Telegraph,* 188
Australian estuarine crocodiles, 176, 187–90
  bite-wound infections, 188
  fatalities from, 187–89
Australian Reptile Park, 83
Australian Venom Research, 27
Aventis (drug company)
  and antitrypanosomal drug shortages, 118–19

B-virus (*Herpesvirus simiae*) infections, 244, 247–48, 249, 250, 255–65
  protocol, 262–65

B-virus Working Group (Emory University/ CDC), 260–61
bacteria from bites
  Capnocytophaga canimorsus, 209–12
  EF-2 bacteria group, 208
  IIj bacteria group, 208
  Pasteurella multocida, 208–9, 215–19
  treatment of, 209, 210–12
  See also rabies
Badumna (black window spider), 27
Baer, Harold, 15
Barnes, Jack H., 47–52
Barss, Peter G., 237
Bassoe, Peter, 93–94
bats and rabies, 194, 205
Bayer Pharmaceuticals, 115
  and antitrypanosomal drug shortages, 118–19
bedbug (*Cimex lectularius*)
  and the transmission of kala azar, 135–36
  See also leishmaniasis
Bidenknap, J. H., 238
big cat
  African lion, 215
  and *Pasteurella multocida,* 208, 217–19
  tiger, 218
bird attacks, 240–43
birds, and West Nile virus, 153, 156, 160–61
black-bellied swamp snake (*Hemiaspis signata*), 83
black fire ant (*Solenopsis ricteri*), 6
black snake, 79
black widow spider (*Latrodectus mactans*), 20, 27, 32
black window spider (*Badumna*), 27
blood donors and recipients
  screening tests, 164
  and West Nile virus, 163–64
Borovsky, Alfred, 130–31, 134, 139
Bothrops jararacussu (jararacuçu), 70–71
Bothrops moojeni, 75
Bourrel (army veterinarian), 201

box jellyfish (*Chironex fleckeri*), 46, 54
Brackenridge Field Laboratory
　(University of Texas in Austin),
　8
Brand, Margaret, 228–29
Brand, Paul, 228–29
Brazil
　and *Aeromonas hydrophila* infections,
　75
　jararacuçu attacks in, 70–71
　spiders in, 32–33
Brebner, William B., 245
Brewis, Alexander, 274
Bristol Myers Squibb, 119
British Medical Journal, 108, 122, 133,
　184, 237
Bronstein, Phil, 169–70, 176
brown recluse spider (*Loxosceles reclusa*),
　21–24
　fatalities from, 23
　venom of, 22
brown snake, 79
Bruce, Sir David, 104–6, 111–12, 121
Brucella melitensis, 105
brucellosis, 105
Bundy, Theodore "Ted," 284
Buren, Dr. W. F., 11
Burma
　Japanese soldiers, crocodile attacks
　on, 187
bushmaster (*Lachesis muta muta*), 67,
　71–72
Butler, Dr., 209
Butler, Kevin, 241–42

calcium gluconate
　as treatment for black widow spiders
　bites, 31–32
California, black widow spiders in,
　28
California Department of Health
　Services, 224
California Institute of Technology, 62
camel bites, 234–36
Canadian Department of Agriculture,
　89

Canadian Medical Journal, 89
Capnocytophaga canimorsus, 209–12
　treatment of, 210–12, 219–20
Carey, Harry, 31
Carson, Rachel, 12
Carukia barnesi (Irukandji agent), 49
Carukia (jellyfish), 49–50
Castellani, Aldo, 111
cat bites, 214–16
　and *Pasteurella multocida*, 208,
　215–17
　treatment of, 219–20
　See also bacteria from bites; big cats;
　dog bites
cat
　ancient Egyptians and, 215
　evolution of, 214
　See also big cat
Centers for Disease Control and
　Prevention (CDC), 145, 157,
　162–63, 165, 222
　B-virus Working Group, 260–61
　preventing dog bites, 212–14
Central African Republic
　sleeping sickness epidemic in,
　122
Chandler, Asa, 140
cherry spider (*araña capulina*), 27
Chickene, Thomas, 180
Chile, spiders in, 20–21
Chilean brown spider (*Loxosceles laeta*),
　20–21
chipmunks and rabies, 205
Chironex fleckeri (box jellyfish), 46, 54
Christy, Cuthbert, 111
Chulalongkorn University Hospital
　(Bangkok, Thailand), 81
Churchill, Winston, 115
Cimex lectularius (bedbug)
　and the transmission of kala azar,
　135–36
　See also leishmaniasis
Clinical Infectious Diseases, 281
Clostridium tetani, 277–78
Cloth of Gold cone snail
　(*Conus textile*), 57

cobra, 67, 74, 78–79
  king cobra, 68
  and snake charmers, 81–82
  venom of, 81
cockatoo as witness to murder, 241–42
College of Veterinary Medicine
  (Michigan State University), 208
Collier, Michael, 144
common viper (*Vipera berus*), 69–70
cone sail bites, 56–65
  attacks and fatalities, 56–59, 64
  treatment of, 64
  venom and toxins of, 57, 59–61,
    62–64
cone snail, 56–59
  Cloth of Gold (*Conus textile*), 57
  Conus cedonulli ("matchless" cone),
    64–65
  Conus geographus, 57–58, 60, 62
  evolution of, 58–59, 61–64
  Glory of the Sea (*Conus glorimaris*),
    56
  in Hawaii, 61
  as living drug factories, 65
  shells, value of, 64–65
Congo Free State, 110
Conrad, Joseph, 113
Conus cedonulli ("matchless" cone),
    64–65
Conus geographus, 57–58, 60, 62
Conus glorimaris (Glory of the Sea
    cone), 56
Conus textile (Cloth of Gold cone
    snail), 57
Cook, Albert, 111
Cook, Jack, 111
Cooktown News, 189
copperhead snake, 67
coral snake, 67, 74
Corsica, widow spiders in, 27
Costa, Joseph A., 94
cottonmouth snake, 67
Cousins, Norman, 227–29
coyotes and rabies, 205
crab-eating macaque
    (*Macaca fascicularis*), 254

crocodile attacks, 184–87
  bite-wound infections, 188
  fatalities from, 183, 185, 186–87,
    187–90
  superstitions concerning, 184–85
  and the tourist industry, 184–85
crocodile, 176–77, 182–90
  alligator, distinguished from, 177
  American crocodile (*Crocodylus
    acutus*), 183–84
  ancient Egyptians and, 182
  Australian estuarine crocodiles, 176,
    187–90
  coexisting with, 186
  diet, 177
  habitat, 177
  life span, 182
  Nile crocodile, 171, 176, 182
  protection of, 184
  saltwater crocodile (*Crocodylus
    porosus*), 186–87
  See also alligator
Crocodylus acutus (American crocodile),
    183
  Lacey Acts and, 184
Crocodylus niloticus (Nile crocodile),
    176
  life span, 182
  monitor lizards and, 171
Crocodylus porosus (saltwater crocodile),
    186–87
Crotalus horridus horridus (timber
    rattlesnake), 77
crow attacks, 241
crows and West Nile virus, 153, 160–61
cul rouge (red-tail spider), 27
Culley, James, 37
Cunningham, D. D., 130
Currie, Dr. Bart, 54
cutaneous leishmaniasis. *See*
    leishmaniasis

Daniels, C. W., 108–9
Datubo-Brown, D., 273
de Lafontaine, Agnes 60–61, 62
de Lafontaine, Frédéique, 59–61

De Morbis veneris (Astruc), 250
de Shazo, Dr. Richard, 10
Demerol
  as treatment for black widow spiders
    bites, 31–32
Democratic Republic of Congo
  sleeping sickness epidemic in, 121
Department of Agriculture
  Methods Development Laboratory
    (Gulfport, MS), 12
Desowitz, Robert, 121, 135, 137
Dimetapp (antihistamine)
  fire ant sting and, 3
dog bites, 207–14
  bite-wound infections, 208
  and *Capnocytophaga canimorsus,*
    209–12
  fatalities from, 207
  and *Pasteurella multocida,* 208–9
  preventing, 212–14
  treatment of, 209, 210–11, 219–20
  See also bacteria from bites; cat bites;
    rabies
donkey bites, 234–35
Donovan, C., 133–34, 139
doxycycline and *Pasteurella multocida,*
  208
Doyle versus State (of Texas), 284
"Dum Dum fever." *See* leishmaniasis
Dutton, Joseph Everett, 108, 112–13, 124

ear, human bites on, 272–73, 273–74
East African Standard, 184
eastern diamondback rattlesnake, 67
Eber's Papyrus, 79
EF-2 bacteria group, 208
eflornithine
  shortages of, 118, 119
  as treatment for sleeping sickness,
    116–17
Egyptians. *See* ancient Egyptians
Ehrkich, Paul, 13, 115
Eiken, Dr., 270
Eikenella corrodens, 268, 270–73, 277
Emergency Medicine Animal Bite
  Infection Study Group, 215

Emerging Disease Lab (University of
  California at Irvine), 158
Emerging Infectious Diseases journal,
  265
Environmental Protection Agency
  (EPA), 12
Epi-pen and anaphylaxis, 15
epinephrine and anaphylaxis, 15
Evans, Griffith, 104

Federal Drug Administration (FDA),
  145
fer-de-lance, 67
ferret bites
  attacks and fatalities, 221, 222–24
  and rabies, 222–23
Ferret Friends, 223
ferret (*Mustela putorius*), 221–22
  and medical research, 222
fire ant. *See* black fire ants; red fire ants
Flecker, Dr. Hugo, 45, 46, 47, 58
Florida and "nuisance alligators,"
  181
Florida Game and Fresh Water Fish
  Commission, 181
"Fly Who Would Be King, The"
  (Desowitz), 121
Forde, R. M., 107–8
Fox, Roger, 2–3
foxes and rabies, 205
Freeman, Graham, 189
funnel web spider (*Atrax robustus*),
  33–38
  antivenin for, 37–38
  fatalities from, 34, 37, 95

gaboon viper, 67
Garbutt, Charles, 58
garfish bites, 236–37
Gibbes, Dr. J. Heyward, 92–93
Gila monster, 171
Giuliani, Rudolph W., 155–56
Glory of the Sea cone snail (*Conus
  glorimaris*), 56
Glucantime, 148
Goldstein, Ellie, 74, 215, 268

Gonzalez, Thomas A., 246
Grancher, Jacques, 204–5
Gray, Lieutenant, 123
Grice, Gordon, 28–29, 76
Griffin, Elizabeth, 261–64
Gruby, David, 104
Gubler, Daniel J., 157
Guillain-Barré syndrome, 87, 164–65

Hadwen, Seymour, 89
hares and rabies, 205
Harlow, Harry, 254
Haverhill fever, 229–31
Hawaii, cone snails in, 61
Heart of Darkness (Conrad), 113
Hemiaspis signata (black-bellied swamp snake), 83
Hensley, George, 77
hepatitis, human bites and, 279–81
heptachlor (chlorinated hydrocarbon heptachlor)
    and chemical control of fire ants, 12
Hermitte, Dr. L. C. D., 59–61
Herodotus, 182
herpes
    acyclovir (antiherpes drug), 256–57
    genital herpes, 249–50
    herpes simplex, 249–51
    See also B-virus
Herpes simplex, 164
Hilliard, Julia, 263, 266
Hinde, B., 57
Hiribae, Nathan, 184
Histories (Herodotus), 182
HIV. *See* AIDS/HIV
Hoare, C. M., 131
hobo spider (*Tegenaria agrestis*), 24–26
Holmes, Gary, 266
Holyfield, Evander, 272–73
Horn, Roy, 218
horse bites, 233–34
Hospital Vital Brazil, 33, 70–71
human African trypanosomiasis (sleeping sickness), *xi*, 101–25
    drug therapies, shortages of, 118–19

epidemics of and fatalities from, 112, 119–20, 121–24
Dr. Livingston and, 103–4
nagana's relationship to, 105, 106–7, 112
Stanley's expedition and, 112
symptoms of, 112–13, 114–15
treatment of, 107–8, 115–21
Trypanosoma brucei gambiense (West African or Gambian sleeping sickness), 112, 115, 117, 122
Trypanosoma brucei rhodesiense (Rhodesian or East African sleeping sickness), 114–15, 119, 122
tsetse flies as transmitters, 102, 106, 112, 121
Zulus and, 103–4, 106
human bites, 268–86
    and AIDS/HIV, 281–83
    on the armpit, 278
    bite-wound infections, 268–73, 278–79
    on the calf, 277
    clenched-fist infections, 271–72
    "coital love bites," 275–76
    on the ear, 272–73, 273–74
    Eikenella corrodens, 268, 270–73, 277
    fatalities from, 269–70
    on the finger, 278
    and forensic dentistry, 283–86
    and hepatitis, 279–81
    on the nose, 274–76
    on the penis, 276–77, 278–79
    as ritual and punishment, 274–75, 278
    and tetanus, 277–78
Hymenoptera, 3

IIj bacteria group, 208
immunotherapy and anaphylaxis, 15–16
"In Search of Kala Azar" (Desowitz), 135
"Incurable Wound, The" (Roueché), 193

India
  crocodile attacks in, 186
  See also kala azar
Indian Kala Azar Commission, 137
Infectious Disease Unit (Massachusetts
  General Hospital), 208
insects
  mosquitoes and West Nile virus,
    155–56, 161, 167–68
  mosquitoes and yellow fever, 167
  red fire ant, 1–17
  sandflies and leishmaniasis, *xi,*
    126–52
  spider, 18–39
  ticks and tick paralysis, 87–88,
    88–100
  tsetse flies and sleeping sickness, *xi,*
    101–25
Instituto Butantan (São Paulo, Brazil),
  32
International Convention on
  Endangered Species, 184
Irukandji syndrome, *xi,* 45–46, 48–54
  See also Carukia barnesi
Isbister, Dr. Geoffrey, 83

Jackson, F. L., 270
Jacobson's organ, 172
Jamaica, crocodile attacks in, 186
James's Powders, 147
Jannin, Jean, 119
jararacuçu (*Bothrops jararacussu*), 70–71
jellyfish bites, 40–55
  antivenin for, 50–53
  attacks and fatalities, 40–41, 41–42,
    43–45, 50 55
  Irukandji syndrom, *xi,* 45–46, 48–54
  treatment of, 40–41, 50–55
jellyfishes
  in Australia, 43–45, 54–55
  box jellyfish (*Chironex fleckeri*), 46, 54
  Carukia, 49–50
  carybdeid medusa, 48
  Portuguese man-o'-war (*Physalia*),
    40, 42–43
John of Rupescissa, 146

Jonson, Ben, 177
Journal of Forensic Pathology, 286
Journal of Hand Surgery, 238
Journal of Emergency Medicine, 224
Journal of Experimental Medicine, 247
*Journal of the American Medical
  Association,* 179, 217, 223
Journal of Tropical Medicine and Hygiene,
  84

Kaire, Dr. G. H., 97
Kakadu National Park (Australia), 188
kala azar (visceral leishmaniasis), 132,
  134, 135–36, 137, 139–40, 147
  See also leishmaniasis
Kelly (human African trypanosomiasis
  victim), 107–8, 124
Kenya, crocodile attacks in, 184
Kesteven, Dr. Leighton, 95
King, John, 189
king cobra, 68
King Kong toxin, 64
knoppiespinnekop (shoe-button spider),
  27
Knowles, Robert, 136
Koch, Robert, 105
Kohn, Alan J., 61
Komodo dragon (*Varanus komodoensis*),
  169–70, 170–76
  bite-wound infections, 175–76
  fatalities caused by, 174–75
  humans, attacks of, 169–70, 173–74
  name, derivation of, 171
kraits, 67, 74, 79

L. hasseltii (redback spider), 27, 31
Lacey Acts, 184
Lachesis muta muta (bushmaster), 67,
  71–72
Lake Victoria, crocodile attacks at,
  185
Lampona (white-tailed spider), 26–27
Lancet report, 274, 275, 277, 281
Lankester, Sir Ray, 111
latrodectism (widow spider bite)
  antivenin for, 31

Iatrodectism (*continued*)
    attacks and fatalities, 28, 29–31,
      31–32
    symptoms of, 28, 29–31
    treatment of, 30, 31–32
    venom of, 29–30
Latrodectus. See widow spiders
Latrodectus mactans (black widow
    spider), 20, 27, 32
Lauer, Brian, 223
Layton, Marcelle, 154–55
Leishman, W. B., 132–34, 139
Leishmania braziliensis (protozan),
    141
Leishmania donovani (protozan), 130–32,
    133–34
Leishmania tropica (protozan), 134, 140
leishmaniasis, *xi,* 126–52
    Antimony and, 146–48
    epidemics of, 132–33, 137–38, 139
    espundia (mucocutaneous
      leishmaniasis), 141
    and HIV, 138–39
    and Operation Desert Strom,
      140–41
    symptoms and effect of, 128–20,
      139–40
    Pentostam, 145–46
    transmission, 134–38
    treatment ("Alfred Eliah"), 142–52
Leopold II of Belgium, 110
leprosy (Hansen's disease), 227–29
Linda (nurse), 144
Lipkin, W. Ian, 158
Liverpool School of Tropical Medicine,
    124
Livingston, David, 103–4, 109
Loir, Adrien, 203–4
London Humane Society, 224
long tom bites, 236–37
Louis XIV, 147
Low, G. C., 111
Loxosceles laeta (Chilean brown spider),
    20–21
Loxosceles reclusa (brown recluse spider),
    21–24

    fatalities from, 23
    venom of, 22
Ludbey, Don, 49
Lunsford, Mary, 284

Macchiavello, Dr., 20–21
McLeod, Lee, 188
McMamara, Tracey S., 153, 156–58
macaques, 252
    and scientific research, 253–55
    See also crab-eating macaque; rhesus
      monkeys
magpie attacks, 241
Maguire, Dr., 148
Mala, crocodile attacks in, 186
malarial parasite, 133
Malathion spraying, 155
Malawi, crocodile population in,
    184
mambas, 67, 79–81
    black mambas, 80–81
Manson, Dr., 134
Manson, Sir Patrick, 108–9, 111,
    112–13
Masters, Dr. Edwin, 21–22
Meadows, Ginger, 188
Médecins Sans Frontières, 119, 139
Medical Journal of Australia, 35, 45, 50,
    53, 56
Meister, Joseph, 202–3, 204, 206
melarsoprol
    shortages of, 118
    as treatment for sleeping sickness,
      116
Mexico, widow spiders in, 27
mice and rabies, 205
mirex (chlorinated hydrocarbon mirex)
    and chemical control of fire ants,
      12–13
Mississippi Allergy Clinic (Jackson,
    MS), 16
Monash Medical Center (Australia), 27
monitor lizard. *See* Komodo dragon;
    Nile monitor
monkey bites. *See* rhesus monkey bites
Monticone, C. A., 34–35

Morbidity and Mortality Weekly Reports,
165, 197, 257
mosquitoes
abatement and control, 156, 161, 166
and yellow fever, 167
and West Nile virus, 155–56, 161,
167–68
mucocutaneous leishmaniasis (*espundia*),
141
See also leishmaniasis
Mwakamba, Elipba, 185
Mycoplasma phocacerebrale, 239–40

Nagami, Pamela, 142–45, 244, 265–67,
286
Napoleon, 86
National Institute of Health, 199, 200
needle-fish bites, 236–37
Neill, Wilfred T., 183
Neumann, Arthur H., 183
Neurex as a pain inhibitor, 64
New York Times, 157
New England Journal of Medicine, 21, 31,
88, 138, 215, 241
New York City
Malathion spraying, 156, 161
West Nile virus outbreak, 153–58,
160, 161–62
New York City Health Department, 154
New York Herald, 109
New York State Health Department,
154, 158
New Zealand cassowary attack, 241
Nicholls, Amy, 184–85
Nile crocodile (*Crocodylus niloticus*), 176
life span, 182
monitor lizard and, 171
Nile monitor, 171
Northern Territories (Australia)
crocodile attacks in, 188–90
nose, human bites on, 274–76
Nosema (bedbug parasite), 136
Novak, Susan, 143

Olivera, Dr. Baldomero, 61–64
Ollapallil, Jacob, 274

oriental sore, 131, 135, 140, 147
See also leishmaniasis
Orkneyinga Saga, 269–70
ostrich attacks, 241
Ostrowski, Stephanie, 265
owl attacks, 242–43

Paisley, John, 223
Panama, crocodile attacks in,
186–87
Pantanal flood plain and red fire ants,
5–6
Paracelsus, 146
Pasha, Emin (Eduard Schnitzer), 110
Pasteur, Louis, 208
and rabies vaccine, 200–204, 206
Pasteurella multocida, 208–9, 215–17
treatment of, 209
Patton, W. S., 135–36
Paul of Aegina, 249
Pelletier, Louise, 204, 206
Pendeh sore, 131 135
See also leishmaniasis
penicillin and *Pasteurella multocida,*
208
penis, human bites on, 276–77, 278–79
pentamidine
shortages of, 118
as treatment for sleeping sickness,
116
Pentostam, 145–46, 148–51
side effects, 148
Peru, 126–27
Peters, James A., 66
Peterson, Lyle, 162
pets. *See* cat bites; dog bites
Phillips, Dr. Charles M., 85
Phlebotomus argentipes (sandfly)
and the transmission of kala azar,
136–38
See also leishmaniasis
Phoneutria nigriventer (wandering
spider), 32–33
phorid flies
as natural enemy of red fire ants, 6,
13

Physalia (Portuguese man-o'-war), 40, 42
  venom of, 42–43
pit vipers, 70, 74
Pittman, "Crocodile Mike," 190
Pliny the Elder, 86
Polio
  West Nile virus resemblance to, 165
Pope, Max, 188
Porter, Sanford, 8
Portuguese man-o'-war (*Physalia*), 40, 42
  venom of, 42–43
Posadas Amazonas Lodge (Peru), 127
priapism (spontaneous erection)
  spider bites and, 33
Primate Freedom Project, 255
Psylli people as snake shamans, 86
puff adders, 67

Queensland (Australia), crocodile
  attacks in, 189
Quetzalcoatl, 77

rabbits and rabies, 205
rabies, 191–206
  fatalities from, 192, 194, 198–99, 200, 204
  ferrets and, 222–23
  human-to-human transmission, 199–200
  immune globulins, 204
  raccoons and, 194
  treatment of, 204
  See also bacteria from bites; rabies vaccine
rabies: agitated (furious), 194
  aerophobia and, 195
  hallucinations and, 195, 196
  hydrophobia and, 194–95, 196
  symptoms, 194–97
  treatment, 196
rabies: paralytic (dumb), 194
  fatalities from, 198–99, 200
  symptoms, 197–200

rabies vaccine, 200
  Louis Pasteur and, 200–204, 206
raccoons
  and *Pasteurella multocida,* 208
  and rabies, 194, 205
Raleigh, Sir Walter, 177
Ramani, Dr., 209
rats
  rat-control programs, 225
rat bites, 225–32
  fatalities from, 231
  and Haverhill fever, 229–31
  leprosy (Hansen's disease) and, 227–29
  and *Pasteurella multocida,* 208
  poverty and, 225–26
  and rabies, 205
  and *sodoku* (rat-bite fever), 229, 231–32
  Spirillum minus, 231
  Streptobacillus moniliformis, 229–30
  treatment, 230, 232
rattlesnake round-ups, 76
rattlesnakes, 77–78
  eastern diamondback rattlesnake, 67
  fatalities from, 77–78
  timber rattlesnake (*Crotalus horridus horridus*), 77
  western diamondback rattlesnake, 66–67
red fire ant bites
  anaphylactic reaction to, 3–4, 14–15
  attacks and fatalities, 1, 3, 4–5, 10–11
  immunotherapy and, 15–16
  nervous system, venom and, 2–3
  treatment of, 3, 4–5, 14–16
red fire ant mounds, 5
  in the U.S., 6, 8
red fire ant (*Solenopsis invicta*), 1–17
  adaptability and mutations of, 5–6, 7–8, 11–12
  agriculture, menace to, 5, 8–9
  chemical control, attempts at, 12–13
  description and origins of, 1–2, 5–6
  ecological disruption by, 8

electrical current, attraction to, 9–10
eradication, attempts at, 11–13,
    16–17
fish, danger to, 9
home and apartment infection, 10
natural enemies of, 6, 13
other species, competition from, 6
rural roads, destruction of, 9
U.S., invasion of, 6–7
venom of, 2–3, 13–16
See also black fire ant
Red Hourglass, The (Grice), 28–29, 76
Red River (movie), 31
red-tail spider (*cul rouge*), 27
redback spider (*L. hasseltii*), 27, 31
religious snake-handling, 76, 77
reptile bites
    alligator, 176–77, 178–81
    crocodile, 176–77, 182–90
    Komodo dragon, 169–70, 170–76
    See also snake bites
rhesus monkey bites
    B-virus (*Herpesvirus simiae*)
        infections, 244, 247–48, 249, 250,
        255–65
    fatalities from, 245, 255–60
    treatment of, 245, 256–57, 264–66
    rhesus monkey (*Macaca mulatta*), 245,
        252–53
    illegal traffic in, 264–65
    and scientific research, 253–55
Rhoades, Robert, 4, 5
Robinson, Ansil, 284
Rogers, Sir Leonard, 135
Roizman, Bernard, 265
Ross, I. C., 97
Ross, R., 133
roster attacks, 240–41
Roueché, Berton, 193
Roux, Emile, 202, 203
Rumphius, G. E., 57

Sabin, Albert, 247
Sadler, Ross, 83
St. Louis encephalitis virus, 154
Salk, Jonas, 165

saltwater crocodile (*Crocodylus porosus*),
    186–87
San Francisco Chronicle, 169
sandfly (*Phlebotomus argentipes*)
    and the transmission of kala azar,
        136–38
    See also leishmaniasis
Savignano, Dolores, 8
School of Public Health and Tropical
    Medicine (Sydney, Australia), 46
Schottmüller, H., 229
Science journal, 20–21, 62
Scientist, The, 262, 265
seal finger, 238–40
serum sickness, 74, 77
Shebane (crocodile victim), 183
Shiffer, Jeffrey, 144
shoe-button spider (*knoppiespinnekop*),
    27
Shortt, Henry Edward, 137
Shuman, Stewart, 211–12
Sidney funnel web spider (*Atrax
    robustus*), 33–38
    antivenin for, 37–38
    fatalities from, 34, 37
Sigurd the Powerful, 269–70
Silent Spring (Carson), 12
Sinton, John, 136
sleeping sickness (human African
    trypanosomiasis), xi, 101–25
    drug therapies, shortages of, 118–19
    epidemics of and fatalities from, 112,
        119–20, 121–24
    Dr. Livingston and, 103–4
    nagana's relationship to, 105, 106–7,
        112
    Stanley's expedition and, 112
    symptoms of, 112–13, 114–15
    treatment of, 107–8, 115–21
    Trypanosoma brucei gambiense (West
        African or Gambian sleeping
        sickness), 112, 115, 117, 122
    Trypanosoma brucei rhodesiense
        (Rhodesian or East African
        sleeping sickness), 114–15, 119,
        122

sleeping sickness (*continued*)
  tsetse flies as transmitters, 102, 106,
    112, 121
  Zulus and, 103–4, 106
skunks and rabies, 205, 222
snake bites, 66–86
  Aeromonas hydrophila infection,
    74–76
  antivenin for, 73–74, 80–81
  attacks and fatalities, 66–67, 67,
    69–71, 71–73, 75–76
  Australia and, 82–83
  and bite-wound infections, 73–74,
    74–76
  rattlesnake round-ups and, 76
  religious snake-handling and, 76, 77
  serum sickness, 74, 77
  treatment of, 72–74, 80–81
  United States, victims in, 79
  venoms, 68–69
  See also reptile bites
snake charmers, 81–82
snake-venom detection kit, 82–83
snakes, 66–86
  and ancient Egypt, religion of, 79, 86
  diet of, 68
  evolution of, 67–68
  and the human imagination,
    85–86
  rattlesnake round-ups, 76
  religious snake-handling and, 76, 77
snakes (Elapidae family), 78–83
  and ancient Egypt, religion of, 79, 86
  black snake, 79
  brown snake, 79
  cobra, 67, 74, 78–79
  coral snake, 67, 74
  king cobra, 68
  krait, 67, 74, 79
  mamba, 67, 79–81
  species of, 78
  tiger snake, 79
snake (sea snake family), 67, 78, 84–85
  attacks, 84–85
  venom of, 84
snake (viper family), 69–72

black-bellied swamp snake
  (*Hemiaspis signata*), 83
Bothrops moojeni, 75
bushmaster (*Lachesis muta muta*), 67,
  71–72
common viper (*Vipera berus*), 69–70
copperhead, 67
cottonmouth, 67
eastern diamondback rattlesnake, 67
fer-de-lance, 67
gaboon viper, 67
jararacuçu (*Bothrops jararacussu*), 70–71
pit viper, 70, 74
puff adder, 67
timber rattlesnake (*Crotalus horridus
  horridus*), 77
water moccasin, 75
western diamondback rattlesnake,
  66–67
Smith, R. O., 137
sodoku (rat-bite fever), 229, 231–32
Solenopsis invicta. See red fire ant
Solenopsis ricteri. See black fire ant
South America, spiders in, 20–21
Southcott, Dr. R. V., 45, 47, 50
Southern Medical Journal, 15–16, 75
spider bites
  antivenin for, 31, 37–37
  attacks and fatalities, 23, 27, 31, 33
  treatment of, 31–33
  venom of, 20
spider (Araneida), 18–39
  black widow (*Latrodectus mactans*), 20,
    27, 32
  black window (*Badumna*), 27
  brown recluse spider (*Loxosceles
    reclusa*), 21–24
  Chilean brown spider (*Loxosceles
    laeta*), 20–21
  hobo spider (*Tegenaria agrestis*), 24–26
  red back spider, 95
  Sidney funnel web spider (*Atrax
    robustus*), 33–38, 95
  species, 19–20
  wandering spider (*Phoneutria
    nigriventer*), 32–33

white-tailed spider (*Lampona*), 26–27
widow spider (*Latrodectus*), 27–32
Spirillum minus, 231
spontaneous erection (priapism)
spider bites and, 33
squirrels and rabies, 205
Stanley, Sir Henry Morton, 109–11,
125
Staphylococcus hyicus, 234
Stephens, J. W., 113–14
Steurer, Frank, 143, 144–45, 150
Stone, Sharon, 169–70
Strauss, Stephen, 262
Streptobacillus moniliformis, 229–30
Sudan, sleeping sickness epidemic in, 119
suramin
shortages of, 118
as treatment for sleeping sickness,
115–16
Sutherland, Dr. Struan K., 33, 35–38,
94–95
Swaminath, C. S., 137

Taelman, Henri, 117
Tambopata Research Center
(Tambopata Candano National
Reserve), 127–28
Tanzania, crocodile attacks in, 184
Tegenaria agrestis (hobo spider), 24–26
tetanus, 277–78
Thelohania as natural enemy of red fire
ants, 6
Thomas, Peter, 271
Tib, Tippu, 110
tick bites, 87–100
fatalities from, 94–95, 95–96
and Rocky Mountain spotted fever,
88
and tick paralysis, 87–88, 88–100
treatment of, 97–98
ticks
bush tick (*Ixodes holocyclus*), 95–96
Dermacenter, 88
evolution of, 90–91
removing, 98–99
as a veterinary problem, 91–92

tiger snake, 79
tigers and *Pasteurella multocida,*
218
timber rattlesnake (*Crotalus horridus
horridus*), 77
Time Magazine, 170
Todd, Dr. John Lancelot, 88–89,
124–25
Topsell, Edward, 182
Torres, Daniel, 241–42
Trehy, Liam, 38
Triplett, Dr. R. Faser, 15–16
Truman, Harry S., 179
Trypanosoma brucei gambiense (West
African or Gambian sleeping
sickness), 112, 115, 117, 122
Trypanosoma brucei rhodesiense (Rhodesian
or East African sleeping sickness),
114–15, 119, 122
trypanosome. *See* human African
trypanosomiasis
tsetse flies. *See under* African
trypanosomiasis (sleeping sickness)
Tulloch, Forbes, 123–24
Turnier, Jocelyn, 148
twenty-four hour spiders (*veinte cuatro
horas*), 27
Tyson, Mike, 272–73

Uganda
crocodile attacks in, 185
sleeping sickness epidemic in, 112,
119–20, 122
West Nile virus and, 158
"Unidentified Gram-negative Rod
Infection" (Butler/Weaver/
Ramani), 209
United States
black widow spider in, 27, 28, 32
and rabies, 205
snakebite victims in, 79
and tick paralysis, 92
venomous snakes in, 67
United States Army Medical Research
Institute for Infectious Diseases
(USAMRIID), 157–58

University Hospital (São Paulo, Brazil),
70
Uruguay, spiders in, 20

Valentin, Gabriel, 104
van Hensbroek, Steyn, 172
Vaniqua, 119
veinte cuatro horas (twenty-four hour
spider), 27
Venomous Life, A (Sutherland), 37
Venomous Reptiles (Minton/Minton), 79
Vest, Dr. Darwin K., 24
Viala (Loir's colleague), 203–4
Vinson, S. Bradley, 9
Vipera berus (common viper), 69–70
viral encephalitis, 154
visceral leishmaniasis (kala azar), 132,
134, 135–36, 137, 139–40, 147
See also leishmaniasis
Von Jordan, Isabel, 188

Walton, Bryce, 147
wandering spider (*Phoneutria
nigriventer*), 32–33
water moccasin, 75
Weaver, Dr., 209
Webber, David J., 208
Weber, Dr., 202
West, George, 242
West Indies, widow spiders in, 27
West Nile virus, 153–68
birds as transmitters of, 160
blood donors and recipients, 163–64
experimental vaccines, 166
fatalities from, 155, 163–64
Malathion spraying and, 156, 161
mosquito abatement and control,
156, 161, 166
mosquitoes and, 155–56, 161,
167–68
New York City outbreak, 153–58,
160, 161–62
polio, resemblance to, 165
recovery from, 167
transmission and origins of,
158–60

western diamondback rattlesnake,
66–67
Westmead Hospital (Sidney, Australia),
96
white-tailed spider (*Lampona*), 26–27
widow spider bites
antivenin for, 31
attacks and fatalities, 28, 29–31, 31–32
symptoms of, 28, 29–31
treatment of, 30, 31–32
venom of, 29–30
widow spider (*Latrodectus*), 27–32
black widow (*Latrodectus mactans*), 20,
27, 32
cherry spider (*araña capulina*), 27
red-tail spider (*cul rouge*)/twenty-four
hour spider (*veinte cuatro horas*), 27
redback spider (*L. hasseltii*), 27, 31
shoe-button spider
(*knoppiespinnekop*), 27
wild animal exposure
and *Pasteurella multocida,* 208
rabies and, 194, 205
See also individual animals
Williams, Dr. David, 10, 11
Winterbottom, Thomas Masterman,
103
Wolf, Stuart, Jr., 276
Wolfish, Paul, 144
wolves and rabies, 205
Wood, Dr. Yvonne, 54
World Health Organization (WHO),
119, 137
and rabies, 194
World War II
Japanese soldiers, crocodile attacks
on, 187
Wright, Arthur, 247
Wright, Bruce, 187
Wright, James Homer, 134

yellow fever, mosquitoes and, 167
Yerkes Regional Primate Center, 261

zidovudine (AZT), 282
zoonotic infections, 251–52, 278